D1207217

CONTEMPORARY ISSUES *in* HEALTHCARE LAW & ETHICS

Dean M. Harris

CONTEMPORARY ISSUES *in* HEALTHCARE LAW & ETHICS

FOURTH EDITION

AUPHA

Health Administration Press, Chicago, Illinois

Association of University Programs in Health Administration, Arlington, Virginia

Your board, staff, or clients may also benefit from this book's insight. For more information on quantity discounts, contact the Health Administration Press Marketing Manager at (312) 424–9470.

18   17   16   15   14   5   4   3   2   1

Library of Congress Cataloging-in-Publication Data

Harris, Dean M., 1951–author.
Contemporary issues in healthcare law and ethics / Dean M. Harris. — Fourth Edition.
    pages cm
  Includes index.
  ISBN 978-1-56793-637-7 (alk. paper)
  1. Medical care—Law and legislation—United States—Popular works. 2. Medical ethics—Popular works. I. Title.
  KF3825.H25 2014
  344.7303'21—dc23
                         2013040247

The paper used in this publication meets the minimum requirements of American National Standard for Information Sciences—Permanence of Paper for Printed Library Materials, ANSI Z39.48-1984. ∞™

Acquisitions editor: Tulie O'Connor; Project manager: Amy Carlton; Cover designer: Marisa Jackson; Layout: Cepheus Edmondson

Found an error or a typo? We want to know! Please e-mail it to hapbooks@ache.org, and put "Book Error" in the subject line.

For photocopying and copyright information, please contact Copyright Clearance Center at www.copyright.com or at (978) 750–8400.

Health Administration Press
A division of the Foundation of the American
  College of Healthcare Executives
One North Franklin Street, Suite 1700
Chicago, IL 60606–3529
(312) 424–2800

Association of University Programs
  in Health Administration
2000 North 14th Street
Suite 780
Arlington, VA 22201
(703) 894–0940

Dedicated to

Deborah McLaughlin Harris

BRIEF CONTENTS

DETAILED CONTENTS

LIST OF EXHIBITS

LIST OF ACTIVITIES

PREFACE TO THE FOURTH EDITION

Since the third edition of this book was published 2008, healthcare law has changed significantly. The Patient Protection and Affordable Care Act (ACA), signed by President Barack Obama in March 2010, is often described as the most significant change in healthcare law since 1965, when Congress established the Medicare and Medicaid programs. The legislation is long and complex, and it changes existing healthcare laws in many ways.

For example, the ACA makes extensive changes to the laws about health insurance, including instituting a tax on individuals who fail to have health insurance, increasing responsibilities for employers, establishing insurance exchanges, and regulating health plans and health insurance companies. In addition, the ACA makes important changes to Medicare and Medicaid, including such issues as eligibility and coverage, payments and financial incentives, program administration, and the prevention of fraud and abuse. Other important provisions of the ACA address abortion, medical malpractice, patient safety, and the legal obligations of tax-exempt hospitals.

Since the adoption of the ACA, many legal issues have arisen regarding its implementation, interpretation, and constitutionality. On June 28, 2012, the U.S. Supreme Court held in *National Federation of Independent Business v. Sebelius* that the individual mandate to buy health insurance is not a valid regulation of interstate commerce, but the penalty for failure to do so is valid under Congress' power to tax. In addition, the Supreme Court held that the federal government cannot withdraw existing Medicaid funds from states that decline to participate in the ACA's expansion of Medicaid. Thus, expansion of Medicaid is optional for the states, and some state governments have refused to participate.

As of this writing, courts are considering ongoing legal challenges to mandated contraceptive coverage and whether federal subsidies may be provided for coverage that is purchased through a federally operated exchange. Legal issues and requirements in the ACA are not limited to health insurance, and, therefore, those issues are addressed throughout the fourth edition. Those issues include the ACA's legal obligations for tax-exempt hospitals (Chapter 4), the impact of the ACA on Medicare and Medicaid (Chapter 8), initiatives for reform of medical malpractice laws (Chapter 10), mandated contraceptive coverage and limitations on federal funding for abortion in health insurance purchased through an exchange (Chapter 13), and health insurance provisions of the ACA and the 2012 Supreme Court decision (Chapter 15).

Healthcare law has changed in many other important respects since publication of the third edition. For example, some states have joined Oregon in permitting physician-assisted suicide, and changes have been made to the laws that protect the privacy of medical information. These developments and others are addressed in this new edition.

This edition also places increased emphasis on the relationship between healthcare law and ongoing changes in the healthcare system. Specifically, when the healthcare system begins to undergo significant change, how do existing laws respond to, promote, or maybe even interfere with or prevent that change?

Sometimes, we can apply or adapt existing legal rules to new factual situations. For example, as discussed in Chapter 7, a set of rules existed for many years to govern the relationship between physicians and hospitals. When physicians began to develop relationships with other types of healthcare organizations, such as networks and preferred provider organizations, the law applied existing rules to these new relationships.

In other situations, we need to develop new laws to address new types of problems in a changing healthcare system. For example, to prevent fraud and abuse of government payment programs, the law had developed a complex set of rules to regulate financial incentives to provide more tests, treatment, referrals, and admissions, as discussed in Chapter 8. When the Medicare program transitioned from a system of retrospective, cost-based reimbursement to a system of prospective payment, a new law was needed to prevent hospitals from giving financial incentives to physicians to *reduce* the level of care provided to Medicare patients.

Sometimes, existing laws pose a barrier to change in the healthcare system or an impediment to solving a particular problem. As discussed in Chapter 8, the ACA promotes development of accountable care organizations (ACOs) under Medicare's Shared Savings Program, in which groups of healthcare providers work together deliver coordinated care. However, participation in an ACO raises potential problems under antitrust law and the law of fraud and abuse. As discussed in Chapters 8 and 9, the federal government recognized that some waivers or exceptions from existing laws would be needed in order to facilitate the development of ACOs. In that type of situation, the task is to tailor the waiver or exception so that the existing laws do not pose a barrier to change, without eliminating other important functions of those laws.

The fourth edition includes updated information and new readings, while outdated materials have been eliminated. In addition, former Chapters

14, 15, and 16 have been consolidated into an updated and more concise Chapter 14, on the legal issues in healthcare cost containment. The former Chapter 17 of the third edition is now Chapter 15, describing legal issues in health insurance and health reform

Finally, this new edition expands the use of activity-based learning by adding additional activities to the text. Other than the three introductory chapters, every chapter in the fourth edition includes an activity that applies the legal principles in that chapter to a specific set of facts. This textbook and the accompanying instructor manual are designed to facilitate discussion and learning. The instructor manual contains a model answer to each activity and a PowerPoint presentation for each chapter as a teaching aid. For access information, e-mail hapbooks@ache.org.

ACKNOWLEDGMENTS

I am grateful to many people for their assistance with various aspects of this project. I appreciate the support and encouragement of my colleagues on the faculty and staff of the Department of Health Policy and Management, Gillings School of Global Public Health, University of North Carolina at Chapel Hill.

I want to thank my research assistant, Natalia Botella, for her excellent work on this book. In addition, I want to acknowledge Lydia Stewart for her excellent work.

I am very grateful to the staff at Health Administration Press for their hard work throughout the entire process. In particular, I want to thank Tulie O'Connor, Amy Carlton, and Beth Shomin.

Most important, I thank Deborah, David, and Devon Harris for their patience, good humor, and support.

THE ROLE OF LAW IN THE U.S. HEALTHCARE SYSTEM

1

USING THE LAW TO PROMOTE OUR POLICY GOALS AND ETHICAL PRINCIPLES

The study of law is more than simply memorizing a list of activities that are illegal, such as Medicare fraud or price-fixing. It is more than memorizing the penalties for particular violations, such as the number of years in prison one can receive for a class B felony or the fine for driving 50 miles per hour in a 35-mile-per-hour zone. It is more than trying to remember the names of court cases or the citations to statutes and regulations. Instead, law is a policy discipline and a social science.

Moreover, the law is not cast in stone but is subject to change. For hundreds or perhaps thousands of years, people have reconsidered and changed the rules that govern their activities. In a democratic society, we have the power to make further changes in the laws by which we live. Therefore, as students and teachers of law, we not only study the current state of the law, but also what we think the law should be. In particular, we consider how we can use the law to accomplish our goals of public policy.

We begin this type of analysis by identifying a practical problem. For example, we may want to focus on discrimination, environmental pollution, or inadequate access to healthcare services. Then we try to figure out how to use the law and the legal system to solve that particular problem, by creating a new law or by changing an existing law.

"There Ought to Be a Law!"

When we talk about reforming the healthcare system, we are really saying we should change the laws that regulate that system. For example, if we think health insurance companies should be required to provide coverage for everyone without regard to health status, we are really arguing for a particular type of law that governs the operation of insurance companies. If we think insurance companies and health maintenance organizations should be required to authorize potentially lifesaving care for patients dying of cancer or should be held liable in damages for the harm caused by their refusal to authorize care, we are really arguing in favor of laws that would make those changes to the existing rules of law. Thus, when we say we want to reform the healthcare system to achieve our policy goals, what we really are saying is, "There ought to be a law."

Coming to this conclusion is the relatively easy part. The harder—and more interesting—part is figuring out what kind of law to create and what that law should provide. Several alternatives will arise, and each will have its own advantages and disadvantages. The task is to choose the alternative that will be most effective and most efficient in achieving the particular policy goal.

The first set of alternatives to consider is whether the problem can best be handled by a single federal law or a series of separate state laws. As discussed in Chapter 2, one of the underlying themes of healthcare law and policy is determining the appropriate roles for the federal government and state governments in regulating healthcare providers and third-party payers. Each level of government has its own legal powers and its own practical advantages. The federal government has the power to create laws that establish uniform standards throughout the country and has greater resources than the states to finance and enforce its laws. The states, however, may be more aware of and responsive to local needs and may be able to experiment with new approaches for which a national consensus has not yet developed. Of course, regulation by one level of government does not necessarily preclude regulation by the other, and many activities are subject to overlapping regulation by federal, state, and even local authorities.

In addition to choosing local, state, or federal law, the next step is to select an approach or combination of approaches to using the law as a way to solve a particular problem. For example, several different approaches to using the law as a means of promoting quality of patient care and reducing medical errors are available. Under a regulatory approach, a governmental body would prohibit certain activities or require that those activities only be performed under governmental supervision. One example of this regulatory approach is licensure of healthcare professionals, in which state governments prohibit unqualified persons from practicing a specific healthcare profession and provide governmental supervision over those persons who are permitted to practice. A different approach would be to allow or create a private right of action in civil court for monetary damages by an injured patient against the healthcare provider who allegedly caused the injury. In a combination of these different approaches, our legal system attempts to promote quality of care by requiring a physician to obtain a license to practice medicine from a state licensing board, but also permits an injured patient to sue the licensed physician for medical malpractice in a civil action for monetary damages. A third approach would be to use the government's power as a large-scale buyer of healthcare services to impose legal requirements on those healthcare facilities and professionals who elect to serve the beneficiaries of government payment programs.

Once we decide on the best approach or combination of approaches, the next step is to decide where to draw the line between lawful and unlawful conduct. It may be obvious that certain bad conduct should be against the law and that certain good conduct should be lawful. However, most activities in the real world fall somewhere in the middle. In creating a law, we have to draw a line and say that everything on one side of the line is lawful and everything on the other side is unlawful. As a matter of fundamental fairness, that line must be clear and understandable, so that people will have fair notice of what is prohibited and will be able to conform their behavior to the requirements of the law.

In deciding where to draw the line, we want to choose the point at which the law will be most effective in stopping the bad conduct without inhibiting socially useful activities. If the rules of law are too weak, they will not be effective in achieving the policy goal. If the rules are too restrictive, however, they will be impractical to follow, difficult to enforce, and prohibitively expensive for society as a whole. We also need to avoid, or at least minimize, the unintended consequences that are almost certain to occur when we create a new law or revise an existing law. Thus, the challenge is to create or revise a law that will accomplish our policy goals effectively with minimal adverse consequences.

Ethics in the Healthcare Field

When people talk about ethics in healthcare, they may be speaking about a variety of topics, including bioethics, professional ethics, and business or organizational ethics. Depending on the context, this book will address each of these different aspects.

Sometimes the term *ethics* is used to refer to the moral quandaries of bioethics, such as defining the extent of a patient's right to refuse treatment or the right to a natural death. We might conclude, for example, that a competent adult patient should have the right to refuse a lifesaving blood transfusion on the ground of religious belief. Under those circumstances, an individual's right to religious freedom may outweigh society's interest in keeping its members alive. However, if the patient's death would leave the patient's child as a ward of the state, we might conclude that the interests of society should take precedence over the rights of the individual in those circumstances. In either case, our view of the appropriate ethical solution is *not* a question of what is required or allowed by the laws of the state. Rather, our view of what is right and wrong is an expression of our moral philosophy and our beliefs about the proper relationship between the individual and society.

In other situations, the concept of ethics in healthcare refers to the professional standards of medical practitioners, such as the Principles of Medical Ethics adopted by the American Medical Association (AMA). These principles do not have the force of law and do not purport to dictate how society as a whole should resolve difficult questions of morality. Rather, the AMA's Principles of Medical Ethics only set forth the standards of ethical conduct for physicians.

For example, the ongoing debate over physician-assisted suicide involves several aspects of healthcare ethics. Apart from the legal issue of criminal prosecution for causing the death of a human being, an ethical issue arises as to whether it is morally right to cause the death of another person. In addition, a separate issue of professional ethics exists about whether a member of the medical profession should participate in the suicide of a patient. In that regard, the AMA Council on Ethical and Judicial Affairs has indicated that physicians should *not* assist terminally ill patients in committing suicide, whether or not suicide is justifiable in a moral sense or permissible under the laws of the state.[1] This example shows the importance of distinguishing among the legal, moral, and professional issues in this type of debate, as well as the importance of clarifying how the term *ethics* is being used.

Aside from the moral issues of bioethics and the professional standards of medical ethics, the term may refer to business or organizational ethics in the context of the healthcare industry. As one author has explained, "[b]usiness ethics is the study of how personal moral norms apply to the activities and goals of commercial enterprise."[2] As in any other enterprise, each organization in the healthcare industry must determine what it considers to be appropriate conduct for its officers and employees. The Joint Commission (formerly the Joint Commission on Accreditation of Healthcare Organizations), for example, has required accredited healthcare facilities to operate in accordance with a "code of ethical business and professional behavior."[3] Moreover, because of the unique importance of healthcare services for individuals and society, organizations in the healthcare industry and the people who work in those organizations have additional ethical duties to the people and communities they serve.

The Relationship Between Law and Ethics

Contrary to popular notions, the law is not totally separate from ethics. In fact, the rules of law are based on ethical beliefs that are commonly held in our society. These basic ethical principles include respect for individual autonomy, beneficence (helping others), nonmaleficence (not harming others), and justice or fairness.[4] Regardless of whether these ethical duties are derived from religious faith, natural law, or a social contract, these principles form the basis for the legal rules of our society. For example, the legal prohibitions against violence and theft are expressions of the ethical principle of nonmaleficence.

In some cases, however, these ethical duties require us to do more than what is currently required by law. As discussed in Chapter 11, U.S. law generally imposes no duty to help a stranger in distress, even though most people believe an ethical obligation exists to do so. Therefore, it is reasonable to ask at this point why the law does not always go as far as ethics in requiring particular conduct.

Creating rules of law to implement the principle of nonmaleficence, such as prohibiting one person from attacking another or stealing the property of another, is relatively easy. Members of our society generally agree that attacking other people in any way or stealing any amount of their money or property is morally wrong. In contrast, creating rules of law that would require us to help others, in accordance with the ethical principle of beneficence, is more difficult.

No consensus can be reached on precisely how far each of us should be required to go in giving our time and money to help other people or how much sacrifice and risk we should be required to incur in doing so. In addition, developing clear rules in advance that would put people on notice of how much help they are required to provide to others to avoid violating the law is difficult. If we cannot reach a consensus or draw clear lines between lawful and unlawful conduct, we cannot hold people legally liable for failing to act as we would have preferred.

The disparity between ethical principles and legal obligations can be particularly acute with regard to providing healthcare services to people in need. According to the President's Commission for the Study of Ethical Problems in Medicine and Biomedical and Behavioral Research, society has a moral obligation to provide access to an adequate level of healthcare for all of its members, even though there is no comprehensive legal right to healthcare at the present time.[5] Under these circumstances, the ethical duty of beneficence requires us to do more than is currently required by law. In the meantime, we can also work to change the law in ways that would provide greater access to care.

This dynamic interaction between healthcare law and ethics can be seen in the tragic case of a 15-year-old boy who died outside the door of Ravenswood Hospital in Chicago. On May 16, 1998, Christopher Sercye was playing basketball when he was shot twice in the stomach. His friends helped him get to the bottom of the entrance ramp of the private hospital's emergency department, but Christopher collapsed outside the door. Although his friends and police officers pleaded with hospital employees to help him, the emergency department employees refused to leave the building because of hospital policy. Eventually, a police officer took Christopher in a wheelchair to the emergency department, where he died. Later, the director of the Illinois Department of Public Health spoke to the *Washington Post* about this tragic case:

"It's important for people in healthcare to be first and foremost care-givers and not lawyers," complained John Lumpkin, director of the Illinois Department of Public Health, whose office mailed letters to that effect to all hospitals licensed by his regulatory agency. "First and foremost, you do what's right for the patient. There is no legal obligation for them to provide care outside their doors but morally we would expect them to do the right thing."[6]

In fact, if Christopher was on the hospital's property, the hospital was legally obligated to provide the necessary emergency care. In 1986, Congress enacted the Emergency Medical Treatment and Active Labor Act (EMTALA), which is also known as the Consolidated Omnibus Budget Reconciliation Act (COBRA) antidumping law.[7] That law requires all hospitals that have an emergency department and participate in the Medicare program to provide certain emergency services, regardless of a patient's ability to pay. The law applies to any individual who "comes to the emergency department."[8] Under regulations that had been issued by the U.S. Department of Health and Human Services (HHS), a person was considered to have come to the emergency department if he was "on the hospital property."[9] Therefore, if Christopher was on the property of the hospital, the hospital was legally required to provide emergency services.

As a result of this incident, Ravenswood Hospital changed its policy. In addition, without admitting that it did anything wrong, the hospital paid $40,000 in a settlement with the HHS Office of Inspector General (OIG).[10] Morality may have required more than the law in that case, but it does appear that some legal obligations were already in effect at that time.

These events also caused HHS to clarify or change the law on a prospective basis. In its amended regulations, HHS explicitly provided that the hospital property includes "the entire main hospital campus . . . including the parking lot, sidewalk, and driveway."[11] In addition, HHS defined the term "campus" to include areas within 250 yards of the main hospital buildings.[12] These amendments remind us that we have the ability to change the law over time to become more consistent with our ethical principles.

Moreover, the OIG, which reached the settlement with Ravenswood Hospital, has encouraged all healthcare organizations to adopt effective compliance programs. According to the OIG, those compliance programs should not be limited to ensuring compliance with the law; they should also be designed to encourage ethical business behavior.[13] Each healthcare organization should strive for a standard of ethical behavior that exceeds the current requirements of law. In addition, each organization should encourage its officers, employees, and trustees to consider the ethical implications of their decisions, and should develop policies and systems that encourage people to act in the best interest of the patient and of society in general.

In figuring out how to do "the right thing," you should *not* begin your analysis by asking what the law requires you to do. That would be like the tail wagging the dog. Instead, determine what act or decision would be the most ethical. Then, find a way to do that in a manner that complies with the law and minimizes the risk of liability. In addition, you may decide that advocating for a change in the law is necessary to encourage or require people to act in an ethical manner.

The Goals of This Book

One of the goals of this book is to help you to stay out of jail and reduce the risk of civil and criminal liability. In fact, you *can* be sent to prison for breaking some of the laws in the healthcare industry, such as those against price-fixing and Medicare fraud. In addition, healthcare providers can be held liable for millions of dollars in damages, and can be excluded from participation in government payment programs. From a positive perspective, knowing what the laws permit you to do—not merely what the laws prohibit—is important.

However, memorizing every one of the potentially applicable laws or creating a complete list of legal "dos and don'ts" is impossible. Even if that could be done, it would not be particularly helpful, because laws change every day with the issuance of new statutes, regulations, and court decisions.

Moreover, legal consequences depend on the unique facts of each particular case, and every case is different. For example, we may know that factors A, B, and C would make an arrangement between a hospital and a physician lawful, but that factors X, Y, and Z would make it unlawful as a violation of the federal Medicare Anti-Kickback Statute.[14] The problem is that your situation will never be exactly like A, B, and C or exactly like X, Y, and Z but rather will be somewhere in the middle. Under these circumstances, the lawyer's job is to analyze the particular set of facts, apply the rules of law to those facts, and form a professional opinion or prediction as to whether a court or government agency is likely to find your facts more similar to A, B, and C or to X, Y, and Z. In fact, that is precisely what lawyers are trained to do.

In contrast, managers and healthcare professionals need to learn how to identify situations that raise potential legal issues. In that way, they will begin to develop a good intuitive sense for avoiding legal problems and for knowing when to consult their lawyers. Therefore, another goal of this book is to help managers and healthcare professionals learn how to identify potential legal problems that they are likely to encounter in the healthcare industry.

Another important objective is to understand how legal rules have changed over time and how they continue to change to promote the underlying goals of an evolving public policy. As discussed earlier, the laws regulating the U.S. healthcare system are the result of the collective desire of society to change the previous laws for reasons of policy and ethics. By studying the underlying policy goals and ethical principles, you can gain a better understanding of the existing laws that regulate the healthcare system. Moreover, by understanding the policies on which the laws are based, recognizing a situation that raises a potential legal issue will be easier. In other words, you will be able to recognize when something *should* be against the law.

Understanding what the law currently requires of participants in the healthcare field is important, but that alone is not sufficient. You should also understand how to change the law. In that way, you will be able to achieve your policy objectives, promote your ethical standards, and make progress toward the common goal of healthcare reform.

In many ways, the study of health reform is the study of law, particularly healthcare law. The Patient Protection and Affordable Care Act (ACA)[15] is a law that was enacted by Congress in 2010 in two parts, as Public Law No. 111-148 and Public Law No. 111-152. The ACA creates some new federal laws and makes significant changes to some existing federal laws on subjects such as Medicare, fraud and abuse, and the obligations of tax-exempt hospitals. In addition, the ACA requires federal agencies to issue many new federal regulations, which also are a type of law. Finally, the U.S. Supreme Court, which is a court of law, rendered a decision on the extent to which the ACA meets the requirements of the U.S. Constitution, which is our highest law.[16] Under these circumstances, studying and understanding healthcare law is necessary to understanding health reform.

Notes

1. Council on Ethical and Judicial Affairs, American Medical Association, "2.211," in *Code of Medical Ethics: Current Opinions with Annotations* (1996–1997).
2. L. L. Nash (1990). *Good Intentions Aside: A Manager's Guide to Resolving Ethical Problems*. Boston: Harvard Business Review Press: 5.
3. Joint Commission on Accreditation of Healthcare Organizations (1997). "New Standards Seek to Protect Integrity of Clinical Decision Making." *Joint Commission Perspectives*, Jan./Feb.: 18–19.
4. National Commission for the Protection of Human Subjects of Biomedical and Behavioral Research, *The Belmont Report: Ethical Principles and Guidelines for the Protection of Human Subjects of Research* (1979). www.hhs.gov/ohrp/humansubjects/guidance/belmont.html.

5. President's Commission for the Study of Ethical Problems in Medicine and Biomedical and Behavioral Research (1998). *Securing Access to Health Care: A Report on the Ethical Implications of Differences in the Availability of Health Services*, no. 5, vols. 1–3.

6. J. Jeter (1998). "Chicago Cringes at Teen's Death; Hospital Wouldn't Treat Gunshot Victim 35 Feet from Its Door," *Washington Post*, May 20, A2.

7. Emergency Medical Treatment and Active Labor Act of 1986 (EMTALA), 42 U.S.C. § 1395dd (2005).

8. *Id.* § 1395dd(a).

9. 42 C.F.R. § 489.24 (2001).

10. L. Meckler (1999). "Ravenswood Hospital Is Fined $40,000 in Boy's Death," *Chicago Sun-Times*, March 13, 4.

11. Office of Inspector General; Medicare Program; Prospective Payment System for Hospital Outpatient Services, 65 Fed. Reg. at 18434, 18548 (April 7, 2000).

12. *Id.* at 18538 (adding a new 42 C.F.R. § 413.65).

13. See Publication of the Office of Inspector General Compliance Program for Hospitals, 63 Fed. Reg. at 8987, 8988 (Feb. 23, 1998).

14. 42 U.S.C. § 1320a–7b (2000).

15. Patient Protection and Affordable Care Act, Pub. L. No. 111-148, 124 Stat. 119 (2010), amended by Health Care and Education Reconciliation Act of 2010, Pub. L. No. 111-152, 124 Stat. 1029 (2010).

16. *National Federation of Independent Business v. Sebelius*, 132 S. Ct. 2566 (2012).

THE AMERICAN LEGAL SYSTEM

Who Makes the Laws, and Who Changes the Laws?

In some societies, the law is simply what the king says it is. However, in the U.S. system, laws are created by the legislatures, courts, and administrative agencies.

Under the doctrine of *separation of powers*, the legislative, executive, and judicial branches of government perform different functions. Moreover, each branch of government creates laws in different ways. Therefore, saying that legislatures make the laws, courts interpret the laws, and the executive branch enforces the laws oversimplifies the issue. It is true that one function of the judicial branch is to interpret some laws, and one function of the executive branch is to enforce the laws. However, the judicial and executive branches have other functions as well, and all three branches make laws.

The Judicial Branch

The judicial branch makes laws by deciding particular cases brought before the court. In deciding the case, the judge may not merely do what she thinks is right, just, or fair in each individual case. Instead, the judge is required to decide each case in a manner consistent with the legal precedents that were established in similar cases. That body of precedents is known as the **common law**.

As it is developed by the courts, the common law is constantly changing. The court's decision in each new case is added to the existing body of precedents and thereby becomes a part of the common law. The judicial branch also has the power to change the common law to accommodate the changing values and policies of our society. For example, at one time a traditional common-law doctrine of charitable immunity provided that nonprofit hospitals could not be held liable for negligence. However, courts in many states decided that charitable immunity was no longer appropriate because of changes in the nature of hospitals and the ability to purchase insurance. Therefore, some courts acted on their own to change the law in their respective states, without the need for any action by the legislative or executive branches.

Common law
The body of legal principles and precedents that were established by courts in a particular jurisdiction, modified by those courts over time, and subject to change by those courts in the future.

The Legislative Branch

Of course, legislatures have the power to enact their own sets of laws, which are referred to as **statutes** or **acts**. The legislature that enacted a statute has the power to change it by adopting an amendment or by repealing the old statute and enacting a new and different statute. Moreover, a statute enacted by the legislature will take precedence over a rule of the common law. Therefore, if the judicial branch is unwilling to change a traditional rule of the common law, the legislature in that jurisdiction may take action on its own to change the situation by enacting a statute.

For example, the rules that apply to medical malpractice suits have been developed over many years by the courts of each state as rules of the common law. However, state legislatures in many states became convinced that malpractice awards against healthcare providers should be limited, and they enacted tort reform statutes, which took precedence over the common-law rules. In California, the state legislature enacted a statute known as the Medical Injury Compensation Reform Act, which imposed a maximum limit or "cap" on the damages a patient could recover for pain and suffering in a medical malpractice case.[1] Because statutes take precedence over common law, judges in California were obligated to follow the new statute, even if they thought it was unwise as a matter of public policy or unfair as applied in a particular case. When a statute exists that applies to the facts of the case, the court is required to decide the case in accordance with that statute.

Some statutes are ambiguous, in the sense that the words of those statutes are susceptible to more than one plausible interpretation. In some situations, legislatures tolerate a degree of ambiguity in enacting their statutes because some issues are too complex or too controversial to resolve in the legislative process. In other situations, legislatures are unable to anticipate all of the circumstances in which a statute might be applied in the future, and therefore the words of the statute do not clearly indicate how it should be applied in those unforeseen circumstances. Interpreting an ambiguous statute is the role of the courts. In that sense the judicial branch does indeed interpret the law, although that is only one of its functions. If any question exists about the meaning of a statute, the court must interpret it in a way that will carry out the intent of the legislature. Courts attempt to determine the intent of the legislature by considering factors such as the purpose of the statute and its legislative history, including hearings, debates, and committee reports.

A court has the power to overrule a statute in one situation, although that power is rarely used. If the court determines that a statute is unconstitutional, it is not limited to merely carrying out the intent of the legislature. For example, a court might rule that a state statute imposing a cap on malpractice damages violates the state's own constitution and therefore cannot be enforced.[2] Similarly, the U.S. Supreme Court ruled in 2012 that the

Affordable Care Act's individual mandate to buy health insurance was not within the power of Congress to regulate interstate commerce, although the court also ruled that the act's penalty for failure to have health insurance was a valid exercise of Congress' power to assess taxes.[3] Thus, legislatures can supersede the common law by enacting a statute, but courts retain the important power to declare that a statute is unconstitutional, in whole or in part.

The Executive Branch

Because of the complexity of government regulation, legislators have neither the time nor the expertise to develop all of the details of the law. Therefore, legislatures create administrative agencies and delegate authority to the agencies to develop the specific requirements of the law. Administrative agencies have no inherent power of their own, only the specific powers that were delegated to them by the legislature. For example, Congress enacted statutes to establish the Medicare and Medicaid programs and set forth the broad outlines of those programs, but it delegated authority to the secretary of the U.S. Department of Health and Human Services (HHS) to develop many of the details. Similarly, state legislatures enacted statutes to require healthcare facilities and practitioners to obtain licenses before providing services in the state, and the legislatures created administrative agencies or licensing boards with authority to hire staff, adopt rules, and regulate the providers. Some agencies have been given the authority to impose fines, while other agencies do not have that authority.

In addition to enforcing the laws enacted by the legislature, administrative agencies make laws of their own. Through a process referred to as **rulemaking**, agencies adopt rules or regulations, such as the Medicare regulations of HHS or state licensing regulations, that flesh out the details of the regulatory scheme established by the legislature. (For this purpose, the terms *rule* and *regulation* are interchangeable.) If the agency's regulations are within the scope of its statutory authority as delegated by the legislature, and if the agency followed the appropriate rulemaking procedures as specified by law, the agency's regulations have the force of law.

Rulemaking
The procedure by which administrative agencies propose and adopt regulations to implement a statute enacted by the legislature.

For example, the U.S. Food and Drug Administration (FDA) had attempted to regulate tobacco products in 1996, but the U.S. Supreme Court held that Congress had not delegated to the FDA any authority to regulate tobacco.[4] According to the Supreme Court, "we believe that Congress has clearly precluded the FDA from asserting jurisdiction to regulate tobacco products."[5] Subsequently, Congress amended the relevant statute to delegate that additional authority to the FDA.[6] In other situations, courts may hold that an agency's rules are invalid, on the grounds that the agency failed to comply with all of the formalities of rulemaking procedure, such as providing appropriate notice of the proposed rules.

Adjudication
The procedure by which administrative agencies decide cases that involve a specific party, such as whether to revoke a license or impose an administrative penalty.

Exhaustion of administrative remedies
The doctrine that a person opposed to a specific action of an agency must go through that agency's internal review process before challenging the agency in court.

Separation of powers
The division of authority among legislative, executive, and judicial branches of government, at both the federal and state levels.

Federalism
The relationship between federal and state governments, in which the powers of each level of government are subject to constitutional principles.

In addition, through the process of **adjudication**, the agencies decide individual cases that arise under the regulatory scheme, and thereby make a type of administrative common law. For example, when a medical licensing board conducts a hearing to consider whether to revoke a physician's license, the board's decisions in prior cases may provide a set of precedents for resolving the pending case.

Under the doctrine of **exhaustion of administrative remedies**, a person who objects to the action of an agency, such as the proposed revocation of a license, must go through the agency's own internal process of administrative review before challenging the agency's action in court. After the agency has completed its process of internal administrative review, a person who is dissatisfied with the agency's final decision may seek judicial review of the agency's action in the courts. In theory, the process of internal administrative review provides an opportunity for an agency to reconsider its proposed action and builds a complete record for subsequent review by the court. In practice, it is unlikely that an agency will change its proposed action as a result of its own internal administrative review, and the process of exhausting administrative remedies can require substantial time and expense.

Even after pursuing all of the administrative remedies, obtaining a reversal of an agency's decision by means of judicial review may be difficult, especially when the issue involves an agency's judgment or disputed questions of fact. Courts will not reevaluate all of the evidence as if the case was starting over from the beginning, nor will they weigh the persuasiveness of the evidence that was introduced by each party. Rather, courts ordinarily will defer to the judgment and expertise of an agency and will uphold the agency's decision if it is supported by substantial evidence in the record as a whole. Nevertheless, a court might reverse an agency's final decision if the agency failed to follow all of the procedural requirements for adjudication, such as providing adequate notice of its intended action and properly adopting all of the rules on which the agency's decision was based. Thus, a challenge to agency action by means of judicial review is more likely to prevail on issues of legal procedure than on the substantive merits of the agency's decision. By reviewing the decisions and regulations of the agency, the court will provide a safeguard against arbitrary action.

Federal and State Governments

Under the doctrine of **separation of powers**, each branch of government provides checks and balances against the other branches and contributes to the ongoing development and refinement of the law. Separation of powers can be seen among the three branches of state government, as well as among the three branches of the federal government.

In addition, an important relationship called **federalism** exists between the 50 state governments and the federal government. Under the

Supremacy Clause in Article VI, Clause 2 of the U.S. Constitution, laws enacted by the federal government are the supreme law of the land and take precedence over any contrary provisions of state law. For example, the federal government has chosen to regulate employee health plans under the federal Employee Retirement Income Security Act of 1974.[7] As a result of this clause in the Constitution, state laws on the same subject are often preempted—or displaced—by the federal law. Although the Supremacy Clause provides for federal preemption of state laws, the Tenth Amendment to the U.S. Constitution reserves certain powers to the states.

In the healthcare field, one of the underlying issues of law and policy is determining what should be regulated by the federal government as opposed to state government. For example, some people have argued that the laws should be changed to give the federal government a more active role in controlling medical malpractice litigation and regulating the licensure of healthcare professionals. However, others believe states should continue their traditional role in governing those particular issues. Similarly, some people have argued that the federal Medicaid law should be changed to allow the states more flexibility in operating their own Medicaid programs, whereas others believe we should retain the law that provides minimum federal standards for all state Medicaid programs. Other examples include whether we should regulate health insurance at the state or federal level and whether we should have one uniform federal law of patient privacy or different state privacy laws that may exceed federal standards. As indicated by these examples, the appropriate roles of the federal and state governments will be a recurring theme in the analysis of healthcare policy and law.

Substantive Areas of Law

Important distinctions must be made within the overall framework of the law, such as the difference between civil and criminal law. **Criminal law** refers to wrongs against society as a whole, even if the wrong consists of harming an identifiable member of society. Regardless of whether the victim pursues a private claim for damages against the perpetrator, society has been wronged by a violation of its criminal law. Therefore, society may impose punishment in the form of fines, imprisonment, or, in some places, execution.

Of course, strict procedures have been established for determining a person's guilt or innocence in a criminal case, such as the constitutional right to trial by jury. Moreover, the accused cannot be forced to testify against himself, and the prosecution is required to prove the guilt of the accused beyond a reasonable doubt. A criminal case will be prosecuted by a district attorney in state court or a U.S. attorney in federal court and will be described by a caption such as *People v. Jones*, *[State name] v. Jones*, or *U.S. v. Jones*.

Criminal law
Legal prohibitions and penalties for wrongs against society as a whole, even if the wrong harms an individual member of that society.

The healthcare field is experiencing a trend toward expanding the application of criminal law to healthcare facilities and practitioners. Historically, criminal law has been used to prohibit abortion, and criminal penalties are still in effect for performing abortions not authorized by law. In addition, criminal law has been used for many years to prevent the unlicensed practice of medicine. In 1889, a West Virginia statute prohibited the unlicensed practice of medicine, and the U.S. Supreme Court upheld a criminal conviction for violating that statute.[8]

However, the modern trend has been to expand the application of criminal laws to other types of conduct by healthcare providers. In cases of Medicare fraud and abuse, providers are subject to criminal prosecution and not merely civil or administrative remedies. In addition, criminal law has been applied against providers in several cases involving harm to their patients. For example, Dr. Gerald Einaugler, a New York physician, was convicted of the crimes of reckless endangerment and willful neglect of a patient.[9] In another case, a Wisconsin district attorney charged a laboratory company with homicide for alleged recklessness in reading Pap smears, which apparently caused the deaths of two women.[10] The Michigan attorney general brought a criminal case against a nursing home company for charges that included alleged patient abuse and alteration or destruction of medical records.[11] Although each case is unique, these and other cases appear to indicate a shift toward greater use of criminal charges against healthcare practitioners and organizations.

Despite this increase in the use of criminal law, most legal issues in the healthcare field still involve matters of **civil law**, such as contracts or torts. A civil case involves the private rights and obligations of specific parties. For example, if Mrs. Jones attacked Mr. Smith, the victim (Smith) could sue the attacker (Jones) in a civil suit for battery and seek monetary damages as compensation for losses, such as pain and suffering, medical expenses, and lost wages. The civil case would be captioned *Smith v. Jones*, which means Smith is the plaintiff who filed the suit and Jones is the defendant who is being sued. As a civil case, it would be pursued by Mr. Smith and his attorney rather than by a public prosecutor. To prevail, Mr. Smith would not need to prove his case beyond a reasonable doubt. Rather, Mr. Smith would merely need to prove that the greater weight of the evidence (i.e., more than 50 percent) is in his favor.

Many civil cases are based on a **contract**, which is a voluntary agreement between two or more parties. If people fail to meet their obligations as set forth in a contract—called **breach of contract**—the court may use the power of government to force them to pay monetary damages to the other party to the contract.

In the healthcare industry, contracts are used to construct buildings, purchase equipment and supplies, hire administrators, and sell services to

Civil law
In contrast to criminal law, these legal rules cover the private rights and obligations of specific parties, as in contracts, torts, or some violations of statutes.

Contract
A voluntary agreement between two or more parties that meets the requirements for a binding and legally enforceable obligation.

patients and third-party payers. Some of the specialized types of contracts in healthcare are physician recruitment contracts, management contracts for operating a facility, exclusive contracts to provide medical coverage for a department of a hospital, and preferred provider contracts with managed care organizations. In addition, the physician–patient relationship is based on a contract, which may be in writing or implied from the actions of the parties.

In contrast, a **tort** is a wrong committed by one person against another, without the need for any contract between the parties. For example, a driver who carelessly injures a pedestrian has committed a wrongful act, even though the driver had no preexisting contractual relationship with the pedestrian. Regardless of whether the state elects to prosecute the driver for a criminal offense such as reckless driving, the injured pedestrian may sue the driver for monetary damages in a civil action under the law of torts. Similarly, if a physician fails to meet the applicable standard of care in providing services to a patient, the patient may sue the provider for medical malpractice, which is based on the tort of negligence.

Breach of contract
Failure to meet the obligations of a contract.

Tort
A civil wrong committed by one person against another for violation of a legal duty other than a contract between the parties.

State and Federal Court Systems

Each state has its own system of courts, and the federal courts constitute a separate system. Within each system, the most important distinction is between the trial courts and the appellate courts.

A **trial court** determines the facts of a particular case, such as which driver caused an accident. If a jury is involved, its members will determine the facts, and the role of the trial judge will be limited to controlling the proceeding, instructing the jury about the law, and ruling on objections made by the lawyers. Alternatively, many cases are tried by a judge without a jury, in which case the judge will act as the finder of fact and the judge of the law.

Trial court
The court that hears a case first and determines the facts, before any appeal to a higher court.

Although trial courts are often referred to as *lower courts*, they have important powers that cannot be exercised by the so-called *higher courts*. The higher courts are referred to as **appellate courts** because they hear appeals from decisions of the lower courts. The appellate courts are higher in the sense that they have the power to reverse decisions of the lower courts, and they may establish legal precedents that are binding on the lower courts within their territorial jurisdiction. However, the appellate courts do not have the authority to conduct their own trials and cannot even hear a case until it has been heard or rejected by the lower court.

Appellate court
A court that hears appeals from decisions of lower courts. It has the power to affirm, reverse, or modify the decisions of those lower courts, and may establish legal precedents that are binding on the lower courts in a particular jurisdiction.

When a higher court considers an appeal, it does not conduct a new trial or listen to the witnesses. An appeal is a review of documents in the record and transcripts of the prior testimony, together with the written and oral arguments of the lawyers for each side. The purpose of the appeal is to determine whether the trial judge made errors of law in conducting the trial, such as mistakes in instructing the jury or ruling on the admission of evidence. The appellate court may affirm, reverse, or modify the decision of the trial court. In some cases, the appellate court may determine that the trial judge's mistakes were sufficiently serious to require a whole new trial of the case. In that event, the appellate court cannot conduct the new trial, but rather must send the case back to the lower court for retrial.

In the federal system, the trial courts are called *federal district courts*.

The United States has 94 federal district courts, and some of the larger states have more than one district. For example, the state of Illinois has three federal district courts: the Northern District, the Southern District, and the Central District. In addition, some specialized federal courts handle matters such as bankruptcy, taxes, and international trade. At the appellate level, the federal system has 13 intermediate appellate courts. These include 12 regional courts of appeal with jurisdiction over particular geographic areas, or *circuits*. Also, the U.S. Court of Appeals for the Federal Circuit has jurisdiction throughout the entire country over appeals in particular kinds of cases, including trademarks, patents, and international trade. The highest court in the federal system is the U.S. Supreme Court.

State court systems have a similar structure, with trial courts and appellate courts, although the names of the courts vary widely. For example, the Supreme Court of California is the highest court in that state, but the Supreme Court of New York is the trial court in that system. New York's highest court is the Court of Appeals, which is the name of the intermediate appellate court in North Carolina. Some states refer to their trial courts as superior courts, district courts, or circuit courts, and some states have specialized courts for probate, juvenile, and family law cases. To evaluate the significance of a court decision, understanding the level of the court that rendered the decision is crucial.

In one sense, the authority of federal courts is more limited than the authority of state courts. State governments have substantial power over matters that occur within their states, and state courts have general jurisdiction over cases in their respective states. In contrast, the powers of the federal government are limited by the U.S. Constitution, even though federal law is the supreme law of the land. Thus, federal courts may only exercise jurisdiction in particular types of cases.

To understand the decision of a federal court, the first step is to determine why the federal court had jurisdiction of that particular case.

Cases Arising Under Federal Statutes

For example, federal courts have jurisdiction over cases arising under federal statutes. If a patient claims that a hospital failed to provide emergency services as required by the Emergency Medical Treatment and Active Labor

Act,[12] which is a federal statute, the patient may sue the hospital in federal court, as discussed in Chapter 11. Similarly, many cases involving Medicare, antitrust law, and employment discrimination arise under federal statutes, and therefore may be filed in federal district court.

Protecting Constitutional Rights

Aside from federal statutes, another basis for federal court jurisdiction is the protection of rights under the U.S. Constitution. Sometimes people believe their state government has violated their rights under the federal constitution. The Fourteenth Amendment to the U.S. Constitution provides that no *state* may "deprive any person of life, liberty, or property, without due process of law; nor deny to any person within its jurisdiction the equal protection of the laws."[13] Therefore, a person may ask the federal court to order the state government to stop violating the person's rights under the federal constitution.

In this context, the U.S. Supreme Court addressed the issue of abortion in the famous case of *Roe v. Wade.*[14] Jane Roe is the fictitious name of a woman who was unmarried and pregnant and who wanted to obtain an abortion in Texas. The legislature of the state of Texas had enacted statutes that made obtaining an abortion a crime, except when necessary to save the life of the mother. Because Roe did not fit within that exception, the criminal statutes enacted by the state prevented her from obtaining an abortion.

According to Roe, the state of Texas was violating her rights under the U.S. Constitution, including her right of personal privacy. Roe filed a case in federal court against the district attorney of Dallas County, who was an official of the state. Specifically, she asked the federal court to prevent the state official from enforcing the state's criminal abortion statutes. In its decision, the U.S. Supreme Court agreed that the Texas criminal abortion statutes violated Roe's rights under the U.S. Constitution.

In this type of case, it is important to recognize the limited nature of a federal court's decision. In *Roe v. Wade*, the U.S. Supreme Court did *not* purport to decide the ethical issue of abortion. Nor did the federal court decide any issues of Texas law, which can only be decided by the courts of that state. Moreover, the U.S. Supreme Court recognized that the state of Texas and other states may continue to prohibit abortion under some circumstances. Because the role of the federal courts in this type of case is limited to deciding the constitutional issues, the decision of the federal court will be limited to those issues.

Another example of the limited role of the federal court in this type of litigation involved the termination of treatment for Nancy Cruzan.[15] In that case, Ms. Cruzan had been injured in an automobile accident and was in a persistent vegetative state. Her parents wanted to terminate her artificial nutrition and hydration. However, she had never made any formal advance directive and had not expressed her desires clearly with regard to continuing or terminating life-sustaining treatment. The highest state court in Missouri had refused to order nutrition and hydration to be terminated because there was no clear and convincing evidence of the patient's desires, as required by Missouri law. Thus, Cruzan's parents asked a federal court to order the treatment terminated.

Under those circumstances, the federal court had no authority to determine whether Cruzan's case had met the requirements of Missouri law. The highest state court in Missouri had already determined that there was no clear and convincing evidence, and an issue of Missouri law could only be decided by the state courts of Missouri. Therefore, the only issue for the U.S. Supreme Court in that case was whether Missouri's requirement of clear and convincing evidence violated Cruzan's rights under the U.S. Constitution. After hearing the case, the U.S. Supreme Court merely held that Missouri's requirement did not violate the U.S. Constitution. That was a limited ruling in accordance with the limited role of the federal courts.

Diversity Jurisdiction

In addition to cases involving federal statutes and constitutional rights, federal courts have jurisdiction to hear cases between citizens of different states. Thus, federal courts may decide cases involving contracts or torts, provided that the dispute is between citizens of different states. For example, a federal court could decide a medical malpractice case, provided that the patient and physician are citizens of different states.

At the time the U.S. Constitution was adopted, a concern arose that citizens of one state would not be treated fairly in the courts of another state. For example, if a citizen of Georgia had to sue a citizen of Vermont in the state court of Vermont, the plaintiff from Georgia might be treated as an outsider in the Vermont state courtroom, and the local defendant might have a "home court advantage." Therefore, the U.S. Constitution permits the Georgia plaintiff to sue the Vermont defendant in a federal district court, although the federal court might be located within the state of Vermont.

Diversity jurisdiction
The authority of a federal court to hear a civil case on the ground that the parties are diverse in citizenship (e.g., citizens of different states), even if the case does not arise under a federal statute or protect a constitutional right.

This authority of the federal court is referred to as **diversity jurisdiction**, because the federal court may only hear the case if a diversity of citizenship exists between the parties. When the federal court hears a case under its diversity jurisdiction, it acts as if it were a court of the state. Therefore, the federal court would apply the statutes and common law of a particular state rather than the federal law.

The Process of a Civil Lawsuit

Regardless of whether a civil suit is filed in state or federal court, the process for handling the case will be essentially the same. Although some variations exist in the civil procedure of each state and between state and federal procedure, one basic format is used for civil cases in almost every U.S. jurisdiction.

The plaintiff generally begins the case by filing and serving a complaint, and the defendant files and serves an answer (see Exhibit 2.1). After an exchange of information, known as **discovery**, takes place, a trial, posttrial motions, and appeals may ensue. Under some circumstances, the court may terminate the case on legal grounds at an early stage of the proceedings. Many cases are also resolved by some type of negotiated settlement before the entire process is completed.

The Plaintiff's Complaint and Summons

The **complaint** is a document that sets forth the basis for the plaintiff's suit. It begins with a caption identifying the parties and the court, and it tells the plaintiff's side of the story in numbered paragraphs. By separating each of the

Discovery
The procedure for pretrial exchange of information in a civil lawsuit, in which each party may compel the disclosure of information from another party.

Complaint
The document that sets forth the plaintiff's allegations and requests particular types of legal relief.

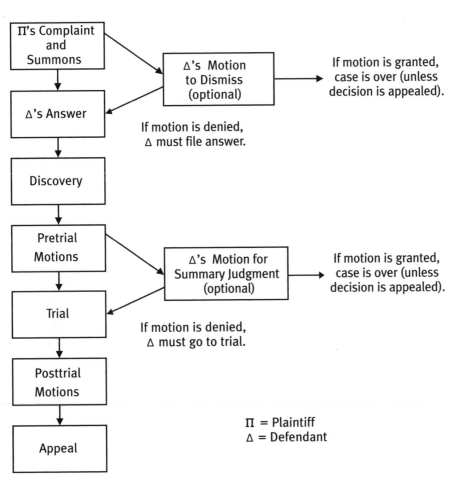

EXHIBIT 2.1
The Process of a Civil Lawsuit

Π = Plaintiff
Δ = Defendant

plaintiff's allegations into numbered paragraphs, the defendant will be able to respond to each specific allegation, thereby clarifying the issues on which the parties agree and the issues that remain in dispute. Finally, the complaint asks the court to grant particular types of legal relief, such as ordering the defendant to pay monetary damages or issuing an injunction against some action by the defendant.

The plaintiff will file the complaint in the office of the clerk of court and will serve a copy of the complaint on the defendant. In addition, the plaintiff will serve a **summons**, which officially notifies the defendant of the suit and the deadline for the defendant to respond. Distinguishing between the functions of filing and service is important. To file a document, it must be delivered to the office of the clerk by hand or by some other permissible means, and it will be stamped as received with the date and time by the personnel in that office. In contrast, a document is served by delivering it to the opposing party or to an authorized agent by handing it to them or by some other manner permitted by law.

Summons
The document that notifies the defendant about the suit and the deadline for the defendant to respond.

The Defendant's Answer or Motion to Dismiss

The defendant ordinarily responds to the complaint by filing and serving an **answer**, which contains the same caption as the complaint. In the answer, the defendant is required to admit or deny each of the numbered paragraphs of the complaint or state that she lacks sufficient knowledge to be able to admit or deny that particular allegation.

Answer
The document that sets forth the defendant's response to the complaint.

Distinguishing among denials, defenses, and counterclaims in the defendant's answer is important. Denials are disputes about the facts set forth in each paragraph of the complaint, such as denying that the defendant was negligent or denying that plaintiff suffered all of the damages alleged in the complaint. As mentioned, the defendant must admit or deny each allegation or indicate a lack of knowledge about that allegation. In contrast, defenses are legal reasons the plaintiff would not be entitled to recover damages from the defendant, such as the defendant being too young to have entered into a legally binding contract. Thus, denials are disputes about the facts alleged in the complaint, whereas defenses raise issues of law. The answer may also include a counterclaim, by which the defendant asserts her own claim against the plaintiff for damages allegedly suffered by the defendant as part of the same incident or transaction described in the complaint. Finally, the answer will request particular types of relief from the court, such as dismissing the complaint or requiring the plaintiff to pay the defendant's costs.

Motion
An oral or written request for a particular action from the court.

As indicated in Exhibit 2.1, the defendant may take the optional step of filing a **motion** to dismiss the plaintiff's complaint. A motion is simply a request for a particular action from the court. The motion to dismiss is a type of safety valve through which the court could dispose of certain cases at an early stage in the proceedings without the need to go through the time and expense of a trial.

Generally, plaintiffs want to get their cases to a jury, which they hope will be sympathetic to injured parties, such as patients or their survivors. In contrast, defendants generally want the cases against them to be thrown out of court as soon as possible to avoid the time and expense of further litigation and the possibility of losing at trial. Our legal system is designed to accommodate the legitimate interests of both parties, by allowing certain types of cases to be terminated at an early stage while requiring other types of cases to be pursued all the way to a jury trial.

As discussed, the role of the jury is to determine the facts of a case, such as which party is telling the truth, while the role of the judge is limited to deciding issues of law. Therefore, a case cannot be terminated at an early stage on the basis of a judge's decision about which party is telling the truth, because that is an issue of fact that can only be decided by a jury. Instead, the safety valves for early termination of a case must be based on situations in which resolving issues of fact is not necessary, and therefore there is no need for a trial. One example is the situation that gives rise to a motion to dismiss.

In a motion to dismiss, the defendant is *not* disputing the factual allegations in the complaint. Rather, for the purpose of the defendant's motion to dismiss, all of the facts alleged by the plaintiff in the complaint are assumed to be true. By making a motion to dismiss, the defendant argues that, *even if* all of the plaintiff's allegations were true, the plaintiff could not win the case as a matter of law. For example, the complaint may disclose on its face that the plaintiff waited too many years to file the suit, and therefore the claim is foreclosed by the statute of limitations. Under those circumstances, even if all of the plaintiff's allegations were true, he could not prevail, and the case should be dismissed before wasting any more time and money.

Similarly, a case should be dismissed if the allegations of the complaint do not constitute a legally valid claim. For example, a plaintiff who was born with severe birth defects might try to assert a claim against a physician or laboratory for alleged negligence in genetic testing or counseling of the plaintiff's parents. Under that theory, if the plaintiff's parents had been properly tested and advised, they could have obtained an abortion, in which case the plaintiff would have never been born and would have never suffered the terrible birth defects. In some states, courts would allow the plaintiff to pursue a claim for negligence or malpractice under those circumstances. However, some states refuse to recognize a claim for "wrongful life." If the particular jurisdiction does not consider wrongful life to be a legally valid claim, the plaintiff could not prevail, even if all of the allegations are assumed to be true. There would be no need to prolong the proceedings or to waste the time of a jury. Instead, the court would grant a motion to dismiss and would terminate the case, unless the claim is reinstated by a higher court on appeal.

If the court denies the defendant's motion to dismiss, that does not mean the plaintiff wins the case. Rather, denial of the motion merely means the case will not be dismissed at that point. The defendant will be required to file and serve an answer in the manner described previously, and the case can proceed to the process of discovery.

Discovery

In the movies and on television, trials appear to be won at the last minute with the help of a secret document or surprise witness. In reality, few surprises occur in a civil trial.

Long before the trial begins, each side has the right to obtain information about the other side's witnesses, exhibits, and arguments. In addition, each side has the right to question the other side's witnesses under oath in advance of the trial. The process of exchanging information before trial is referred to as *discovery.*

Each party is required to disclose information before the trial for several reasons:

1. The process of discovery reduces the element of surprise. Although surprise is dramatic and exciting, civil litigation is not a game. Rather, the process is a serious search for truth, and that search is advanced more by disclosure than by surprise. By being well prepared for trial, each side will be able to introduce its best evidence and make its best arguments.
2. Pretrial discovery helps speed up the trial and avoids wasting time while the judge and jury are present. Each party can distill its case down to the most important issues and evidence and avoid lines of questioning that turn out to be unproductive.
3. The discovery process may facilitate settlement of the case without the need for a long and expensive trial. If each side knows the strengths and weaknesses of the other side's case, it can analyze the likelihood of success, the risks of trial, and the value of the claims for purposes of settlement.

Several methods are used for pretrial discovery, including depositions, written interrogatories, and requests for production of documents. Each party has the right to choose the methods it wishes to use and may use all of those available. For example, parties may be required to provide documents and answer written interrogatories with regard to the issues in the case. As an ethical matter, parties and their lawyers must respond honestly and provide the information and documents to which the other party is entitled. Moreover, a court may impose legal sanctions, such as financial penalties, for failure to respond to discovery in good faith.

In a deposition, lawyers have the opportunity to question opposing parties or their witnesses under oath. This includes depositions of individuals who have knowledge of the facts, individuals who are designated to answer questions on behalf of their employer, and experts who may testify at trial in support of a particular party. Generally, a deposition is held in a lawyer's office or conference room, without the presence of a judge or jury. A court reporter will make a verbatim transcript of the deposition and will make copies available to each party.

Pretrial Motions

After conducting discovery and before beginning the trial, a party may file a motion to obtain an advance ruling on the admissibility of particular evidence. Some issues about the admissibility of particular evidence could significantly affect the outcome of a trial, and resolving those issues in advance is preferable.

In addition, a defendant might file a motion for **summary judgment** to resolve the case without the need for a trial or limit the issues on which a trial would be held. A motion for summary judgment is another type of safety valve for situations in which determining the facts is not necessary, and therefore the case can be terminated without the need for a trial. In a motion for summary judgment, the moving party argues that no genuine issue of material fact exists for determination at a trial, and the moving party is entitled to judgment in its favor as a matter of law.

A motion for summary judgment is different from a motion to dismiss. In a defendant's motion for summary judgment, the allegations of the plaintiff's complaint are *not* assumed to be true. The process of discovery has been completed, and the parties have had ample opportunity to gather all the facts that support their respective positions. If the defendant makes a motion for summary judgment, the plaintiff is required to provide a preview of the evidence that she would introduce at trial in support of each of her allegations. The plaintiff has the burden of proof on each essential element of her claim, and she would need to introduce some evidence on each of those essential elements to prevail at trial. Those elements are specified by the substantive law that governs the particular type of claim, such as the law of contracts or the law of torts. By making a motion for summary judgment, the defendant argues that the plaintiff has no evidence to support one of the essential elements of her claim. If the plaintiff cannot show any evidence on one of those essential elements, even after completing discovery, a trial would be futile, and the court would grant the defendant's motion for summary judgment.

Summary judgment
An order of a trial court that no genuine issue of material fact exists for determination at trial, and, therefore, the party that filed the motion is entitled to judgment in its favor as a matter of law.

For example, to prevail in a suit for medical malpractice, the plaintiff must be able to introduce some evidence on all four of the essential elements of a negligence case:

1. Duty
2. Breach of duty
3. Causation
4. Damages

Even if the plaintiff could prove the first three elements, no recovery could occur without at least some evidence that the plaintiff suffered damages. If the plaintiff cannot produce any evidence of damages, the defendant should not be required to endure the time and expense of a trial that the plaintiff cannot possibly win. Therefore, the defendant would make a motion for summary judgment in an effort to terminate the case without the need for a trial. If the court grants the defendant's motion for summary judgment, the case is over unless that decision is reversed on appeal. However, if the court denies the defendant's motion for summary judgment, that does *not* mean that the plaintiff wins the case. Rather, it merely means the case will not be terminated at that stage, and a trial must be held to determine the facts.

The Trial

All the documents and other exhibits that a party wants to use at trial must be listed and provided to the other party before the trial begins. Similarly, each party must provide a list of the witnesses it may call to testify at the trial.

Each party will have the opportunity to make an opening statement, introduce evidence, call witnesses to testify on direct examination, question the witnesses for the other party on cross-examination, and make a closing argument.

The judge will control the proceedings, decide matters of scheduling, and determine who may speak at any particular time. During the trial, the judge will make legal decisions about the admission or exclusion of evidence that is offered by each party. The lawyer for each party may argue for or against the admission of particular items of evidence, under the applicable rules of evidence in that jurisdiction. The trial judge will make decisions about objections to the use of evidence, and those decisions might provide grounds for a subsequent appeal by the party that loses at trial.

In addition, the judge will instruct the jury by explaining the law that applies to the case before the jury retires to deliberate and make its decision. Each party might give the judge a set of proposed jury instructions, which are phrased in a manner that is favorable to that party. The judge will make a legal decision about the most appropriate way to instruct the jury on each legal issue, and those decisions could also provide the basis for a subsequent appeal. If no jury is used in a particular case, the judge will act as the finder of fact as well as the judge of the law.

Posttrial Motions

After a decision has been rendered, the losing party has the right to ask the trial judge to reject the decision of the jury and substitute a different decision in favor of the losing party. In addition, the losing party may ask the judge to reduce the amount of damages awarded by the jury or order a new trial of the case. Even if the trial judge is unlikely to grant these motions, they may be made by the losing party as the next step before filing an appeal to a higher court.

The Appeal

As discussed earlier in connection with the role of an appellate court, the appeal is not a new trial. Rather, it is a review of the written record and transcript of testimony from the trial court, together with the written briefs and oral arguments of the lawyers for each side.

The purpose of the appeal is not to reevaluate the facts but rather to determine whether the trial judge made errors of law in conducting the trial or ruling on particular issues. For example, the party that lost the trial might argue that the trial judge had incorrectly instructed the jury about the law or made erroneous decisions to admit or exclude certain items of evidence According to the party that lost at trial, those errors of law by the trial judge caused the jury to reach a decision in favor of the other party.

Some errors in a trial are so minor that they would not have affected the outcome of the trial, and those are described as "harmless errors." However, if the appellate court decides that the trial judge made serious errors of law, the appellate court may reverse the decision of the trial court or grant the losing party an entirely new trial.

Notes

1. Cal. Civ. Code § 3333.2 (West 1997).
2. See, e.g., *Lucas v. United States*, 757 S.W.2d 687 (Tex. 1988).
3. *National Federation of Independent Business v. Sebelius*, 132 S. Ct. 2566 (2012).
4. *FDA v. Brown & Williamson Tobacco Corp.*, 529 U.S. 120, 126 (2000).
5. *Id.* at 126.

6. Family Smoking Prevention and Tobacco Control Act, Public Law No. 111-31 (2009) (codified at 21 U.S.C. §§ 387 *et seq.*). See also 111th Congress, House Report 111-058 – Part 1 (regarding H.R. 1256-background and need for legislation).

7. Employee Retirement Income Security Act of 1974 (ERISA), 29 U.S.C. §§ 1001 *et seq.* (2005).

8. *Dent v. West Virginia*, 129 U.S. 114, 128 (1889).

9. *People v. Einaugler*, 208 A.D.2d 946, 618, N.Y.S.2d 414 (N.Y. App. Div. 1994), *aff'd, Einaugler v. Supreme Court of the State of New York*, 109 F.3d 836, 839–41 (2d Cir. 1997).

10. E. Felsenthal (1995). "Chem-Bio Charged with Homicide over Pap Smears," *Wall Street Journal*, April 13, B4.

11. M. Moss (1998). "Criminal Probes Target Abusive Nursing Homes," *Wall Street Journal*, May 28, B1.

12. Emergency Medical Treatment and Active Labor Act of 1986 (EMTALA), 42 U.S.C. § 1395dd (2005).

13. U.S. CONST. amend. XIV, § 1.

14. 410 U.S. 113 (1973).

15. See *Cruzan v. Director, Missouri Department of Health*, 497 U.S. 261 (1990).

HOW TO CONDUCT LEGAL RESEARCH

A certain mystique that is justified in some respects and unjustified in others surrounds the complexities of legal research. Using the techniques of legal research to locate a particular court decision, statute, regulation, or bill is relatively easy. In that situation, you are looking for something specific that you already know to exist. For example, assume that you have read about the decision of the U.S. Supreme Court in *Cruzan v. Director, Missouri Department of Health*,[1] which was discussed in Chapter 2. Now, you may want to find a copy of the actual opinion of the court in that case to read yourself. After completing this chapter, you will have a working knowledge of the skills required to find that case, as well as other types of legal materials.

However, a different type of legal research exists that is beyond the scope of this book. As discussed in Chapter 1, lawyers are trained to apply the law to the facts of a particular case and reach a conclusion as to the likely consequences of a particular situation. In performing that analysis, lawyers need to identify *all* of the sources of legal authority that might apply to a particular situation or else perform sufficient research to determine with confidence that no controlling legal authority exists.

For that purpose, merely finding a case that deals with the particular subject, such as the *Cruzan* case, would not be sufficient. Rather, finding all of the applicable precedents under the common law of a particular jurisdiction would be necessary, as would determining whether and to what extent those common-law rules have been changed by subsequent cases, modified by statutes, or affected by constitutional decisions. If an applicable statute exists, one must identify all of the judicial opinions that interpret the statute or address its constitutionality, as well as any regulations that supplement the statutory requirements.

Obviously, that type of comprehensive legal research requires extensive training, experience, and judgment, and that type of research ordinarily should be left to the professionals. Nevertheless, nonlawyers can learn to use legal research techniques to locate and obtain important materials, such as court decisions, statutes, regulations, and proposed legislation. To learn how to find these materials, the first step is to understand the citation format by which legal materials are identified, labeled, and categorized. The next step is to learn how to find the materials in the easiest possible way.

As your skills improve, finding documents and information will become easier. Like a treasure hunt, it can be both frustrating and gratifying. So, happy hunting!

Understanding Legal Citation Form

Citation form
The standardized method of identifying and labeling sources of legal authority, such as court decisions, statutes, and rules.

As in other disciplines, the law has developed a standardized method of identification and labeling. In the law, this method is referred to as **citation form**. Every court decision, statute, and rule can be distinguished from every other by means of its label. Moreover, for those who have learned to read the "secret code," the labels provide a great deal of information about the particular law. For example, the label will indicate the type of law; the identity of the court, legislature, or agency that issued the law; and the date on which it was issued. Most important, the labels provide the easiest way to find a particular law, regardless of whether you are using books in a library or doing research on the Internet.

Citations to Court Decisions

Citations to court decisions begin with identification of the parties from the caption of the case, such as *Roe v. Wade*. Ordinarily, the plaintiff is listed first. However, in some jurisdictions, the defendant is listed first in an appellate decision if the defendant had filed the appeal to the higher court.

Reports, reporters
Books or sets of books that contain decisions of particular courts.

After identifying the parties, the citation identifies the court that decided the case by reference to a particular set of books, which are called **reports** or **reporters**. For example, the *United States Reports* (abbreviated "U.S.") contain only the decisions of the U.S. Supreme Court. Thus, the identity and level of the court that decided the case can be determined by reference to the particular set of reporters that are mentioned in the citation.

In addition, the citation will include a volume number *before* the abbreviated name of the reporter and a page number *after* that abbreviated name. The first number is the volume of that reporter in which the court's opinion can be found, and the subsequent number is the page on which the opinion begins. For example, the citation to *Roe v. Wade*, 410 U.S. 113 (1973), indicates that the opinion can be found in the *United States Reports*, which means that the case must have been decided by the U.S. Supreme Court. The citation also indicates that the opinion can be found in volume 410 of that reporter and begins at page 113. Finally, the date of 1973 in parentheses at the end of the citation is the date on which the court rendered its decision.

In addition to the official *United States Reports*, which are published by the federal government, decisions of the U.S. Supreme Court are published commercially in the *Supreme Court Reporter* (abbreviated "S.Ct.") and the *Lawyer's Edition* (abbreviated "L.Ed."). Regardless of the publisher, the abbreviation of the reporter will be preceded by the volume number and followed by the page number at which the court's opinion can be found.

Decisions of a federal court of appeals are published in the *Federal Reporter*, which is abbreviated simply as "F." Because so many volumes of that reporter have been published, the publisher began a second and third series, which are abbreviated as "F.2d" and "F.3d," respectively. The inclusion of a case in any series of the *Federal Reporter* will indicate that it was decided by a federal court of appeals, but does not indicate which specific court of appeals decided the case. Therefore, the citation includes a parenthetical notation that identifies the particular court, such as the U.S. Court of Appeals for the Ninth Circuit, as well as the date of decision.

For example, the case of *Spain v. Aetna*, which is discussed in Chapter 14, is cited as *Spain v. Aetna Life Insurance Company*, 11 F.3d 129 (9th Cir. 1993), *cert. denied*, 511 U.S. 1052 (1994). This citation indicates that the case can be found in volume 11 of the third series of the *Federal Reporter* and begins at page 129. It was decided by the federal Court of Appeals for the Ninth Circuit in 1993. The term "cert. denied" indicates that, after the decision by the Ninth Circuit in 1993, the U.S. Supreme Court refused to hear the case in 1994. Because the U.S. Supreme Court refused to hear the case, the decision of the court of appeals is still the law within the geographic boundaries of the Ninth Circuit. However, no conclusion can be drawn about the view of the Supreme Court from its decision to deny "cert." in a particular case. The Supreme Court only accepts a small percentage of the cases that are filed, and its decision not to hear a case does not necessarily mean that it agreed with the decision of the lower court.

Cert. denied
The designation in citation form to indicate that the U.S. Supreme Court declined to hear that case. Abbreviation of "the petition for writ of certiorari is denied."

Decisions of the federal district courts are reported in the *Federal Supplement*, which is abbreviated as "F.Supp." or "F.Supp.2d." To identify the particular district court that rendered the decision, the parenthetical notation containing the date will also contain an abbreviation for the court. For example, "S.D.N.Y." is the federal district court for the Southern District of New York. The citation to *Owens v. Nacogdoches County Hospital District*, 741 F.Supp. 1269 (E.D. Tex. 1990), which is discussed in Chapter 11, indicates that the case was decided by the federal district court for the Eastern District of Texas in 1990.

State court decisions are reported and cited in similar fashion. The official reporters are identified by the abbreviation of the state, such as "Mass." or "Va." In addition, there are unofficial reporters for state court decisions within a particular region, such as the *Pacific Reporter* ("P." or "P.2d") or the *North Eastern Reporter* ("N.E." or "N.E.2d"), and there are unofficial reporters specifically for California ("Cal.Rptr." or "Cal.Rptr.2d") and New York ("N.Y.S." or "N.Y.S.2d"). Sometimes, a citation will include a parallel cite, which indicates where to find the case in the unofficial as well as the official reporter.

Regardless of which reporter is used, the citation will indicate the level of the state court that rendered the decision, such as a trial court, an intermediate appellate court, or the highest court in the state. For example, a famous medical malpractice case is cited as *Darling v. Charleston Community Memorial Hospital*, 211 N.E.2d 253 (Ill. 1965), *cert. denied*, 383 U.S. 946 (1966). The first parenthetical notation contains the date of decision and the abbreviation of a state, which in this case was Illinois. The abbreviation of a state without any other letters indicates that the decision was rendered by the highest court of that state. In contrast, a citation to "Ill. App." would indicate that the decision was rendered by an appellate court, which is *not* the highest court in Illinois.

Citations to Statutes and Regulations

Federal statutes are enacted as public laws by a particular session of Congress and can be identified by their public law (Pub. L.) number. For example, the National Organ Transplant Act was enacted in 1984 by the 98th Congress. It was the 507th public law passed by that session of Congress. Therefore, the law is identified and cited as Pub. L. No. 98-507 (1984).

After public laws are enacted, they are compiled into the *United States Code* (U.S.C.), which is a codification of statutes by title and section (§). As explained by the U.S. Government Printing Office (GPO), "The United States Code is the codification by subject matter of the general and permanent laws of the United States. It is divided by broad subjects into 51 titles and published by the Office of the Law Revision Counsel of the U.S. House of Representatives. The U.S. Code was first published in 1926. The next main edition was published in 1934, and subsequent main editions have been published every six years since 1934. In between editions, annual cumulative supplements are published in order to present the most current information."[2]

For example, the National Organ Transplant Act was codified in Title 42 of the U.S.C., which contains many of the federal statutes relating to public health and welfare. An important provision of that act, which prohibits buying or selling human organs, was designated as section 274e of Title 42 and may be cited as 42 U.S.C. § 274e.

For easier reference, the sections of the U.S.C. are divided into subsections, which are labeled by letters in parentheses, such as subsection (a) of § 274e. However, distinguishing a letter that is part of the *section* from a letter that indicates a *subsection* is extremely important. To include additional sections in the U.S.C. or to insert new sections between existing sections,

Congress may add a lowercase letter *without parentheses* after a number as the designation for a new section of the Code. For example, Title 42 has a § 274 as well as § 274a, 274b, 274c, 274d, and 274e, each of which are separate sections and not merely subsections of section 274. Thus, the prohibition against buying or selling human organs in the National Organ Transplant Act is codified as § 274e, *not* subsection (e) of § 274. Similarly, the definitional section of the federal Medicare statute is 42 U.S.C. § 1395x, not § 1395(x). However, there is also a subsection (x), which is labeled as 1395x(x).

Another aspect of U.S.C. section numbering that may confuse people is the use of multiple letters as additional code sections. In addition to § 1395x, the Medicare law contains a separate § 1395xx, although mercifully § 1395xx is too short to have its own subsection (x). After using § 1395x, 1395y, and 1395z, the Code will begin a new series of sections as 1395aa, 1395bb, and so forth. Similarly, after using up § 1395zz, the next available section number would be 1395aaa. In each case, these duplicated letters are *not* in parentheses, and therefore they signify separate sections, *not* subsections.

A final point on section numbering in the U.S.C. is to recognize that sections of the Code are *not* the same as sections of the act by which Congress adopted the statute. For example, provisions of the Medicare and Medicaid laws are often referred to as specific sections of the Social Security Act. However, those section numbers of the Act are not the same as the section numbers of the U.S.C. in which those provisions have been codified.

At the state level, statutes are also enacted as public laws, session laws, or acts and are later codified into titles and sections. For example, in 1989 the legislature of the state of Maine enacted statutes on the legal effect of clinical practice guidelines in medical malpractice cases. Those statutes were adopted as Chapter 931, § 4 of the laws of 1989, and were later codified in Title 24, § 2971 through 2979 of the Maine Revised Statutes Annotated.

Viewed in isolation, each section of a statute may appear to stand on its own. In fact, one of the first sections of the U.S.C. provides that "[e]ach section shall be numbered, and shall contain, as nearly as may be, a single proposition of enactment."[3] However, each section of a statute should be read in the context of the larger article, chapter, or title of which it is a part. Terms that are used in a specific section might not be used in their ordinary meaning. Instead, those terms might be defined in a particular manner in a separate section for purposes of all of the related sections. For example, one section of a statute might specify the obligations of healthcare facilities, but a separate section might define the term *healthcare facilities* for purposes of all of those related sections. In addition to having a definitional section, some statutes are limited by an introductory section that specifies the applicability of the entire group of sections.

Like statutes, regulations of the federal and state governments, which are often referred to as "rules," are codified after their adoption. Federal regulations are published first in the daily *Federal Register* (Fed. Reg.) in proposed or final form. If the federal regulations are adopted in final form, they will be codified in the *Code of Federal Regulations* (C.F.R.), which is categorized by title, part, and section. For example, safe harbor regulations under the Medicare/Medicaid anti-kickback statute were published on January 29, 1992, in volume 57, page 3330 of the *Federal Register* and are codified at 42 C.F.R. § 1001.952. Similarly, regulations of a state government will be codified in the state's administrative code and can be identified and located by means of their citation.

How to Find Legal Materials in the Most Efficient Way

You have many ways to find legal materials, but the goal of legal research is to find those materials efficiently with as little time and effort as possible. Finding things the easy way depends on what you are seeking and what you already know.

Traditionally, legal research was performed in a law library by using bound sets of federal and state reporters, statute books, and regulatory codes. For modern computer-assisted legal research, some companies offer useful proprietary services. However, those proprietary services can be expensive or impractical for other reasons. Therefore, the following discussion focuses primarily on information that is available to the public on the Internet and easily accessible without charge.

Finding a statute, regulation, or court decision is relatively easy if you already have the citation in the form previously described. If you do not have the citation, you will need to search by the name of a party to the case, the date of a statute or regulation, the subject of the law, or some other means.

As with any type of research, online legal research requires creativity, and the optimum techniques will vary depending on the type of material for which you are searching. In particular, different techniques and different sites can be used for federal and state legislation, regulations, and court decisions.

Most importantly, the goal is to avoid reinventing the wheel. Before you begin your research, try to figure out who has looked up this information before and where you can find the results of their research. For example, the authors of a treatise on healthcare law, such as *Health Law* by Furrow and colleagues,[4] would have already identified most of the important court decisions, statutes, and regulations on each specific topic. The names of cases may be listed alphabetically in a table of cases in the front or back of the treatise, together with the citation of each case, and a treatise may also include tables of statutes and regulations.

Similarly, an article on a particular subject in a law journal or law review may be a good place to start because it would contain citations to the relevant cases, statutes, and regulations on that subject. You can find articles on particular subjects through an index, an online catalog, or a search engine. Articles and treatises may contain a useful explanation of the law on a specific subject, but remember that the law may have changed since the date of publication.

You need not duplicate others' efforts by starting from scratch. In fact, even Sir Isaac Newton attributed his success to "standing on the shoulders of giants."[5]

Court Decisions

As with other types of legal materials, the easiest way to search for court decisions is through the citation. If you do not know the citation to the case, you could search by the name of one of the parties. In a case involving an agency of government, such as the hypothetical case of *Federal Trade Commission v. Jackson*, many cases likely exist in which that agency was a party. Therefore, searching under the name of the other party would be more efficient.

Decisions of the U.S. Supreme Court can be found on the court's website.[6] The website provides links to recent decisions as "slip opinions" with access by the names of parties, date, or docket number. Earlier decisions are available for a few years as opinions by the term of court, and even older opinions are available online as bound volumes. In addition to the court's official website, decisions of the U.S. Supreme Court can be located on the website of the Oyez Project of Chicago-Kent College of Law, which is part of the Illinois Institute of Technology (IIT).[7]

The Legal Information Institute (LII) at Cornell University Law School[8] and Justia.com[9] provide mechanisms for online access to decisions of lower federal courts as well as decisions of the U.S. Supreme Court. Those sites also provide access to many decisions of state courts. In addition, many state courts maintain their own websites that provide access to information and documents.

In searching for court decisions about current controversies in healthcare law, some of the most useful tools are the websites maintained by stakeholder organizations and advocacy groups. Begin by thinking about which organizations or types of organizations are likely to be involved in a particular controversy or have a strong interest in that controversy. The websites of those stakeholder organizations and advocacy groups often provide information about pending litigation as well as links to recent court decisions on those issues. Remember that the descriptions of cases and explanatory material on the website will be affected by that organization's views and its position with regard to the specific controversy. Nevertheless, that type of website can be useful in finding information about pending cases and links to the decisions of courts in those cases.

Statutes and Regulations

For federal legislation, the Library of Congress has developed an excellent system for obtaining information on the Internet.[10] The system is called "Thomas," in honor of Thomas Jefferson, who believed in the importance of an educated population. This site is an excellent gateway to pending legislation as well as to statutes enacted by Congress.

Each session of Congress lasts two years. For example, the 113th session was held in 2013 and 2014. For the current session of Congress, you can find pending bills by searching with a word or phrase or, if you know it, by the number of the bill. In searching by bill number, each number is preceded by the letter "S" for Senate bills and "H" or "H.R." for bills in the House of Representatives.

After a session of Congress has adjourned, you can still use Thomas to locate legislation from that particular session. For example, former Representative Pete Stark (D-CA) introduced a bill in the 105th Congress with a working title of "No Private Contracts To Be Negotiated When the Patient Is Buck Naked Act of 1997." By searching under the 105th session of Congress and using phrase "buck naked" in the "word/phrase" window, you will find, not surprisingly, that only one bill in Congress contained that phrase exactly as entered. That bill was H.R. 2784, which was not ultimately enacted. You could read a summary of the bill, obtain information about its history and status in the legislative process, and even read the text of the bill. In addition, Thomas provides links to any reports of Congressional committees that considered a bill. That type of report is part of the legislative history, and can be helpful in understanding the intent of Congress with regard to a particular law.

Even if you do not know the title or number of a bill, you could find that bill by searching in other ways, such as by its sponsor or by a descriptive word or phrase. For example, the alphabetical listing of members of the House of Representatives in the 105th session of Congress includes former Congressman Stark, and it lists all of the bills that he sponsored in that session. On that list, only the summary of H.R. 2784 refers to "private contracts during periods in which the patient is in an exposed condition."

If a bill was enacted into law, you can find it through Thomas by using its public law number. For example, the Health Insurance Portability and Accountability Act of 1996 (HIPAA) was enacted in the 104th Congress as Public Law No. 104-191. On the Thomas home page, select "Public Laws," and then select the 104th Congress. The information for Public Law No. 104-191 includes a summary, the text of the legislation, and a link to the Latest Report of the Conference Committee (House Report 104-736).

Once a public law has been codified as part of the U.S.C., you can find it by using its U.S.C. citation. If you do not know the citation, one approach is to use a secondary source, such as a health law treatise or an article as a search aid. When you find the citation to a federal statute in the U.S.C., you can locate that statute in the online system of the U.S. GPO, which is known as the Federal Digital System (FDsys).[11] As explained by GPO, "FDsys contains virtual main editions of the U.S. Code. The information contained in the U.S. Code on FDsys has been provided to GPO by the Office of the Law Revision Counsel of the U.S. House of Representatives. While every effort has been made to ensure that the U.S. Code on FDsys is accurate, those using it for legal research should verify their results against the printed version of the U.S. Code available through the Government Printing Office."[12]

Federal statutes can also be located by using the sites that are provided by the LII at Cornell University Law School[13] as described on page 37. It is important to remember that statutes are often amended and sometimes they are repealed in their entirety. Care should be taken, therefore, to find the current version of the statute including any amendments.

Regulations issued by agencies of the federal government can also be located through FDsys, by searching in the Federal Register or the Code of Federal Regulations. In addition, the websites maintained by federal agencies can be useful in providing links to the regulations of those agencies. For example, the Medicare website maintained by the Centers for Medicare & Medicaid Services (CMS) provides a link to relevant regulations and guidance from the agency.[14] The HHS Office of Civil Rights (OCR) provides online information and links to regulations about the HIPAA privacy rule and related issues,[15] while the HHS Office of Inspector General (OIG) provides links to regulations and other resources about fraud and abuse laws.[16] The website of the Federal Trade Commission (FTC) provides extensive materials about competition in healthcare, including policy statements and guidance about antitrust laws, as well as detailed reports about FTC actions in the healthcare industry.[17] These examples show just some of the useful information that is available on websites maintained by agencies of the federal government.

State governments often provide similar information online, although states may differ in the extent of information available. Many state legislatures and agencies maintain their own websites that provide access to statutes and regulations. As discussed previously, the LII and Justia.com also provide access to state law materials. In searching for examples and trends in state legislation on a particular issue of healthcare law and policy, one of the most useful sources is the website of the National Conference of State Legislatures.[18]

In searching online by word or phrase, or in using the index volumes of bound sets of statutes or regulations, you may need to be creative and try different words to describe the topic for which you are searching. For example, statutes that regulate pig farming for the protection of public health might be listed under pigs, hogs, swine, animals, farm animals, or some other term. If all else fails, you can politely throw yourself on the mercy of the nice people at the reference desk of a law library.

Conclusion

In using websites for legal research, consider who established a particular site and evaluate the reliability of that site. Websites established by stakeholder groups and advocacy organizations can be useful in obtaining information and links to documents, but the information on that type of site may be influenced by the organization's view or its position in litigation. One approach is to use unofficial sources to find names, dates, and citations. Then, that information could be confirmed by checking official sources, such as the websites maintained by legislatures, agencies, and courts. Government websites are very reliable. However, explanatory material on a government agency's website might reflect an interpretation of the law that is subject to dispute or even the subject of pending litigation involving that agency.

Also remember that the interpretation of laws requires professional training and judgment. By analogy, a person who is not a healthcare professional could not possibly diagnose a patient's medical condition by reading one article in a medical journal, or even by reading several articles. Similarly, finding a legal document does not provide a basis to reach a definitive conclusion about the legal consequences of particular conduct.

Over time, more legal materials will become available to the public in free online services. In addition, new methods may be developed to help you find legal materials in the most efficient way.

Notes

1. 497 U.S. 261 (1990).
2. U.S. Government Printing Office, "United States Code." www.gpo.gov/fdsys/browse/collectionUScode. action?selectedYearFrom=-1&go=Go.
3. 1 U.S.C. § 104 (2013).
4. See B. R. Furrow, T. L. Greaney, S. H. Johnson, T. S. Jost, and R. L. Schwartz, *Health Law*, 2nd ed. (St. Paul, MN: West Group, 2000)

(an abridgment of the same authors' *Health Law*, Practitioner Treatise Series).

5. A. Partington (ed.) (1996). *The Oxford Dictionary of Quotations*, rev. 4th ed. New York: Oxford University Press, 493.

6. Supreme Court of the United States, "Home." www.supremecourt. gov.

7. The Oyez Project at IIT Chicago-Kent College of Law, "Home." www.oyez.org.

8. Cornell University Law School, "Legal Information Institute." www. law.cornell.edu.

9. Justia, "Home." www.justia.com.

10. Library of Congress, "Thomas." thomas.loc.gov.

11. U.S. Government Printing Office, "Federal Digital System." www.gpo. gov/fdsys.

12. U.S. Government Printing Office, "About United States Code." www. gpo.gov/help/about_united_states_code.htm.

13. See LII (www.law.cornell.edu) or Justia (www.justia.com).

14. Centers for Medicare & Medicaid Services, "Medicare." www.cms. gov/Medicare/Medicare.html.

15. U.S. Department of Health and Human Services, "Health Information Privacy." www.hhs.gov/ocr/privacy/index.html.

16. Office of Inspector General, "Compliance Education Materials." oig. hhs.gov/compliance/101/index.asp.

17. Federal Trade Commission, "Competition in the Health Care Marketplace." www.ftc.gov/bc/healthcare/index.htm.

18. National Conference of State Legislatures, "Home." www.ncsl.org.

MANAGING AND REGULATING THE HEALTHCARE SYSTEM

THE LEGAL STRUCTURE AND GOVERNANCE OF HEALTHCARE ORGANIZATIONS

This chapter explains the different ways in which healthcare organizations may be established and describes the advantages and disadvantages of each type of legal structure. In addition, the chapter addresses the rights and responsibilities of the people who manage and oversee healthcare organizations, such as the officers, directors, and trustees of healthcare facilities.

This chapter analyzes important issues of public policy as well as significant practical issues. From a policy perspective, what types of organizations do we want to operate our society's healthcare facilities? What legal obligations do we want to impose on tax-exempt healthcare organizations as a condition of granting exemption from taxes?

From a practical perspective, which laws apply to each type of healthcare organization? How can one create a nonprofit organization and become eligible to receive donations that will be tax-deductible for the donors? What are the legal obligations of an officer, director, or trustee of a healthcare organization?

In the wake of corporate and accounting scandals, renewed attention is being paid to issues of organizational ethics, accountability, and the fiduciary duties of officers and directors. Although many of those scandals involved industries other than healthcare, some of the same legal and ethical issues apply to healthcare facilities and even to nonprofit organizations. From a legal perspective, the obligations of officers and directors are derived from the law that governs the particular type of organization, such as business corporation law, nonprofit corporation law, or the law applicable to public bodies. From an ethical perspective, officers, directors, and trustees of healthcare organizations have ethical obligations to manage their facilities for the benefit of their communities. The underlying values of healthcare extend beyond economic efficiency and maximizing profit. Regardless of the type of legal structure, those who manage and oversee healthcare organizations should always remember that they are the stewards of some of society's most important assets.

Healthcare Providers as Legal Entities

Healthcare facilities may be owned and operated by a variety of legal entities. In developing and operating a healthcare facility, providers may choose from several organizational forms that are described in this chapter. Each form of legal organization has advantages and disadvantages for the healthcare provider and for society as a whole.

As shown in Exhibit 4.1, the first major distinction is between publicly owned facilities (government bodies) and privately owned entities. Private entities can be distinguished further between those owned by investors and those owned by nonprofit organizations, such as charitable or religious groups.

Different legal rules and obligations apply to each type of entity. In evaluating the obligations of a specific healthcare facility, the first task is to determine the type of legal entity that is involved in the particular case. This task may be complicated by the fact that some healthcare facilities are hybrid organizations. For example, a government-owned hospital might be managed by a private corporation, or it might be leased to a for-profit or nonprofit corporation that operates the facility. In those cases, evaluating legal obligations is more complex and depends on the applicable laws as well as the terms of the management contract or lease.

EXHIBIT 4.1
Ownership of
Healthcare
Facilities

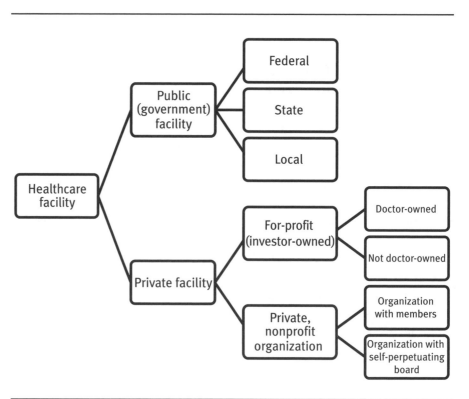

Historically, most hospitals in the United States have been owned by units of government or by private, nonprofit corporations. Recent years have seen a significant increase in for-profit ownership of hospitals and the development of for-profit hospital chains, but most hospitals are still owned by public or nonprofit entities. According to data from the American Hospital Association's 2011 annual survey, aside from 208 hospitals operated by the federal government, the United States had 4,973 short-term, community hospitals, including but not limited to teaching hospitals.[1] Of those 4,973 community hospitals, about 58 percent were owned by private, nonprofit organizations, 21 percent were owned by state or local governments, and about 21 percent were owned by investors in for-profit companies.[2]

In contrast, the majority of skilled nursing facilities or nursing homes are owned by for-profit corporations. Although some skilled nursing facilities are operated by nonprofit hospitals or religious organizations, most are owned and operated by for-profit chains. Similarly, most of the large psychiatric hospital systems are owned and operated by for-profit companies, although there are many public psychiatric hospitals and psychiatric units of public hospitals. In the field of home health, the industry is dominated by large, for-profit chains and franchises, although some home health agencies are operated by hospitals, public health departments, or nonprofit organizations. Physicians and other individual practitioners may operate as sole proprietors or in partnership with others, but many physicians are now shareholders or employees of a professional corporation or similar legal entity.

Public Healthcare Facilities

Government-owned providers are often referred to as public facilities. Many hospitals and other healthcare facilities are owned and operated by units of local government, such as counties, cities, hospital districts, hospital authorities, and local public health departments. However, not only local governments can own and operate healthcare facilities. One of the largest hospital systems in the country is operated by the federal government through the U.S. Department of Veterans Affairs. Many states operate public psychiatric hospitals as well as large teaching hospitals at state universities.

Government ownership provides several advantages from the viewpoint of the operator of a public healthcare facility. First, a public facility may receive direct financial support from a government agency. In addition, the facility will be exempt from income taxes and property taxes and is eligible to receive tax-deductible donations. Therefore, individuals and corporations may be more willing to donate money or property to the facility, because the donor can claim a tax deduction for the donation.

In addition, a public facility can raise money for construction or new equipment by issuing tax-exempt bonds. In that type of financing, people and institutions lend money to the facility by purchasing the bonds, and the facility promises to pay the money back to the bondholders, with interest, over a long period. Because the bonds are tax-exempt, the bondholders will not have to pay federal income tax on the interest they receive on the bonds. Therefore, they will be willing to lend the money to the public facility at a lower rate of interest, which is a significant advantage to the facility. Although a public facility can raise money by tax-exempt bond financing, it cannot raise money by selling shares in the facility to members of the public, which is called equity financing.

A public healthcare facility will be subject to a high degree of public oversight and control. If the facility is operated directly by a unit of government, the administrators of that facility will be appointed by government officials and may also be removed by those officials. If the public facility has a board of trustees, the board of the facility is probably appointed in whole or in part by a government body, such as an elected board of county commissioners. Ordinarily, the board meetings of a public healthcare facility are open to the public and the news media under state open-meeting laws. In addition, most of the public facility's records, other than medical records of individual patients, may be available to the public and the media under state public-record laws. The funds of a public healthcare facility are generally considered to be public funds and thus may be subject to laws that restrict a government agency's use and investment of the public's money. The employees of a public healthcare facility are public employees and therefore often cannot be terminated for cause without long and complex proceedings. Finally, the powers of a public facility are limited to those set forth in the statute or resolution by which it was created, and that statute or resolution might limit the activities of the facility or prohibit expansion into other geographic areas.

From the perspective of the facility's managers, this type of public oversight and control may be seen as a hindrance, particularly if partisan politics are allowed to interfere in the operation of the facility. However, from the point of view of the citizens in the community, public oversight and control of *their* healthcare facility may seem advantageous and appropriate. Most important, many public facilities have a legal obligation to provide access to care for people in their communities, and public oversight may help to ensure that this obligation is fulfilled.

For-Profit Corporations

Corporation
A legal entity whose owners or members have limited liability for its debts.

For-profit or investor-owned facilities are often established as business **corporations** under state corporation law. As explained by Chief Justice John Marshall of the U.S. Supreme Court in 1819, "A corporation is an artificial being, invisible, intangible, and existing only in contemplation of law."[3] Thus, a corporation is a legal being or entity, and it exists as a person in the eyes of the law.

As a legal entity, a corporation is distinct from its owners, who are referred to as shareholders. A corporation could be owned by a single person, in which case the corporate entity would survive after the death of its sole shareholder. Moreover, a corporation has its own rights and responsibilities. A corporation can own property, make contracts, borrow money, and hire employees. In addition, it is required to pay taxes, can be held liable for damages under the civil law of contracts or torts, and can be fined by the government for violating criminal law.

Another important aspect of a corporation is that its owners have limited liability for the entity's debts. Specifically, a corporation's debt is the obligation of the corporation and *not* the obligation of the shareholders, even if it has only one shareholder. If the corporation cannot pay its bills and goes out of business, the shareholders may lose all of their investment in the corporation. However, as a general rule, the creditors cannot make the shareholders pay the corporation's obligations.

Another advantage of the corporate form is that organizational control and decision-making authority are clearly set forth in the state corporation law and the documents that created the corporation. Even if a corporation has many investors, a structure will be in place for making decisions, as will a mechanism for changing who gets to make the decisions.

Thus, the corporate form is an efficient way to pool the efforts and resources of many people, raise capital, conduct operations, and avoid personal liability. To raise capital, for-profit corporations may borrow money, but not by means of tax-exempt bond financing. In addition, for-profit corporations may use equity financing by selling shares in the corporation to members of the public. Those who purchase the shares are referred to as shareholders or stockholders. In equity financing, the shareholders would not own any of the assets of the corporation. Instead, the corporation would own all of the assets, and each investor would merely own some percentage of the shares in the corporation. If one of the shareholders decides to sell her shares to someone else, the corporation continues to exist, and no departing shareholder has the right to take away any part of the assets of the corporation.

Corporations are creatures of state law, rather than federal law. The state provides the right to establish a corporation and gives investors the advantage of limited liability. Therefore, to establish a corporation, the organizers must file a document with a particular agency or official of state government. This official is usually referred to as the secretary of state or the commissioner of corporations. The document to be filed is called the articles of incorporation (or in some states, the certificate of incorporation or corporate charter). That document will set forth the name and purpose of the corporation as well as other information about its structure, governance, and financing. In addition to its articles of incorporation, a corporation will also have a set of bylaws that describe its officers, meetings, and other aspects of its internal operations. To preserve the advantage of limited liability, these corporate formalities must be followed, and the funds of the corporation must not be commingled with the funds of any other person or corporation.

Often, a for-profit healthcare facility will be part of a larger organization or chain that owns many facilities. In that case, all of the facilities may theoretically be part of one large corporation. It is more likely, however, that each facility is separately incorporated, in which case the shares of each subsidiary would be owned, directly or indirectly, by a parent corporation.

The Board of Directors

Under state law, a corporation is governed by its board of directors. "[T]he board of directors has the ultimate responsibility for managing the business and affairs of a corporation."[4] The directors have the power to appoint the officers of the corporation, such as the president or chief executive officer. The directors should not micromanage day-to-day business. Instead, they are responsible for overseeing the corporation and making sure decisions are fiscally responsible and in compliance with the law.

Directors have duties to the corporation and its shareholders, such as duties of care and loyalty. These are called **fiduciary duties**, because they are similar to the duties a trustee owes to the beneficiary of a trust or the duties a guardian owes to a ward. The directors of a corporation are not personally liable for its debts. However, directors can be held liable if they breach their fiduciary duties to the corporation and its shareholders. Under some circumstances, the directors of a healthcare corporation could be held legally liable for failure to ensure that the corporation has an effective program to promote compliance with the law.[5]

Fiduciary duties
Duties imposed by law in specific relationships to serve the interests of another person or organization rather than one's individual interests.

Directors have the power to change the management, policies, and direction of the corporation. Therefore, the fundamental issue of corporate control is determining who chooses the board and who can replace the board. In a for-profit corporation, the shareholders elect the directors. As a general rule, each share of common stock entitles the holder to one vote; thus, some shareholders will have more votes than others. If the holders of a majority of the shares are dissatisfied with the decisions of the current board, they may be able to replace the board by electing different directors. Note that the shareholders do not have the right to vote directly for the officers of the corporation; therefore, they cannot simply vote to remove the current management. However, the shareholders can change the management of the corporation indirectly by electing a new board of directors that would appoint a new set of officers to manage the corporation.

Additional Obligations and Benefits of For-Profit Ownership

Healthcare facilities that are owned by for-profit corporations are required to pay income taxes and property taxes. In addition, donors are unlikely to give money to a for-profit facility, because the contribution would not be tax deductible for the donor.

However, for-profit corporations provide some significant advantages to their owners and managers. First, profits may be distributed to the shareholders, and the value of their investment may increase over time. In addition, for-profit corporations may use stock options to recruit and provide financial incentives for employees. For-profit corporations do not need to adhere to the restrictions on the use of public funds or the rules for tax-exempt organizations, which are described later in this chapter. The employees of a for-profit facility are not public employees. A for-profit healthcare facility is subject to less public oversight and control than a government-owned facility, although corporations that sell their shares on a stock exchange are subject to oversight by securities regulators. Finally, for-profit hospitals provide less charity care than public hospitals,[6] and they may tend to be located in more affluent communities than nonprofit hospitals.[7] Although these factors may be advantages from the viewpoint of the facility's owners and managers, they could present serious problems from the perspective of society as a whole.

As shown in Exhibit 4.1, some for-profit healthcare facilities are owned by physicians, while some are owned by other types of investors. As of 2013, about 275 hospitals in the United States were owned by doctors.[8] The 2010 federal health reform legislation (Patient Protection and Affordable Care Act, or ACA) imposed limitations on new or expanded physician-owned hospitals under the federal Medicare program.[9]

Other Forms of For-Profit Business Organization

As discussed previously, one important advantage of the corporate form is that investors have limited liability for debts of the entity. For the goal of avoiding personal liability, a corporation would be preferable to a general partnership, because general partners are personally liable for debts of the partnership. However, partnerships have a significant advantage in that they are treated more favorably than corporations for purposes of federal tax law. In fact, federal tax law creates a disincentive to choosing a corporation as a form of doing business.

In a corporation, profits are taxed at the corporate level. After paying taxes, the corporation may distribute a portion of the profit to its shareholders in the form of a dividend. Then, the profits are taxed again at the individual level when the shareholder receives the dividend. In that way, the federal government has taxed the profits twice; this is referred to as *double taxation*. In contrast, partnerships are not taxed as entities. Rather, all of the tax consequences simply flow through to the partners, who pay the tax once at the individual level.

These laws create conflicting incentives and disincentives in choosing the most advantageous form of business organization. For the goal of

Subchapter S corporation
A hybrid form of business organization that combines the tax advantages of a partnership and the limited liability of a corporation, as described in Subchapter S of the federal Internal Revenue Code.

Limited partnership
A form of business organization in which some of the partners have limited liability for debts of the organization, but at least one partner has unlimited liability.

Limited liability company (LLC)
A form of business organization in which none of its members are liable for debts of the organization.

Limited liability partnership (LLP)
A form of business organization in which partners are generally not liable for debts of the organization or for actions of other partners.

limiting personal liability of investors, the corporation is the most advantageous form and the general partnership is the least desirable form. However, for the goal of minimizing federal taxes, the general partnership is the most advantageous form and the corporation is the least desirable form.

Under these circumstances, it is not surprising that the law has developed some hybrid forms of business organization in an attempt to achieve the best of both worlds. One such hybrid organization is called the **Subchapter S corporation**, which provides the limited liability of a corporation and the tax advantages of a partnership. However, the use of a Subchapter S corporation has significant restrictions that make it unavailable in many situations, such as limitations on the number and type of permissible shareholders.

Another hybrid form of organization is the **limited partnership**, in which some of the investors are referred to as limited partners. The limited partners are entitled to limited liability as if they were shareholders of a corporation. However, to form a limited partnership, at least one general partner must bear unlimited liability for debts of the entity. Moreover, to maintain limited liability, a limited partner may not participate in the management of the organization.

In recent years, new hybrid forms have been developed, such as the **limited liability company** (LLC) and the **limited liability partnership** (LLP). An LLC is like a corporation in terms of its limited liability, but may be taxed like a partnership. In addition, an LLC is more flexible than a Subchapter S corporation with regard to the limits on investors. An LLP is taxed like a general partnership, but it may register with the state government to avoid personal liability of the partners under some circumstances.

Finally, there are specialized legal entities for professionals, such as physicians, who want to limit their liability by conducting business in a corporate form. Many states had a traditional prohibition against the practice of medicine by corporations. Therefore, state legislatures enacted statutes to explicitly authorize the practice of medicine in the corporate form. These professional corporation laws may require registration with the state medical licensing board and usually limit the ownership of shares in the professional corporation to persons who are licensed to practice medicine in that state. Often, physicians will establish their private practice as a professional corporation or professional association under those specific state laws. In similar ways, physicians in some states may organize their private medical practice as a **professional limited liability company** (PLLC) or a **professional limited liability partnership** (PLLP).

Private, Nonprofit Corporations

In contrast to facilities that are owned by government bodies or by for-profit entities, many hospitals and other healthcare facilities are owned by **private, nonprofit corporations**. These organizations are not operated for the purpose of generating a profit, but they are private entities, as opposed to agencies of government. Therefore, these private, nonprofit organizations and the facilities they own are not subject to the same degree of public oversight and control as facilities owned by the government. In most cases, private, nonprofit hospitals are exempt from state open-meeting laws and public-record laws, and their employees are not considered public employees.

A nonprofit corporation has no stock and no stockholders. As indicated in Exhibit 4.1, some nonprofit corporations have members, but others merely have a self-perpetuating board of trustees. Like the stockholders of a for-profit corporation, the members of a nonprofit are not personally liable for the debts of the corporation.

Under state law, a nonprofit corporation is governed by its board of directors or board of trustees. Like the directors of a business corporation, directors or trustees of a nonprofit organization have fiduciary duties to the corporation, such as the duties of care and loyalty.[10] The board of a nonprofit corporation will appoint the officers, and the officers will hire the employees.

In a nonprofit corporation, the power to elect directors or trustees depends on whether the corporation has members. If it has members, those members elect the directors or trustees of the nonprofit corporation. If the nonprofit corporation has no members, the self-perpetuating board of trustees will simply elect its own successors.

The principal advantage of a nonprofit structure is the ability to apply for exemption from federal and state income taxes, state sales taxes, and local taxes on the ownership of property. In addition, a tax-exempt, nonprofit facility may solicit charitable contributions that will be tax deductible for the donors. Like a public healthcare facility, a private, nonprofit facility may raise money by means of tax-exempt bond financing, but it may not use equity financing through a sale of shares.

To create a private, nonprofit organization, the first step is to create a nonprofit corporation under the state's nonprofit corporation law. That action alone does not make the organization exempt from federal and state taxes, however; thus, the organizers must take the second step of applying for tax-exempt status under federal and state tax law, including **Section 501(c)(3)** of the Internal Revenue Code.

Under Section 501(c)(3), the tax-exempt organization must be organized for a charitable purpose, such as providing healthcare services to the public, and must be limited to that charitable purpose by its articles of incorporation. A tax-exempt organization may not be organized or operated for private benefit but rather must provide a benefit to the community.[11] Moreover, none of the net earnings may inure to the benefit of any private individual. Finally, the articles of incorporation should expressly provide that, if the organization is dissolved, the assets will be distributed to another tax-exempt organization or to an agency of government.

Professional limited liability company (PLLC) or professional limited liability partnership (PLLP)
Specialized forms of LLC or LLP for professionals, such as physicians.

Private, nonprofit corporation
A type of corporation that is not operated for the purpose of profit but is a private organization rather than a government entity.

Section 501(c)(3)
The section of the federal Internal Revenue Code that sets forth the basic requirements for qualifying as a tax-exempt organization.

Nonprofit corporations often make a "profit" in the sense that they have an excess of revenues over expenses. However, that profit must be used to carry out the charitable purposes of the organization and *cannot* be distributed to the members, trustees, or any other private parties. Paying reasonable salaries to officers and employees does not violate the rules against inurement or private benefit. Tax-exempt hospitals may even use some types of incentive compensation arrangements, provided that the compensation arrangement is consistent with the organization's exempt purposes and does not encourage an executive to act in a manner that conflicts with those purposes.

A private, nonprofit corporation is not subject to the restrictions that apply to the use and investment of public funds. However, a nonprofit organization is subject to the requirements of Section 501(c)(3), and must use caution to avoid losing its valuable tax-exempt status. In particular, tax-exempt healthcare providers must carefully review those legal requirements before engaging in such transactions as joint ventures, physician contracts, executive compensation arrangements, and unrelated business activities.

In the past, the only sanction available to the Internal Revenue Service (IRS) for abuse of those rules was to revoke an organization's tax-exempt status. Yet because that sanction is so drastic, it was seldom used. Therefore, Congress amended the law in 1996 to authorize the IRS to impose so-called **intermediate sanctions** without revoking an organization's tax-exempt status.[12] Under the amended statute, the IRS may impose taxes on certain individuals, such as officers or directors of a tax-exempt organization, if the organization provides an excessive economic benefit to those individuals.

Intermediate sanctions
Penalties for violation of the legal requirements for tax-exempt organizations that are less severe than revocation of an organization's tax-exempt status.

Many private, nonprofit healthcare facilities provide substantial amounts of charity care, especially if they are located in a community that has no publicly owned facility. However, some nonprofit facilities provide much less charity care and operate in a manner that is similar to that of for-profit facilities. In recent years, the IRS has not required tax-exempt hospitals to provide charity care as a condition of maintaining their tax exemption.[13] Although tax-exempt organizations must operate for a charitable purpose, the IRS's position has been that promoting health and providing a benefit to the community are sufficient as charitable purposes. Thus, a nonprofit hospital could maintain its tax exemption if its emergency department provides care to everyone, regardless of the ability to pay and if the hospital provides services to everyone in the community who is able to pay.

Many people have argued that tax-exempt hospitals should also be required by law to provide charity care and demonstrate their benefit to the community. In fact, some state legislatures enacted statutes that require tax-exempt, nonprofit hospitals in their states to provide a specific amount or percentage of charity care, or to provide information to state officials about the hospital's benefit to the community. Congress responded to these concerns to some extent by enacting new obligations for tax-exempt hospitals as part of the ACA. However, as explained below, neither Congress nor the IRS have required tax-exempt hospitals to provide a specific level or percentage of charity care.

Section 9007 of the ACA added four new requirements in §501(r) of the Internal Revenue Code for qualification as a tax-exempt, charitable hospital organization. Specifically, a hospital must meet four additional requirements:

1. a **community health needs assessment** (CHNA),
2. a written financial assistance policy,
3. limitations on charges, and
4. limitations on collection practices.

Community health needs assessment
A process for a tax-exempt hospital with significant input from its community to determine and document the health needs of the community it serves.

The 2012 Supreme Court decision on the constitutionality of the ACA left all of these tax-exemption requirements in effect.[14]

In addition to the statutory requirements set forth in Section 9007 of the ACA, the IRS has issued proposed regulations about these issues. One set of proposed regulations addresses the requirements for a CHNA.[15] A separate set of proposed regulations addresses the other requirements for tax-exempt hospitals.[16] However, as of May 2013, those regulations have not been issued in final form, and the specific details are still subject to change. Under these circumstances, understanding the issues and variables is more important than memorizing the details of the regulations. In particular, you should understand the types of requirements that the IRS could impose, the alternatives that the IRS could adopt, and the types of concerns that have been raised by healthcare organizations about those requirements. Of course, understanding the statutory requirements as enacted by Congress in the ACA is also important.

Section 9007 requires tax-exempt hospitals to conduct a CHNA at least every three years. The CHNA must be prepared with input from the community, and it must be disseminated widely to people in the community. In addition, the hospital must adopt an implementation strategy to meet the identified needs. In issuing its proposed regulations on these issues, the IRS explained, "In interpreting the CHNA requirements of Section 501(r)(3), the Treasury Department and the IRS sought to preserve hospital facilities' flexibility to determine the best way to identify and meet the particular health needs of the specific communities they serve while requiring a transparent assessment process with ample opportunity for community input."[17]

In clarifying the requirements for a CHNA, several issues must be resolved. For example, precisely how should a hospital prepare and publicize its CHNA? What type of community input should be required? How should the requirements for a single hospital apply to multihospital organizations? What should be required for the implementation strategy? When will the new requirements take effect, and how should hospitals proceed in the meantime? Finally, how should the IRS deal with various types of failure by a hospital to meet the requirements for a CHNA?

Taken literally, the statute would allow the IRS to revoke a hospital's tax-exempt status for any violation. However, the IRS has indicated that it will take a flexible approach and distinguish among different circumstances.[18] The IRS will consider some mistakes to be sufficiently minor that they will not be deemed failures to comply. Moreover, some failures to comply will be excused if the hospital discloses and corrects the mistake. Finally, the IRS will consider all relevant circumstances in deciding whether to withdraw tax-exempt status.

Section 9007 of the ACA also imposes requirements for written policies about financial assistance and emergency care. For example, the statute requires a tax-exempt hospital to have—and publicize—a written policy that includes the criteria the hospital will use to determine eligibility for financial assistance. However, the ACA and the proposed regulations do not specify any particular eligibility criteria that a hospital is required to use. Moreover, the statute and proposed regulations do not require hospitals to provide a specific level or percentage of indigent care.

The ACA also imposes limitations on hospital charges in some circumstances. These requirements are intended to fix the problem of charging uninsured individuals more than the rates for groups of insured patients that receive volume discounts. According to Section 9007, a tax-exempt hospital must limit "amounts charged for emergency or other medically necessary care provided to individuals eligible for assistance under the financial assistance policy . . . to not more than the lowest amounts charged to individuals who have insurance covering such care. . . ."[19]

According to the proposed IRS regulations, for patients who are eligible for financial assistance under a hospital's policy, the hospital must limit its charges to the "amounts generally billed (AGB)" to insured patients.[20] The proposed regulations would permit a hospital to choose one of two different ways, either retrospective or prospective, to determine its AGB to insured patients. This requirement is not limited to emergency care but also applies to other hospital care that is medically necessary.

Finally, the ACA imposes new requirements for collection practices. Section 9007 provides that a tax-exempt hospital must "not engage in extraordinary collection actions before the organization has made reasonable efforts to determine whether the individual is eligible for assistance under the financial assistance policy. . . ."[21] The proposed IRS regulations define "extraordinary collection actions" to include any legal or judicial process as well as reporting to a credit agency. Moreover, hospitals will have responsibility for the acts of outside debt collectors. If an extraordinary collection action was performed by a collection agency to which the hospital sold or referred the debt, the hospital will be deemed to have performed that action. Therefore, hospitals must obtain and enforce a written agreement with any outside entity to which it sells or refers a patient's debt during the application period.[22]

Even if a healthcare organization is exempt from paying taxes, federal law generally requires filing an annual information return on Form 990. With Form 990, hospitals must submit Schedule H. The ACA has added two new reporting requirements for tax-exempt hospitals on Form 990. First, a hospital must describe how it is meeting the needs identified in its CHNA. Therefore, the IRS will require each hospital to attach its latest implementation strategy to its Form 990. Second, the ACA imposes an excise tax of $50,000 on any hospital that fails to meet the requirements for a CHNA, and requires that hospital to report the imposition of that excise tax on its Form 990.

ACTIVITY 4.1: ALTERNATIVES FOR DEVELOPING A HOSPITAL

Jefferson County has never had a hospital. To obtain acute care services, residents have to travel 20 to 30 miles to a hospital in an adjacent county. For many years, civic leaders have talked about building a hospital and, for more than ten years, the board of county commissioners has been putting its annual budget surplus in its "hospital fund." At the present time, the county commissioners have accumulated $25 million in cash, which is earmarked for a hospital, but the commissioners have been informed that $100 million will be required to build and equip a hospital of the appropriate size.

The county commissioners have considered several proposals for developing a hospital:

1. Establish a public hospital to be owned and operated by the county. Under this plan, the county would use the $25 million in the hospital fund as a down payment and would finance the remaining $75 million by tax-exempt bonds. Once the building is completed, the county would hire an administrator to run the hospital. Commissioner Green likes this idea because she has a nephew who needs a job and thinks running a hospital sounds like a lot of fun.

(continued)

(continued from previous page)

2. Establish a nonprofit corporation and have the county make a grant of $25 million to the nonprofit corporation for the purpose of building a hospital in the community. The nonprofit corporation would use bond financing for the remaining $75 million in capital cost. Once construction is completed, the hospital would be operated by the nonprofit corporation. If the nonprofit corporation ever dissolved or ceased to operate the hospital, it would have to return the entire $25 million grant to the county. Commissioner Blue is strongly opposed to this proposal. According to Commissioner Blue, if everything in the county, including the new hospital, were to be destroyed someday by nuclear war, the county would not be able to get back any of the money that it gave to the nonprofit corporation. Commissioner Brown thinks Commissioner Blue is an idiot.

3. Establish a for-profit corporation that will raise $100 million by selling shares in the new corporation to investors on the open market. This alternative was proposed by Commissioner Black. Because of his success in business, he believes private enterprise can build and operate the hospital in the most efficient manner. Under his proposal, the county will use the $25 million in its hospital fund to buy one-fourth of the shares in the new for-profit corporation. Therefore, the county will be a minority shareholder but will probably be the largest single shareholder in the new corporation. Commissioner Green, who wants the county to build and operate the hospital itself, is opposed to the idea of using a for-profit corporation because of a concern for the uninsured and indigent people in the community.

As you might expect, the board of commissioners has been unable to agree on a proposal, and at the last meeting they almost came to blows. Therefore, the chair has appointed a committee to study the issue and report back at the next meeting. In turn, the committee has hired you as a consultant and wants your advice on the best alternative for the county. The best alternative might be one of the aforementioned three proposals, some combination of those proposals, or a completely different proposal. Before evaluating each alternative, please fill in the chart showing the advantages and disadvantages for each type of legal

(continued)

(continued from previous page)

EXHIBIT 4.2
Pros and Cons of Each Organizational Form for Healthcare Facilities

Issue	Public	Private, Nonprofit	Private, For-Profit
Exempt from income taxes			
Exempt from property taxes			
Eligible for tax-deductible donations			
Able to use tax-exempt bond financing			
Able to use equity financing			
Able to use employee incentives of stock options			
Subject to public oversight and control			
Subject to public employment laws			
Obligated to provide charity care			
Subject to restrictions on use of public funds			
Subject to IRS rules for 501(c)(3) corporations			

structure (Exhibit 4.2). Write a recommendation to the county explaining your reasoning.

Incidentally, as they say on television, this story is purely fictional, and any resemblance to real persons, living or dead, is purely coincidental.

Trends in Change of Ownership

The healthcare field has seen a significant trend toward consolidation of hospitals and other healthcare providers through mergers, acquisitions, and other types of affiliation. Some of these consolidations have involved the acquisition of public or private nonprofit hospitals by for-profit corporations. In fact, some hospitals have been acquired by for-profit entities with the financial support of a private equity firm. Some public hospitals have been transferred or leased to private, nonprofit organizations. In addition, some nonprofit hospitals have combined with other nonprofits to create large multihospital systems, which might be under the ultimate control of a single nonprofit holding company.

In addition to these alliances among similar institutions, another trend shows consolidation or affiliation among different types of providers to establish integrated delivery systems. Some hospitals have purchased physician practices or joined with physicians on the medical staff to create organizations that provide a combined package of hospital and physician services. Other affiliations have combined healthcare providers and payers into integrated organizations that perform multiple functions.

The motivations for this trend toward consolidation include the pressures of healthcare cost containment, the effects of the economic downturn, and the needs of healthcare providers to position themselves for anticipated changes from health reform legislation. By merging or affiliating with other providers, healthcare facilities may be able to reduce their costs through economies of scale. In addition, combined facilities may be able to purchase equipment and supplies at lower prices through volume discounts, as well as improve their bargaining power with large-scale buyers by providing a full range of services at reasonable cost in a broad geographic area.

Not all alliances between healthcare providers are as complete or as permanent as an acquisition of assets or the formation of a multihospital system. Sometimes providers will enter into limited arrangements for specific purposes while retaining their independent existence. For example, providers might enter into contracts with other providers to obtain particular services that are available only at one of the facilities. Alternatively, many healthcare facilities have entered into contracts for management of the entire facility for a specified period of time. Under a contract, each party generally obligates itself for a period of time to perform the tasks set forth in the agreement.

Similarly, a joint venture allows two or more healthcare providers to work together on a particular project, but they retain their independent existence and remain independent competitors for all other purposes. Two hospitals might form a corporation or other legal entity for the sole purpose of jointly owning and operating a magnetic resonance imaging facility or home health agency, but the two hospitals could continue to exist as separate entities in all other respects. Similarly, a hospital and physicians on its medical staff could establish an organization to sell a combined package of physician and hospital services. This type of joint venture could be structured as a corporation or other legal entity, and could be owned jointly by the hospital and the physicians. In fact, the ACA encourages healthcare providers to cooperate by participating in accountable care organizations (ACOs) that take responsibility for a specific group of Medicare patients and provide incentives for efficiency and quality.

Sometimes a nonprofit, tax-exempt hospital enters into a joint venture with a for-profit entity. In that situation, the nonprofit corporation must make sure that it is operating exclusively for a charitable purpose and that the benefit to the for-profit entity is only incidental. If the nonprofit hospital fails to meet these conditions, it could lose its tax-exempt status under Section 501(c)(3). Other legal issues are raised by the formation and operation of combinations between and among healthcare providers, including issues of fraud and abuse, which are addressed in Chapter 8, and issues of antitrust law, which are addressed in Chapter 9.

Purchase of Public and Private Nonprofit Facilities

The acquisition of one entity by another may raise various issues of corporate, tax, securities, and antitrust law as well as a variety of regulatory issues. If the entity to be acquired (the "target") is a public or private, nonprofit healthcare facility, additional issues will arise as a result of the status of the target. Therefore, the nature of the target will affect the structure of the transaction and the issues that must be addressed.

How can a prospective buyer purchase a public hospital or other public healthcare facility? Under state law, the principal methods of acquiring a corporation are merger, acquisition of stock, and acquisition of assets. A merger is a statutory procedure to combine the assets and liabilities of two corporations, in which one corporation survives and the other ceases to exist. However, this technique could not be used to purchase a public hospital, because a public entity cannot simply cease to exist. Similarly, the acquisition technique of purchasing stock could not be used to purchase a public hospital because a public entity has no stock and no stockholders.

In a stock acquisition, the buyer purchases the stock, as opposed to the assets, of the target company. Technically, the purchaser of stock is not buying anything from the target company itself but rather is buying the stock directly from its stockholders.

Under these circumstances, the acquisition of a public hospital would likely be structured as an acquisition of assets. A government entity may not sell a department or agency such as a police department, fire department, or public hospital. However, a government may sell assets such as unneeded police cars, fire trucks, firehouses, and other *assets* of a government agency. In this way, a buyer could use an asset acquisition to purchase a public hospital by paying the government body for the land, buildings, equipment, and other property of the hospital. In an asset acquisition, the purchaser would buy all or substantially all of the assets directly from the target company as opposed to its stockholders. After the asset acquisition of a public hospital, the government body will no longer operate the hospital facilities, and it will use the proceeds from selling the facilities to carry out its other government functions.

In selling the assets of a public hospital, a government body may be required to comply with state statutes that explicitly regulate the sale of public hospitals or with more general state statutes that regulate the sale or disposition of any public property. Moreover, in determining the value of the assets and selecting a buyer, public officials must act in the public interest, as opposed to their own personal interest. For example, a federal investigation was launched in 1995 to determine whether a public hospital executive had undervalued the assets of the hospital to encourage a for-profit chain to buy the hospital and give the executive a job.[23]

Similar issues can arise in the sale of a private, nonprofit hospital. Like a public hospital, a nonprofit hospital has no stock or stockholders. Therefore, the sale of a nonprofit hospital might be structured as a sale of assets. The nonprofit corporation would not be required to comply with state statutes that regulate the sale of public hospitals or the disposition of public property. However, some states have enacted statutes that specifically regulate the sale of private, nonprofit hospitals.

The directors or trustees of a nonprofit corporation are required to meet their fiduciary duty to the corporation by making sure that it receives fair market value for the sale of its assets. Like the directors and officers of a business corporation, the directors, trustees, and officers of a nonprofit corporation must put the interests of the organization ahead of their personal interests, particularly in responding to a proposed change in control.[24] After an acquisition, the acquiring entity will often terminate the executives and board members of the target and replace them with people designated by the acquiring entity. Even in a nonprofit organization, executives and trustees might react negatively to a proposed acquisition that would have the effect of removing them from their current positions. In other situations, executives of the target might be unduly influenced to support a proposed acquisition because of lucrative job offers from the acquiring entity.[25] Under any of these circumstances, the fiduciary duties and ethical obligations of officers, directors, and trustees require them to disclose their conflicts of interest and make decisions in the best interest of the nonprofit corporation.

If a nonprofit hospital is being acquired by another nonprofit hospital or by a nonprofit hospital system, the acquisition could be structured in a variety of different ways. For example, one nonprofit hospital could acquire another by using the structure of a nonprofit membership corporation with only one member.[26] The target hospital would amend its articles of incorporation to become a nonprofit membership corporation of which the sole member would be the acquiring hospital. As the sole member of the target hospital, the acquiring hospital would effectively control the activities of the target. Alternatively, the parties could create a nonprofit holding company that would be the sole member of both of the nonprofit hospitals. By making the two nonprofit hospitals sister companies under the control of a common parent, this alternative would avoid the negative connotation that one hospital was being acquired by the other. Another alternative for a transaction between two nonprofit corporations is to amend the target's articles of incorporation to give the acquiring party authority to appoint directors of the target or approve particular decisions by the target. This technique might also be used when a public entity acquires a private, nonprofit entity.

In the 1980s, many nonprofit hospitals went through corporate reorganizations to establish nonprofit parent companies with control over various nonprofit and for-profit subsidiaries. Each of those subsidiaries performs a particular function that may be taxable or tax-exempt, such as hospital services, long-term care, home health, ownership of real property, or other business activities. In addition, the nonprofit parent company can be used as a vehicle for acquiring other healthcare facilities and developing a multihospital system.

In some states, state attorneys general have challenged particular actions by nonprofit hospitals and systems, such as proposed affiliations and attempts to close a facility and consolidate services. Some cases have involved issues of nonprofit corporation law, such as whether court approval is required for certain amendments to the articles of incorporation or changes in corporate structure.[27] In other cases, state attorneys general have relied on the law of charitable trusts and their traditional authority to protect the assets of a charitable trust.[28] This type of challenge can result in a settlement or a decision to abandon the proposed transaction.

From a policy perspective, we must ensure that a change in control of a nonprofit hospital, by whatever means, does not adversely affect the use of its assets for charitable purposes. As the techniques of acquisition become more complex, our legal system must develop new ways to protect the interest of the public and ensure that legal formalities are not used to evade regulatory requirements that are designed to protect the public health.

Notes

1. American Hospital Association, "Fast Facts on US Hospitals" (January 3, 2013). www.aha.org/research/rc/stat-studies/101207fastfacts.pdf.

2. *Id*.

3. *Trustees of Dartmouth College v. Woodward*, 17 U.S. 518, 636 (1819).

4. *Quickturn Design Systems, Inc. v. Shapiro*, 721 A.2d 1281, 1291 (Del. 1998).

5. See *In re Caremark International, Inc.*, 698 A.2d 959, 970 (Del. Ch. 1996).

6. See generally R. Kuttner, "Columbia/HCA and the Resurgence of the For-Profit Hospital Business," *New England Journal of Medicine* (1996), 335: 362, 446.

7. E. C. Norton and D. O. Staiger (1994). "How Hospital Ownership Affects Care for the Uninsured." *Rand Journal of Economics* 25(1): 171–185, at 172 ("for-profit hospitals may be skimming off the cream by locating in well-insured areas").

8. A. Mundy (2013). "Doc-Owned Hospitals Prep to Fight," *Wall Street Journal,* May 14, B1.

9. Centers for Medicare & Medicaid Services, "Physician-Owned Hospitals" (August 22, 2012). www.cms.gov/Medicare/Fraud-and-Abuse/PhysicianSelfReferral/Physician_Owned_Hospitals.html.

10. See generally N. Ono, "Boards of Directors Under Fire: An Examination of Nonprofit Board Duties in the Health Care Environment," *Annals of Health Law* (1998), 7: 107–38.

11. See, e.g., *Geisinger Health Plan v. Commissioner*, 985 F.2d 1210, 1217 (3d Cir. 1993) ("a nonprofit hospital will qualify for tax-exempt status if it primarily benefits the community").

12. See Taxpayer Bill of Rights 2, Pub. L. No. 104-168, § 1311, 110 Stat. 1452, 1475 (1996) (codified at 26 U.S.C. § 4958 (2006)).

13. See J. R. Horwitz, "Why We Need the Independent Sector: The Behavior, Law, and Ethics of Not-for-Profit Hospitals," *UCLA Law Review* (2003), 50 (6): 1345–1411, 1382–84; T. L. Greaney, "New Governance Norms and Quality of Care in Nonprofit Hospitals," *Annals of Health Law* (2005), 14: 421–36, 427 ("One of the most remarkable aspects of federal tax-exempt organization law is the absence of any specific requirement of charity care in IRS enforcement in the hospital sector").

14. *National Federation of Independent Business v. Sebelius*, 132 S. Ct. 2566 (2012).

15. 78 Fed. Reg. at 20523 (April 5, 2013) (proposed regulations regarding the community health needs assessment). See also Notice 2011-52.

16. 77 Fed. Reg. at 38148 (June 26, 2012) (proposed regulations on financial assistance policies, charges, billing, and collections).

17. 78 Fed. Reg. at 20525.

18. 78 Fed. Reg. at 20527.

19. Patient Protection and Affordable Care Act, Pub. L. No. 111-148, § 9007(a)(5) (2010).

20. 77 Fed. Reg. at 38153–55.

21. Patient Protection and Affordable Care Act, Pub. L. No. 111-148, § 9007(a)(6) (2010).

22. 77 Fed. Reg. at 38158–59.

23. A. Gerlin (1995). "Hospital in Florida Is Focus of Probes Tied to Scuttled Bid by Columbia/HCA," *Wall Street Journal*, May 8, B10.

24. See generally C. T. Moran, "Why Revlon Applies to Nonprofit Corporations," *The Business Lawyer* (1998), 53: 373–95.

25. See "Ethics & the CEO," *Hospitals and Health Networks* (1998), January 20, 28–34.

26. See D. A. Reiser, "Decision-Makers Without Duties: Defining the Duties of Parent Corporations Acting as Sole Corporate Members in Nonprofit Health Care Systems," *Rutgers Law Review* (2001), 53: 979–1026.

27. See, e.g., *Nathan Littauer Hospital Association v. Spitzer*, 734 N.Y.S.2d 671 (N.Y. App. Div. 2001), *motion for leave to appeal denied*, 744 N.Y.S.2d 762 (N.Y. 2002) (rejecting claim by New York attorney general that court approval was required for charter amendments in an affiliation of two nonprofit hospitals).

28. See D. Bellandi, "The Watchdogs Are Biting: State Attorneys General Asserting Authority over Not-for-Profit Hospitals," *Modern Healthcare* (2001), January 29, 22.

GOVERNMENT REGULATION OF PUBLIC HEALTH AND HEALTHCARE SERVICES

Federal and state governments play important roles in protecting the public health and regulating the healthcare system. As discussed in Chapter 2, one of the underlying themes of healthcare law and policy is deciding what activities should be regulated by the federal government as opposed to the government of each state. Each level of government has its own powers and responsibilities, and each relies on its own sources of legal authority.

State authority to promote public health and regulate healthcare providers is based on the **police power**, which is the traditional authority of the state to protect public health, safety, and welfare. "According to settled principles the police power of a State must be held to embrace, at least, such reasonable regulations established directly by legislative enactment as will protect the public health and the public safety."[1] Under the police power, states may require individuals to be vaccinated against disease[2] and may prohibit individuals from providing healthcare services without obtaining a license from the state.[3]

In contrast, the federal government's authority over health and healthcare is based primarily on the power of Congress to regulate interstate commerce. For example, the National Organ Transplant Act,[4] which was discussed in Chapter 3, prohibits the sale of human organs, provided that the sale affects interstate commerce. The concept of interstate commerce is usually interpreted broadly, and courts have held that a wide range of activities can affect interstate commerce. For example, the U.S. Supreme Court held that interstate commerce can be affected by growing wheat on your own land for your own personal consumption.[5] In the healthcare field, the Supreme Court held that an alleged conspiracy to prevent the construction of a local hospital would substantially affect interstate commerce by reducing the interstate flow of supplies, insurance payments, financing, and management fees.[6] Therefore, many activities in the healthcare system would be found to have an effect on interstate commerce and could be subject to federal regulation on that basis.

However, the power of Congress to regulate interstate commerce is not unlimited, as the U.S. Supreme Court emphasized in its 2012 decision on the constitutionality of the federal Patient Protection and Affordable Care

Police power
The authority of state government to protect public health, safety, and welfare.

Conditional spending power
The authority of Congress to impose conditions on the use of federal funds it provides to state governments.

Certificate-of-need (CON) laws
State laws that prohibit development of new healthcare facilities and services unless officials determine that the proposed facilities and services are needed and meet other criteria in statutes or regulations.

Act (ACA). In that case, the Supreme Court held that the individual mandate to buy health insurance is not a valid regulation of interstate commerce, but the penalty for failure to buy health insurance is valid under Congress' power to tax.[7] Thus, the federal government may not use its power to regulate interstate commerce to require all residents of the United States to buy health insurance. In contrast, state governments may use their broad police power to require their residents to buy health insurance, as the State of Massachusetts had done even before enactment of the federal ACA.

Aside from its power to regulate interstate commerce, the federal government can effectively control many aspects of healthcare by using its **conditional spending power**. Under that power, Congress may require states to enact particular laws as a condition of federal aid to the states.[8] If a state objects to the condition, it is free to turn down the federal money. For example, the U.S. Supreme Court held that Congress has the power to require states to enact **certificate-of-need (CON) laws** as a condition of federal grants, even if that type of law would violate the state's own constitution.[9] Similarly, the federal government provides Medicaid funding to states that are willing to enact medical assistance programs that meet specific federal requirements.

Like the power of Congress to regulate interstate commerce, however, the conditional spending power of Congress is not unlimited. In its decision on the constitutionality of the federal ACA, the U.S. Supreme Court also held that the federal government cannot withdraw *existing* Medicaid funds from states that decline to participate in the expansion of Medicaid.[10] The Supreme Court recognized that, under its conditional spending power, Congress may impose conditions on states that go beyond what Congress could otherwise require states to do. Thus, Congress may impose conditions on use of specific federal funds, and may withhold funds from states that refuse to meet the conditions of a particular federal program. However, if a state refuses to meet the conditions of that particular program, Congress may not withhold federal funds that relate to other federal programs. The Supreme Court treated the expansion of Medicaid as a different federal program and held that the federal government may not "penalize States that choose not to participate in that new program by taking away their existing Medicaid funding."[11]

In addition to imposing conditions on federal grants to state governments, the federal government can use its power as a large-scale buyer of healthcare services to impose conditions directly on healthcare providers that choose to participate in the Medicare program. Although participation in Medicare is a practical necessity for most healthcare providers, it is technically voluntary. Therefore, the Medicare program can use voluntary participation as a mechanism or hook to impose requirements on providers, even if those requirements could not be imposed as a regulation of interstate commerce. The federal government also uses voluntary participation by skilled nursing facilities in Medicare and Medicaid as a way to impose requirements for protecting patients' rights in those facilities.

Some activities may be subject to federal and state regulation at the same time. As discussed in Chapter 2, federal laws are the supreme law of the land, and they supersede contrary provisions of state law. In enacting a federal statute, Congress might explicitly provide that the federal law **preempts** all state laws on the same subject. In other situations, Congress might explicitly permit states to adopt additional requirements to regulate the same activities as the federal statute, provided that the state laws do not interfere with the federal regulatory scheme. Under those circumstances, the federal law would establish a floor of minimum requirements that must be met throughout the country, and individual states could impose higher requirements within their respective jurisdictions if they so desire. Sometimes Congress does not clearly state its intent with regard to federal preemption of state authority, and those situations often result in litigation to determine whether the federal law preempts a particular law of the state.

Preempt
The effect of a federal law that supersedes a contrary provision of state law.

In the healthcare system, federal and state regulation can be used to accomplish several important goals:

1. to protect the public health by preventing and reducing communicable and noncommunicable diseases, preventing injuries, and protecting the safety of food, water, medical products, and the environment;
2. to promote the quality of healthcare services provided by facilities and individual practitioners; and
3. to reduce the costs for healthcare services and promote access to care by all members of the community.

These goals of government regulation are addressed in this chapter. Other goals are addressed in other chapters. For example, the goal of protecting privacy of health information is addressed in Chapter 6, and the goal of protecting consumers in the market for health insurance is addressed in Chapter 15.

Government Regulation to Protect the Public Health

In carrying out their police powers, state governments are responsible for traditional public health functions, such as promoting sanitation and controlling communicable disease.[12] As mentioned, the police power of a state includes the power to require individuals to be vaccinated against disease. The control of communicable disease includes an important role for state governments in protecting the public against bioterrorism. In addition, states use government regulation to promote public health by preventing noncommunicable diseases, such as obesity and heart disease.

To protect the public health, state legislatures may delegate power to administrative agencies at the state level and may authorize municipalities or local boards of health to exercise specific powers. For example, states may authorize local public health officials to investigate instances of communicable disease and to isolate or quarantine persons who pose a danger to the public health. States also require healthcare professionals to report outbreaks of communicable disease to state or local agencies, even though that may require a breach of patient confidentiality. In fact, the federal privacy rule that was adopted under the Health Insurance Portability and Accountability Act (HIPAA) contains an explicit exception to permit healthcare providers and other covered entities to disclose individually identifiable health information to public health officials for such purposes as disease control and surveillance.[13] Aside from the federal privacy rule, state laws may authorize disclosure of otherwise confidential information and may provide immunity from liability for those who make reports in compliance with the law.

In contrast to the active role of the states, the federal role in traditional public health functions has been more limited. However, the terrorist attacks on the World Trade Center and the Pentagon on September 11, 2001, as well as subsequent anthrax attacks, led to a discussion about whether we should reconsider the roles of state and federal governments in protecting public health.[14] No simple solution can be offered about the best way to allocate authority and coordinate the efforts of government agencies in responding to a bioterrorist attack.[15] As experts have pointed out, state and local officials are in the best position to identify and respond to an outbreak,[16] but bioterrorist attacks are likely to extend beyond the boundaries of an individual state and may fall within the federal government's authority to protect national security.[17]

One of the interesting initiatives in this area was the development of a model law for consideration by state legislatures. To ensure that states will have the legal authority to respond effectively to bioterrorism, the Centers for Disease Control and Prevention (CDC) and other organizations asked experts in public health law to prepare a model act,[18] known as the Model State Emergency Health Powers Act.[19] The December 21, 2001, version of the model act was a "draft for discussion" rather than a final document for adoption by state legislatures.[20] Thus, legislatures in many states have taken some action on these issues, but have not necessarily incorporated all of the suggested provisions of the model act.[21] In fact, important issues must be considered and policy decisions must be made before adopting this type of law. Aside from the appropriate roles of the state and federal governments, as already discussed, these issues include the appropriate role of law enforcement authorities in responding to a public health emergency, rationing of scarce resources in an emergency, criteria for declaring a state of emergency, and the proper balance between government powers and civil liberties during an emergency.[22]

The issue of preserving civil liberties during a public health emergency has been a source of significant controversy. One prominent author has criticized the model act on the grounds that "draconian quarantine measures would probably have the unintended effect of encouraging people to avoid public health officials and physicians rather than to seek them out."[23] However, other experts, including the principal authors of the model act, have defended their balancing of state power and individual liberty.[24] The drafters have argued that the model act provides more protection of individual rights than many of the earlier state laws, and they have pointed out that "compulsory power has always been a part of public health law, because it is sometimes necessary to prevent or ameliorate unacceptable threats to the common good."[25]

Aside from protecting against communicable diseases and bioterrorism, other public health functions include preventing noncommunicable diseases and injuries as well as protecting the safety of food, water, medical products, and the environment. State governments may take action under their police power to reduce noncommunicable diseases, such as obesity and heart disease, although some of those actions may be controversial. As Thomas R. Frieden, director of the CDC, explained, "Law and public opinion recognize protection of health and safety as a core government function, but public health actions are sometimes characterized as inappropriately intrusive. Such criticism has a long history, but today we accept many public health measures that were once considered misguided, intrusive, or controversial."[26] One example of a controversial public health measure is a rule that limits the size of soft drinks that may be sold in restaurants.[27] When New York City limited "sugary drinks" sold by certain types of "food service establishments" to 16 ounces, a state trial court issued a permanent injunction to prevent city officials from enforcing that rule, and that decision was affirmed by the intermediate appellate court.[28]

Government Regulation for Quality of Care

One of the most important issues in healthcare law is determining whether to rely on government regulation, industry self-regulation, market competition, or some combination of those methods as a means of achieving our policy goals.[29] In America's free-market economy, competition ordinarily improves the quality and reduces the price of goods and services for the benefit of the consumer. For example, in the healthcare field, competition may promote quality and reduce costs as healthcare providers compete among themselves for the opportunity to be "preferred providers" under managed care contracts. It is doubtful, however, that competition alone could ensure the quality of healthcare services. Most consumers lack the specialized knowledge required to evaluate the quality of medical care, and they often have little choice in selecting their providers.

Another possible way to ensure quality in the competitive marketplace is through the tort liability system of medical malpractice. Theoretically, the tort liability system should publicly identify the bad providers and drive them out of business as a result of damage awards, settlements, and higher premiums for malpractice insurance. In addition, the threat of malpractice liability should serve as a deterrent by causing other providers to be more careful. However, in practice, the tort liability system does not necessarily identify negligent providers or drive them out of business. As discussed in Chapter 10, even though a small number of patients receive large damage awards, most patients who are injured as a result of negligence never even file a claim. Therefore, we cannot rely solely on the medical malpractice system to ensure the quality of healthcare services.

Under these circumstances, the remaining alternatives to promote quality of care are government regulation or industry self-regulation. One advantage of government regulation is that a neutral party will establish the rules and inspect the providers. However, some providers resent the interference by government agents and argue that government officials and inspectors have less expertise than people who work in healthcare.

As an alternative, some healthcare providers favor industry and professional self-regulation. Examples of self-regulation include medical peer review and the voluntary accreditation of facilities by The Joint Commission, which is a private, nongovernmental organization. Under industry and professional self-regulation, people with substantial knowledge and experience will establish the standards and inspect the providers. However, there might be a lack of oversight by a truly neutral party. In fact, some people believe that allowing healthcare providers to regulate one another is like letting the fox guard the chicken coop.

For these reasons, our legal system uses a combination of government regulation and industry self-regulation as a means of promoting quality of care. As a policy matter, the issue is not whether to choose one extreme or the other. Rather, the issue is deciding where to draw the line between government regulation and industry or professional self-regulation, or perhaps choosing which strategy is appropriate for which problem. If we decide that we want a particular activity to be subject to government regulation, the further issue of whether the activity will be regulated by the state or the federal government must be settled. That choice will affect not only the selection of the regulatory agency but also the method of regulation. As already discussed, state and federal governments impose different types of regulation and rely on different types of legal authority as the basis for their regulation.

For many years, people involved in the healthcare system have tried to figure out ways to improve the quality of care and promote patient safety. Many different approaches may be used to improve quality, such as research, training, technology, payment incentives, continuous quality improvement, and clinical practice guidelines. In addition, the law can be used in several ways as a means to promote quality of care.

Merely enacting a statute that requires all healthcare professionals and facilities to provide high-quality care or face the consequences would not be effective, but some measures may be taken. We may be able to enact laws to require actions that we think will promote quality of care, such as requiring minimum levels of nurse staffing in healthcare facilities or requiring hospitals to use a computerized system for entering physician orders. We could also adopt new laws or change existing laws to provide incentives that encourage particular actions, such as encouraging medical peer review by providing immunity to participants in the peer-review process. Similarly, we could provide an incentive to encourage the use of clinical practice guidelines by making compliance with guidelines a defense against a claim of medical malpractice. Another alternative is to adopt laws that prohibit or discourage actions we think would be detrimental to quality of care.

When considering each of these alternatives, however, remember that the proposed legal intervention is not an end in itself but merely a means to an end. We also need to recognize our limitations and proceed with caution in using the coercive power of the law to require healthcare professionals and organizations to do things we think are likely to promote quality of care. Like evidence-based medicine, research on the effect of specific healthcare laws would be useful in determining the likely benefits and costs of proposed legal interventions.

One type of legal intervention would require healthcare facilities to report medical errors to a government agency at the state or federal level. In 1999, the Institute of Medicine (IOM) issued its influential report, *To Err Is Human*, stating that up to 98,000 people are killed every year by medical errors in U.S. hospitals.[30] As part of that report, the IOM recommended that Congress establish a system, similar to the existing system in the airline industry, for reporting adverse events in the healthcare industry. The IOM recommended adopting mandatory reporting of adverse events that cause serious harm or death and voluntary reporting of less serious events to help identify weaknesses in the system.

Others, however, have questioned whether a system that works for airlines would work as well for healthcare.[31] Moreover, some healthcare providers are concerned that, if they are required to report medical errors, patients or their lawyers could obtain copies of the medical error reports for use in malpractice cases. Despite these concerns, several states have enacted laws to require some type of mandatory reporting, and those laws may provide some protection against disclosure of patient-identifiable information.[32] At the federal level, Congress has considered some bills that would make reporting mandatory,[33] but it has not enacted a federal requirement. As discussed in Chapter 10, Congress has provided some degree of confidentiality for information that is voluntarily provided to certain safety organizations.[34]

Another way in which the law is used to promote quality of care is the system of licensure for healthcare professionals and facilities. As discussed in the next section, licensure is not the same as accreditation or certification, and distinguishing among those different methods is important.

Licensure of Individual Healthcare Professionals

State governments use their police power to protect public health, safety, and welfare by prohibiting individuals from providing specific healthcare services without a state license. In fact, practicing medicine without a license may violate criminal law.[35] In addition, each state regulates the practice of medicine and other health professions through **licensing boards**, such as a state board of medical examiners. As one commentator has explained, the justification for regulating healthcare practitioners is "market failure, in particular, a failure caused by lack of information in the hands of consumers and the inability of consumers to understand such information as was available to them."[36]

Licensing board
A state agency that regulates practitioners of a specific profession.

Unlike a state medical society, which is a voluntary professional association, a licensing board is an agency of state government. Because of the need for expertise in evaluating professional competence and ethics, state licensing boards are composed primarily of members of the particular profession. However, these boards act with the power of the state, and their actions are subject to the same statutory and constitutional restrictions that apply to other actions of government. State licensing boards are required, for example, to comply with due process of law by giving fair notice and an opportunity to be heard before taking adverse action on a license.

Practice acts
State statutes that regulate provision of specific professional services and create professional licensing boards.

Professional licensing boards operate under state statutes called **practice acts**. Although minor differences are seen in each state and for each profession, these practice acts are developed with a common structure. First, a practice act prohibits the unlicensed practice of a particular healthcare profession within the boundaries of the state. Then, each profession's act defines the practice of that profession by reference to specific types of activities or in relation to the activities that constitute the practice of medicine. Often an act will provide a series of exceptions so that a person will not be unlawfully practicing that profession if she is lawfully practicing a different healthcare profession within the bounds of her license. In addition, a practice act will create a board with the power to grant, deny, suspend, and revoke licenses, in accordance with the standards and procedures set forth in the act and the rules adopted by that board. As a state agency created by the legislature, a board has only those powers that the legislature delegated to it by statute. Finally, a practice act will specify the procedures for administrative appeal and judicial review of the board's licensing decisions.

Professional licensure can be used in a positive way to promote the quality of care and protect the public health. However, it can also be abused as a means of preserving the status quo in situations where medical doctors or dentists have a lucrative monopoly over the performance of certain functions. State licensure can be used to prevent competition from members of other healthcare professions and from other types of healthcare facilities. Licensure can also be used to prevent innovation by practitioners of different methods of treatment, such as homeopathic medicine. Some people argue that nurses and other allied health professionals are capable of safely performing many of the functions that currently are limited by law to licensed physicians or to those who work as employees under the direct supervision of physicians. Under that argument, state licensure interferes with efforts to reduce health-care costs and increase access to care. Finally, some people argue that medical licensing can be used to perpetuate an outmoded system of gender bias against the predominantly female profession of nursing.

As part of its comprehensive proposal for healthcare reform in the early 1990s, the Clinton administration tried to limit the power of the states with regard to professional licensure. Specifically, the administration's proposal would have prohibited states from imposing restrictions on the practice of any category of healthcare professionals unless those restrictions were justified by the training and skill of those professionals.[37] By proposing a federal prohibition of state licensure restrictions that were not "justified," it appears that the Clinton administration would have left the ultimate evaluation of those restrictions to the federal courts. Of course, that reform proposal was not enacted, and licensure remains under the control of the states.

One of the most interesting issues in professional licensure is determining the type of conduct that would justify revocation of a license. According to a 1990 report on state medical boards by the U.S. Department of Health and Human Services' (HHS) Office of Inspector General (OIG), "the great majority of disciplinary actions taken by the state boards concerns the improper use of drugs or alcohol—be it inappropriate prescribing, unlawful distribution, or self-abuse."[38] Even if the abuse of alcohol or drugs had occurred outside the context of medical practice, as in driving under the influence, that conduct may justify revocation of a license to practice medicine. As one court explained in upholding a board's disciplinary action,

> the state can impose discipline on a professional license only if the conduct upon which the discipline is based relates to the practice of the particular profession and thereby demonstrates an unfitness to practice such profession. . . .
>
> Convictions involving alcohol consumption reflect a lack of sound professional and personal judgment that is relevant to a physician's fitness and competence to practice medicine. Alcohol consumption quickly affects normal driving ability, and driving under the influence of alcohol threatens personal safety and places the safety of the public in jeopardy. . . .
>
> Driving while under the influence of alcohol also shows an inability or unwillingness to obey the legal prohibition against drinking and driving and constitutes a serious breach of a duty owed to society. . . .
>
> In relation to multiple convictions involving driving and alcohol consumption, we reject the argument that a physician can seal off or compartmentalize personal conduct so it does not affect the physician's professional practice. . . .
>
> Substantial legal authority provides that conduct occurring outside the practice of medicine may form the basis for imposing discipline on a license because such conduct reflects on a licensee's fitness and qualifications to practice medicine. . . . A physician who commits income tax fraud, solicits the subornation of perjury, or files false, fraudulent insurance claims has not practiced medicine incompetently. Nonetheless that physician has shown dishonesty, poor character, a lack of integrity, and an inability or unwillingness to follow the law, and thereby has demonstrated professional unfitness meriting license discipline. . . .[39]

Thus, boards may impose discipline for conduct outside the bounds of the traditional physician–patient relationship.

However, some issues on the scope of a board's power remain undecided. State boards might have the authority to revoke the license of a physician for giving improper testimony as a medical expert witness in a malpractice case.[40] Moreover, at least one state licensing board took disciplinary action against a physician for a utilization review decision that was made when the physician was medical director of a managed care organization.[41]

Finally, it is important to note that disciplinary action by a licensing board is not the only legal remedy for a serious problem in quality of care. Other remedies exist and are not mutually exclusive. A physician or other healthcare professional who was disciplined by a state licensing board could also be sued by a patient or by the estate of a patient in a civil suit for medical malpractice for the same conduct that resulted in suspension or revocation of the license. In a particularly egregious case, the same conduct could also provide the basis for a criminal charge.

Licensure of Healthcare Facilities

State governments also use their police power to promote quality of care by requiring healthcare facilities to obtain a license to operate. In fact, licensure laws for healthcare facilities are similar to practice acts for healthcare professionals, although the regulatory body for facilities is usually a traditional administrative agency rather than a board composed of professionals.

Licensing statutes generally prohibit a facility from operating without a license; identify the state agency with the authority to grant, deny, suspend, or revoke a license; and provide standards and procedures for disciplinary action, administrative appeals, and judicial review. In addition, the statutes usually authorize the agency to adopt rules for operating a facility, such as requirements for staffing, record keeping, policies, and safety standards.

Under their licensing authority, state agencies have the power to inspect facilities and take disciplinary action. For relatively minor infractions, the agency might impose a fine or require the facility to submit a plan of correction. In more serious cases, the agency might suspend admissions to the facility or even revoke the facility's license. If the matter involved injury to a patient, an adverse licensing action may have negative consequences for the facility in future malpractice litigation. Therefore, even if the agency's disciplinary action is not severe, the facility might contest the agency's decision through the process of administrative appeal and judicial review.

Although this chapter focuses on laws that are specific to the healthcare industry, healthcare facilities are also subject to general laws that apply to all organizations and individuals. For example, as employers, healthcare facilities and medical practices are subject to labor laws that regulate matters such as minimum wages, overtime pay, employee benefit plans, and discriminatory employment practices. Those types of laws are beyond the scope of this book, but information about them is available on the website of the U.S. Department of Labor.[42]

Accreditation of Healthcare Facilities

Unlike licensure of facilities under the police power of the state, **accreditation** is a voluntary process of industry self-regulation. The most prominent accrediting organization for healthcare facilities is The Joint Commission, which is a private, nongovernmental organization controlled by the healthcare industry. The Joint Commission has developed detailed standards for the operation of healthcare facilities, and it surveys each participating facility on a periodic basis.

Although Joint Commission accreditation is voluntary, about 80 percent of hospitals participating in Medicare are accredited.[43] In addition to being an indication of quality and a method of self-improvement, Joint Commission accreditation may provide at least two important practical benefits for a facility. First, hospital licensing agencies in most states rely on Joint

Accreditation
A voluntary process of industry self-regulation, such as evaluation of healthcare facilities by a private, nongovernmental organization.

Commission accreditation for the purpose of licensure. In those states, the hospital may send its Joint Commission survey report to the state hospital licensing agency, and the state will accept that report for licensure without a separate survey by a state inspector. As a second benefit of Joint Commission accreditation, accredited hospitals are automatically deemed by federal law to meet most of the requirements for participating in Medicare,[44] avoiding yet another duplicative survey.

Although the deemed status of accredited hospitals is advantageous for the facilities, it raises an important issue of public policy. In effect, most state licensing agencies and Medicare are saying that if the facility is good enough for the industry's own program of self-regulation, it is good enough for the government. In other industries where human lives are at stake, allowing companies to exempt themselves from regular government inspections merely by producing a "seal of approval" from their own industry association would be inconceivable. Yet that is the way in which our society relies on industry self-regulation for acute care hospitals, and many people think the system works extremely well.

Certification of Healthcare Facilities for Medicare and Medicaid

Certification
The process through which healthcare facilities are accepted for participation in government payment programs. For individual healthcare professionals, certification is a voluntary, nongovernmental process of professional self-regulation, such as the process for designating physicians as board certified in a particular specialty.

In contrast to voluntary accreditation by The Joint Commission and mandatory licensure by the state, **certification** of healthcare facilities refers to the process of acceptance for participation in the Medicare and Medicaid payment programs. Therefore, certification is an exercise of the government's power as a buyer, rather than its power as a regulator.

Although Medicare is a federal program, many of the survey activities are performed by state agencies under contract or other arrangement with the federal government. As discussed previously, facilities that are already accredited by The Joint Commission are deemed to meet most of the requirements for Medicare certification. Therefore, the 20 percent of Medicare-participating hospitals that are *not* accredited go through the governmental process of certification by state agencies acting on behalf of the federal government.

A certified facility will have a written provider agreement with the program, which is a type of contract, and the facility must comply with the conditions of participation. If the facility fails to comply with all of the applicable requirements, the Medicare program could terminate the provider agreement, which would prevent the facility from treating Medicare patients.

As discussed in Chapter 8, the OIG uses its authority under the law of Medicare fraud and abuse to promote quality of care in participating facilities. As part of the settlements in some cases of fraud and abuse, the OIG has required healthcare organizations to implement systems of quality improvement as well as make changes in systems of financial controls. The OIG's authority over Medicare fraud and abuse is not limited to facilities that are surveyed by state agencies on behalf of the federal government but applies as well to facilities that are deemed acceptable by virtue of their Joint Commission accreditation.

The term *certification* has a different meaning for individual practitioners than it does for facilities. For physicians, certification is granted by one of the independent, nongovernmental organizations known as medical specialty boards. This process is the basis for designating physicians as "board certified" in a particular specialty. Similar systems are in place for other types of healthcare professionals. When used to describe individual healthcare professionals, certification is a voluntary, nongovernmental process of professional self-regulation.

Thus, individual healthcare professionals are subject to government regulation in the form of licensure under the police power of the state as well as professional self-regulation by means of specialty board certification. In addition, healthcare professionals are subject to government supervision as participants in federal payment programs as well as professional self-regulation in the credentialing process for medical staff membership and clinical privileges, as discussed in Chapter 7. In a similar manner, healthcare facilities are subject to government regulation in the form of state licensure, industry self-regulation by means of voluntary accreditation, and government supervision as participants in federal payment programs. In these ways, our legal system promotes quality of care by a unique mix of government regulation, industry and professional self-regulation, and market competition.

Government Regulation of Diversified Organizations

Some of the traditional distinctions among different types of entities in the healthcare industry have been blurred by a continuing trend toward diversification. As discussed in Chapter 4, providers of healthcare services, such as hospitals and physicians, have been joining together to form diversified organizations that offer a combined package of services. The 2010 federal health reform legislation is likely to increase this trend, by encouraging healthcare providers to create and participate in **accountable care organizations** (ACOs) which provide incentives for efficiency and quality.

In some cases, organizations of healthcare providers are taking on risk by agreeing to provide services for a group of people at a predetermined price. Depending on the need for services and the cost for providing services, those healthcare providers could make a profit or suffer a loss on that contract. In fact, those healthcare providers might be performing some functions that traditionally were performed by insurance companies and health maintenance organizations (HMOs). As a policy matter, society has an interest in making sure that this type of organization is financially responsible, so that it

Accountable care organization (ACO)
A group of healthcare providers that delivers quality care to patients in a coordinated manner and shares the cost savings resulting from those efforts, such as a group established under Medicare's Shared Savings Program.

will be able to provide the healthcare services for which payment already has been made. Therefore, an organization of healthcare providers that takes on some types of risk will pose a regulatory challenge for society.

A similar regulatory challenge is posed by diversification at the other end of the provider–payer spectrum. Some insurance companies and self-insured employers, which originally had limited their activities to paying for healthcare services, have established their own networks of healthcare providers. Although insurance companies and employers are usually regulated as third-party payers, some of those payers might also be participating in some ways in the delivery of healthcare services. As payers and providers from each end of the spectrum diversify toward the middle, our society must address the important question of how those hybrid entities should be regulated in the public interest.

A system of government regulation is based on fitting each activity into a defined category and applying rules that are appropriate for that category. If an activity has characteristics that fit into more than one category, a decision must be made as to whether it should be licensed and regulated in one category, the other category, both categories, or perhaps an entirely new category for that new type of activity or organization.

An historical example of this phenomenon is the HMO, which not only pays for care but also provides or arranges for care through licensed physicians and other healthcare providers. In most cases, an HMO would not be a medical practice under the regulatory authority of the professional licensing board. Although HMOs perform a payment function, they are different in some ways from insurance companies, which are regulated under specific state insurance laws. Therefore, adopting new laws to create a new regulatory category for HMOs was reasonable.

Like HMOs, other types of hybrid organizations are found in the modern healthcare marketplace. Many of these entities perform diversified functions and do not fit into the traditional boxes of health regulation. As with the regulatory issues discussed above, the challenge of law and policy is to find ways to protect the public interest, without imposing excessive regulatory burdens that would stifle competition and innovation.

Government Regulation for Cost Containment and Access

CON laws prohibit the development of new healthcare facilities and services unless the provider can demonstrate to the satisfaction of state officials that the proposed facilities and services are needed. In most states, government officials have the power to decide which new facilities may be built and which new services may be provided by each facility. Thus, CON regulation goes to the very heart of the ongoing debate between government regulation and free-market competition as the best method of achieving our policy goals in healthcare.

Arguments For and Against CON Laws

CON laws may have an effect on quality of care, although the nature of that effect is subject to debate. For some highly specialized services, a limitation on the number of providers may promote quality by ensuring that all authorized providers will perform a sufficient volume of procedures to develop and maintain their proficiency. Some evidence indicates, for example, that hospitals that perform a large volume of open-heart surgery procedures have better results, in terms of mortality rates, than programs that perform a small number of procedures. However, in other ways, CON regulation may have an adverse effect on quality of care by preventing some facilities from acquiring state-of-the-art equipment. Moreover, by reducing the level of competition, CON regulation limits the need for healthcare providers to compete with each other on the basis of quality.

Although CON laws may have an effect on quality, the primary goals of CON regulation are cost containment and access to care. In regard to cost, the economic theory of CON regulation is that the law of supply and demand does not operate normally in the healthcare field.[45] In most industries, an increase in the supply of goods and services or an increase in the number of competing sellers would cause prices to go down as sellers compete among themselves for business. However, some people think an increase in the supply of healthcare services or an increase in the number of competing providers would cause prices to go up rather than down.

Under that economic theory, the healthcare industry does not respond normally to competitive forces. When healthcare services are covered by insurance, consumers are insulated to a large extent from the costs and do not have to make economic decisions about purchasing those services. In addition, most consumers do not have the specialized knowledge to determine their need for healthcare services or to compare the relative cost and quality of each alternative. Consumers tend to use whatever services are recommended by their physician, provided those services are covered by an insurance plan. Under these circumstances, most consumers do not shop for the lowest price among healthcare providers, and providers generally do not have to compete for the business of individual consumers on the basis of price.

Even if the supply of healthcare services were to increase, providers would not need to cut their prices, as they would in an ordinary competitive market. In fact, as the number of providers increases, providers might even need to increase their prices to compensate for a reduction in volume at each facility.

As an oversimplified example, assume that Hospital A has the only magnetic resonance imaging (MRI) scanner in the area. If it costs Hospital A

$1 million per year in operating costs for the MRI service, and if Hospital A provides 1,000 MRI procedures per year, Hospital A would need to charge $1,000 per procedure to break even. However, if Hospital B were to obtain an MRI scanner in the same area and provide half of the local procedures (500 procedures), Hospital B would need to charge $2,000 per procedure to break even ($1 million annual operating cost divided by 500 procedures = $2,000 per procedure). Meanwhile, Hospital A would need to raise its charge from $1,000 to $2,000 per procedure to spread its costs over a smaller number of procedures or, alternatively, perform additional procedures that might be unnecessary. This type of scenario leads some people to think that society should replace competition with government regulation of the supply of healthcare services and facilities by means of CON laws.

However, a serious question remains as to whether the economic theory of CON regulation is valid. That economic theory was developed in the 1960s and 1970s, when providers encountered little price competition, and the Medicare program paid hospitals on a retrospective, cost-reimbursement basis. Under that system of Medicare reimbursement, hospitals had a perverse incentive to build large and expensive facilities, even if not all of those facilities were really necessary. Arguably, government regulation may have been necessary to control the supply of facilities and equipment at that time. However, as discussed in Chapter 8, Medicare now pays hospitals on the basis of prospectively determined prices rather than retrospectively determined costs. Under the new system of Medicare payment, hospitals generally have an incentive to reduce their costs to maximize net revenue. In addition, under the bargaining process used by many commercial insurance plans, providers now are more likely to compete on the basis of price for preferred provider contracts. That bargaining process might restrain healthcare costs and prices without the need for government regulation of supply. Even if the economic theory of CON regulation was correct at the time it was developed, it might be invalid as applied to a system of prospective payment and preferred-provider contracting. Moreover, empirical research does not prove that CON laws have significantly reduced healthcare costs, and those states that eliminated CON regulation did not experience significant increases in costs after their laws were repealed.[46]

Another argument in favor of CON regulation is that restraining the supply of healthcare facilities is the best way—or perhaps the only effective way—to prevent healthcare providers from performing unnecessary services. Under this theory, the demand for services by patients and physicians is not the same as the need for those services. Thus, demand for additional services will go up whenever the supply of available facilities increases.[47] According to this argument, government experts should determine the need for new facilities, allow only those facilities to be built, and then rely on physicians in those facilities to ration the limited resources to the most appropriate patients.[48]

This rationale for CON regulation can be criticized on several grounds. First, it is paternalistic for government officials to decide what people really need, as opposed to what patients and their physicians really want. Moreover, thinking that government agencies have the ability to determine what people need is probably unrealistic. If physicians are performing unnecessary procedures, other ways exist to deal with that problem, such as utilization review, peer review, and professional discipline. Finally, in light of the ongoing problems of insurance coverage and access to care, it is doubtful that all providers would allocate their limited resources to those patients with the greatest need.

Despite the limitations of those various rationales for CON regulation, CON laws might be justifiable and necessary for promoting access to care. For example, state officials might be able to require CON applicants to provide a particular level of indigent care or service to Medicaid patients as a condition of approval. Moreover, when more than one applicant is competing for a single CON, the state government could choose the applicant that is most likely to provide access to care. The state could also promote geographic access by limiting the development of new facilities to those areas that have the highest level of unmet need. Finally, CON laws can promote access to care by protecting public hospitals from competition for the paying patients that they need for financial survival. Public hospitals and some nonprofit hospitals provide a substantial amount of care to the indigent at a financial loss to the facility. Those hospitals need the revenue from insured patients to offset the loss and remain financially viable. If a for-profit facility were allowed to open in the same geographic area, it would take many of the paying patients and would leave most of the indigent patients to the public or nonprofit hospital. This practice is referred to as "cream-skimming." To prevent this practice, CON laws may be necessary to protect safety net facilities, regardless of whether the economic theory of CON laws is valid.

The System of CON Regulation

In 1974, the federal government decided to encourage the adoption of state CON laws by enacting the National Health Planning and Resources Development Act.[49] That federal statute provided funding to state governments on the condition that states enact CON laws that comply with federal standards. Initially, almost all of the states enacted CON laws. However, the federal statute was repealed in 1986, and some states have eliminated or reduced their CON requirements. Nevertheless, according to the National Conference of State Legislatures, "about 36 states retain some type of CON program, law or agency as of December 2011."[50] In some states, efforts to repeal CON laws have met with strong and successful resistance by existing providers, who like being protected from competition.[51] In addition, it is possible that some state governments use CON laws as a way to limit their expenditures for the Medicaid program by restricting the number of nursing home beds for which the state's Medicaid program would be obligated to pay.

In an unregulated market, competing sellers would decide what services to offer and where to offer them. However, in a system that is regulated by CON laws, state officials decide where new facilities may be built, who may build them, and what services may be offered. In some ways, the healthcare industry under CON regulation resembles the centrally planned economy of the former Soviet Union. However, other U.S. industries have similar regulatory barriers to market entry, such as public utilities and automobile dealerships in some states.

Where CON laws exist, they are not limited to public facilities or facilities that receive government funds. Moreover, CON laws are not limited to services provided to publicly insured patients, such as those covered by Medicare or Medicaid. Rather, CON laws apply to private and public facilities, and they apply to services provided to commercially insured and self-paying patients, as well as to patients who are publicly insured. Therefore, as practical matter, CON laws limit what a private organization may do with its own land, buildings, money, and patients.

However, CON regulation does not require government approval for the continued operation of existing facilities, equipment, and services. A state CON agency can protect existing facilities from competition by refusing to grant a CON to a potential competitor, but ordinarily cannot take away an existing facility's CON even if the existing facility is underutilized. Therefore, the system of CON regulation has a bias in favor of existing providers, which have received what amounts to a permanent franchise from the state.

Under these circumstances, the attitude of existing healthcare facilities and their managers is ambivalent. When CON laws prevent them from developing new facilities or offering new services, they tend to complain bitterly about intrusive overregulation by the government. However, when someone else proposes to compete in their geographic area, they insist that CON laws should be aggressively enforced to prevent "needless duplication" of healthcare facilities and services, on the grounds that it would be bad for society as a whole.

Under a system of CON regulation, the threshold issue is whether a CON is needed for a particular project. By their terms, CON statutes only apply to specific types of facilities, equipment, and services. In some situations, a CON will be required only if the project involves a capital expenditure or annual operating cost that exceeds a level specified in the law. In contrast, some activities listed in the statute will require a CON regardless of the capital or operating expense.

Healthcare facilities may attempt to structure or describe their projects in ways that will avoid the time and expense of applying for a CON. For ethical as well as legal reasons, healthcare providers must honestly represent the costs and nature of a project to a state CON agency. In the meantime, a provider's competitors may argue that the project should be subject to CON review. The competitors will insist, of course, that they are opposing the project out of concern for the interests of society as a whole and not because of any desire to protect their existing market share. Eventually, the CON agency in that state will have to determine whether the project is subject to CON review.

Sometimes healthcare facilities and their advisers are successful in finding a loophole to avoid CON review for a particular project. Then, the CON agency in that state may attempt to close that loophole for the future by amending its regulations or by seeking a legislative amendment to the CON statute. Eventually, the facilities and their advisers will find new loopholes, and the process will begin all over again in a never-ending game of cat and mouse between the regulated industry and the regulators.

The Medical Arms Race

In addition to dealing with an agency of state government, healthcare providers often compete among themselves for valuable CONs as part of what has been called the "medical arms race." Although state laws differ, the basic regulatory pattern is divided into two separate processes: one for statewide health planning and one for the review of specific CON applications.

The statewide health planning process involves conducting an inventory of existing facilities and services in each geographic area of the state and determining the future need for each type of facility and service. These determinations of need are made without regard to any particular applicant, and they result in allocations for which anyone may apply. For example, a state government might determine that a need exists for 30 new skilled nursing facilities, ten new home health agencies, and three new ambulatory surgery facilities in particular counties or regions of the state. Those needs would be reflected in a state health plan or state regulations, which allocate particular numbers of facilities or beds for future CON reviews.

In some states, the determinations of need are made by a Statewide Health Coordinating Council (SHCC), which might include representatives of provider associations, public officials, and consumers. If healthcare providers want to develop facilities or services in the near future, they might ask the SHCC or other state officials to recognize a need for the proposed facility or service and make an allocation for a future CON review. Meanwhile, other providers might urge or lobby the SHCC not to allocate any new facilities or services that might compete with them in the future. As one court explained, adopting and amending a state health plan is a quasi-legislative process of rulemaking, whereas reviewing individual CON applications is a quasi-judicial process of adjudication.[52]

Allocations in a state health plan or state regulations are often based on some quantitative need methodology, which includes factors such as projections of future population, incidence rate for a particular disease, historical and anticipated rates of utilization, and capacity of all existing and approved facilities. State officials use these methodologies to calculate the precise number of beds, operating rooms, machines, or facilities that will be needed at a particular time in the future. However, these methodologies can be based on gross estimates and assumptions that can be manipulated to achieve a particular result. For example, a state government could choose particular assumptions for its need methodology that would result in an allocation of fewer nursing home beds in that state, thereby limiting the state government's future Medicaid expenditure for nursing home services. Thus, states could use the health planning process as a way to ration care by limiting the number of facilities to a level for which their citizens are willing to pay. Moreover, to the extent that quantitative methodologies are based on historical utilization, states might understate the need for services in the future, because of disparities on the basis of race, gender, and other grounds in the number of procedures that were provided in the past.

Regardless of whether the allocations are based on scientific methodology, politics, or budgetary considerations, those allocations play a crucial role in the CON review process. Under the laws of some states, the need determinations in the state health plan are conclusive, and providers can only apply for a CON to develop facilities or services that are allocated by the plan. Other state laws are more flexible, however, and give applicants an opportunity to try to prove a need for more facilities or services than the number identified in the plan.

Ordinarily, all of the applications for a particular service in a particular geographic area will be reviewed by a state agency on a competitive basis as part of a single "batch" or review cycle. Depending on the state's procedure, opportunities may be provided for a public hearing and written comments about the pending applications. Eventually, the state CON agency will decide whether to approve, deny, or conditionally approve each application on the basis of review criteria set forth in the state statute and regulations. In addition to general statutory criteria, such as need, access, and financial feasibility, many state agencies have adopted specific regulatory criteria that set forth quantitative standards for approval of particular types of services and equipment. These quantitative criteria are designed to ensure sufficient utilization of the proposed service or equipment as well as to prevent adverse effects on existing providers. Unless the applicable state law provides an exception, a CON application must be consistent with all of the general and specific criteria to be approved.

After the state CON agency has made its initial decision, a disappointed applicant or other affected party generally has the right to an administrative appeal. When all administrative remedies have been exhausted and the agency has made its final decision, a party may request judicial review in the courts. In some states, CON litigation can be time consuming and expensive. However, cases are often settled at some point between the state agency and an applicant or among the competing applicants. For example, a settlement may provide for the approval of an application subject to specific conditions.

After a CON is awarded, healthcare providers will have some continuing obligations. First, a CON holder will be required to develop and operate the facility or service in accordance with the representations in its application. Second, the holder must comply with any conditions that the state agency imposed on the award of the CON, such as providing a specified level of care to the indigent or charging no more than specified rates.

Depending on the particular state law, these obligations may also apply to a future buyer of a healthcare facility that obtained a CON. Therefore, a prospective buyer should use due diligence before purchasing a healthcare facility to determine whether he will inherit any legal obligations as the new owner and operator. Moreover, the laws of some states prohibit the transfer of a CON or require the state agency's prior approval for a transfer. Finally, if a facility fails to comply with the law, the state agency may have the authority to withdraw the CON.

ACTIVITY 5.1: CON FOR OPEN-HEART SURGERY

To whom it may concern:

Jackson County Hospital needs your help!

As chief executive officer of Jackson County Hospital, I am issuing this request for professional assistance. We have a big problem, and we are willing to pay whatever is necessary to any outside consultants who can help us solve it. Alternatively, I would be happy to offer the full-time position of executive vice president of the hospital to anyone who can solve it for us.

We desperately need to establish an open-heart surgery service at the hospital, but the state government denied our application for a certificate of need (CON). We still have time to appeal the decision, but I do not know whether we would have a good case. Even if we file an appeal, I do not know whether we could convince the state agency or a court that we comply with all of the regulations for granting a CON.

(continued)

(continued from previous page)

Please review the enclosed facts and regulations, which set forth all you need to know to help us with this problem. Then, please answer the questions attached to this memorandum. I look forward to reading your answers and to rewarding the best responses.

THE FACTS

Jackson County Hospital (County) is a 400-bed, general, acute care hospital in a medium-sized city, owned and operated by Jackson County. County offers most types of sophisticated healthcare services, including MRI, lithotripsy, neonatal intensive care, and cardiac catheterization. However, County does not provide open-heart surgery and must refer all patients for open-heart surgery to other hospitals.

County's primary competitor is Doctor's Hospital, which is the only other hospital in Jackson County. Doctor's Hospital, a private, nonprofit hospital with only private rooms, is the hospital of choice for most of the commercially insured patients in the area. However, Doctor's provides very little care for the indigent. Most of the uninsured patients and Medicaid patients in the area are treated at County.

Doctor's developed an open-heart surgery service about eight years ago when there were fewer regulatory restrictions on acquiring medical equipment and developing new healthcare services. At the present time, Doctor's has the only open-heart surgery service within a 100-mile radius of the city in which we are both located.

County desperately wants to develop an open-heart surgery service for several reasons. First, the new service would generate revenue to support its other operations. Second, to attract more commercially insured patients for all of our services, County needs to change its image as a second-class hospital that lacks the modern facilities and equipment available at Doctor's. Third, because County cannot perform open-heart surgery on those patients who require it, physicians are reluctant to refer patients to County for other cardiac services, such as cardiac catheterizations. Fourth, County has had difficulty obtaining preferred provider contracts with managed care organizations because it is unable to provide the full range of services the patients may require. For all of these reasons, County's top strategic goal is establishing an open-heart surgery service.

(continued)

(continued from previous page)

However, we have been unable to obtain approval for an open-heart surgery service under the state's CON law. Although County applied for a CON, our application has just been denied by the state CON agency.

THE STATE CON REGULATIONS FOR OPEN-HEART SURGERY SERVICES

Following are the state CON regulations that apply to County:

SECTION .1700—CRITERIA AND STANDARDS FOR OPEN-HEART SURGERY SERVICES AND HEART-LUNG BYPASS MACHINES[53]

.1713 Definitions

The following definitions shall apply to all rules in this Section:

(1) "Capacity" of an open-heart surgery room means 400 adult-equivalent open-heart surgical procedures per year. One open-heart surgical procedure on persons age 5 and under is valued at two adult open-heart surgical procedures. For purposes of determining capacity, one open-heart surgical procedure is defined to be one visit or trip by a patient to the open-heart surgery room for an open-heart operation. . . .

(4) "Open-heart surgery service area" means a geographical area defined by the applicant, which has boundaries that are not farther than 90 road miles from the facility, except that the open-heart surgery service area of an academic medical center teaching hospital designated in 10 NCAC 3R. 3050 shall not be limited to 90 road miles.

(5) "Open-heart surgery services" is defined in G.S. 131E-176(18b).

(6) "Open-heart surgical procedures" means highly specialized surgical procedures which:

   (a) utilize a heart-lung bypass machine (the "pump") to perform extracorporeal circulation and oxygenation during surgery;

   (b) are designed to correct congenital and acquired cardiac coronary disease; and

   (c) are identified by Medicare Diagnostic Related Group (DRG) numbers 104, 105, 106, 107, and 108.

(continued)

(continued from previous page)

(7)   "Open-heart surgery room" means an operating room primarily used to perform open-heart surgical procedures, as reported on the most current hospital licensure application.

(8)   "Open-heart surgery program" means all of the open-heart surgery rooms operated in one hospital.

(9)   "Primary open-heart surgery service area" means a geographical area defined by the applicant, which has boundaries that are not farther than 45 road miles from the facility, except that the primary open-heart surgery service area of an academic medical center teaching hospital designated to 10 NCAC 3R. 3050 shall not be limited to 45 road miles.

.1715 Required Performance Standards

The applicant shall demonstrate that the proposed project is capable of meeting the following standards:

(1)   each open-heart surgery room shall be utilized at an annual rate of at least 50 percent of capacity, measured during the twelfth quarter following completion of the project. . .

(3)   a new or additional heart-lung bypass machine shall be utilized at 200 open-heart surgical procedures per year, measured during the twelfth quarter following completion of the project. . .

(5)   each existing open-heart surgery program in each facility which has a primary open-heart surgery service area that overlaps the proposed primary open-heart surgery service area operated at a level of at least 80 percent of capacity during the 12-month period reflected in the most recent licensure form on file with the Division of Facility Services.

THE STATE AGENCY'S DECISION TO DENY COUNTY'S APPLICATION

The state agency recognized that County would provide access to the medically underserved and that its project would be financially feasible. However, the state agency denied the application because the agency believed County failed to meet some of the quantitative criteria set forth in the regulations.

1. Nonconformity with § 1715(1)

First, the state agency found that County's projected utilization of open-heart surgery procedures did not meet the level required by the

(continued)

(continued from previous page)

regulation at § 1715(1). In its CON application, County proposed to develop only one open-heart surgery room. In addition, County made the following quarterly projections of adult and pediatric (aged 5 years and younger) open-heart surgery procedures for the first 3 years (12 calendar quarters) of operation after completion of the project.

Quarter	Adult Open-Heart Procedures	Pediatric Open-Heart Procedures
1	5	1
2	8	1
3	11	1
4	14	1
5	17	2
6	20	2
7	23	3
8	26	3
9	29	3
10	32	4
11	36	4
12	40	5

In its decision, the state agency found that County's application was nonconforming with the regulatory criterion at § 1715(1), on the grounds that County's projected utilization was less than 50 percent of capacity measured during the 12th quarter after completion of the project. The state agency reasoned that the capacity of one open-heart surgery room is defined by the regulation at § 1713(1) as 400 procedures. Therefore, 50 percent of capacity would be 200 procedures. The regulation at § 1715(1) requires a projected utilization of at least 50 percent of capacity (200 procedures) but allows the projected utilization to be measured by annualizing the utilization that was projected for the 12th quarter of operation. Therefore, the applicant must project a utilization of at least 50 procedures during the 12th quarter of operation because that would

(continued)

(continued from previous page)

annualize at 200 procedures, which is 50 percent of the capacity of 400 procedures. In this case, the agency found that County projected a total of only 45 procedures in the 12th quarter, which failed to meet the requirement of § 1715(1).

2. Nonconformity with § 1715(5)

In addition, the state agency found that the level of historical utilization at Doctor's existing open-heart surgery program was not high enough to permit approval of another open-heart surgery program in the same geographic area under the agency's regulation at § 1715(5). Not surprisingly, the administrator of Doctor's had opposed the County application for a CON on the grounds that there was no need for an additional open-heart surgery service in the same geographic area.

Because Doctor's is located in the same city as County, it is clear that Doctor's primary open-heart surgery service area overlaps County's proposed primary open-heart surgery service area. In fact, Doctor's is the only facility whose primary service area overlaps County's proposed primary service area for open-heart surgery. During the 12-month period reflected in the most recent licensure form that Doctor's filed with the Division of Facility Services, Doctor's performed a total of 610 adult open-heart surgery procedures and 20 pediatric open-heart surgery procedures in its open-heart surgery program, which consists of two open-heart surgery rooms.

In its decision to deny the County application, the state agency found that County's application was nonconforming with the agency's regulatory criterion at § 1715(5). Specifically, the agency found that Doctor's existing open-heart surgery program had not operated at a level of at least 80 percent of capacity during the 12-month period reflected in its most recently filed licensure form. As discussed earlier, Doctor's open-heart surgery program had two open-heart surgery rooms. Therefore, the state agency reasoned that, pursuant to the regulation at § 1713(1), the capacity of each of Doctor's open-heart surgery rooms was 400 procedures and the total capacity of Doctor's open-heart surgery program was 800 procedures. Therefore, according to the agency, the regulation at § 1715(5) required Doctor's to operate at a level of at least 640 procedures, which is 80 percent of the capacity of 800 possible procedures. Because Doctor's had only operated at a level of 630

(continued)

(continued from previous page)

procedures in the past year, the agency reasoned that Doctor's had not operated at 80 percent of capacity and County's application for a CON could not be approved.

3. Nonconformity with § 1715(3)

Finally, the state agency found that County's application was nonconforming to the regulation at § 1715(3) because County's proposed new heart-lung bypass machine would not be used at a rate of 200 procedures per year as measured during the 12th quarter. As discussed, County projected to perform a total of only 45 procedures during the 12th quarter, which would annualize at 180 procedures, rather than the 50 procedures needed to annualize at the required level of 200 procedures.

QUESTIONS

1. Was the state agency correct in finding that County's application was nonconforming with the criterion at § 1715(1)? Why or why not?
2. Was the state agency correct in finding that County's application was nonconforming with the criterion at § 1715(5)? Why or why not?
3. On what basis could County argue that it is conforming with the criterion at § 1715(3)? On what basis could the state agency argue that County's application is nonconforming with that criterion? In your opinion, which side has the more persuasive argument? Why?
4. If County's application is not conforming with all of the current regulations, what could it do in an effort to develop an open-heart surgery program?

Notes

1. *Jacobson v. Massachusetts*, 197 U.S. 11, 25 (1905).
2. *Id.*
3. *Dent v. West Virginia*, 129 U.S. 114, 128 (1889) (upholding conviction for violation of West Virginia statute that prohibited unlicensed practice of medicine).
4. 42 U.S.C. § 274e (2006).

5. *Wickard v. Filburn*, 317 U.S. 111, 127–28 (1942).

6. *Hospital Building Co. v. Rex Hospital Trustees*, 425 U.S. 738, 744 (1976).

7. *National Federation of Independent Business v. Sebelius*, 132 S. Ct. 2566 (2012).

8. See generally *South Dakota v. Dole*, 483 U.S. 203 (1987).

9. *North Carolina ex rel. Morrow v. Califano*, 445 F. Supp. 532, 534 (E.D.N.C. 1977), *aff'd mem.*, 435 U.S. 962 (1978).

10. *National Federation of Independent Business v. Sebelius*, 132 S. Ct. 2566 (2012).

11. *Id.*, 132 S. Ct. at 2607.

12. See L. O. Gostin, *Public Health Law: Power, Duty, Restraint* (Berkeley: University of California Press; New York: The Milbank Memorial Fund, 2000): 47–51.

13. 45 C.F.R. § 164.512(b) (2006).

14. See, e.g., W. E. Parmet, "After September 11: Rethinking Public Health Federalism," *Journal of Law, Medicine & Ethics* (2002), 30 (2): 201–11.

15. See, e.g., J. G. Hodge, "Bioterrorism Law and Policy: Critical Choices in Public Health," *Journal of Law, Medicine & Ethics* (2002), 30 (2): 254–61.

16. Parmet, *supra* note 14, at 201.

17. Hodge, *supra* note 15, at 258.

18. See *id.* at 254–55.

19. The Centers for Law & the Public's Health: A Collaborative at Johns Hopkins and Georgetown Universities, "The Model State Emergency Health Powers Act (MSEHPA)," (draft as of December 21, 2001). www.publichealthlaw.net/ModelLaws/MSEHPA.php.

20. See G. J. Annas, "Bioterrorism, Public Health, and Civil Liberties," *New England Journal of Medicine* (2002), 346 (17): 1337–42, at 1340 ("No one any longer considers the act a 'model.' Instead, it is now labeled a 'draft for discussion'").

21. The Centers for Law & the Public's Health: A Collaborative at Johns Hopkins and Georgetown Universities, "The Model State Emergency Health Powers Act (MSEHPA): Legislative Status Update" (as of July 15, 2006). www.publichealthlaw.net/ModelLaws/MSEHPA.php.

22. Hodge, *supra* note 15, at 255.

23. Annas, *supra* note 20, at 1340.

24. L. O. Gostin, et al. (2002). "The Model State Emergency Health Powers Act." *Journal of the American Medical Association* 288 (5): 622–28.

25. *Id.*

26. T. Frieden (2013). "Government's Role in Protecting Health and Safety." *New England Journal of Medicine* 368: 1857–59.

27. *Id.* at 3.

28. *New York Statewide Coalition of Hispanic Chambers of Commerce v. New York City Department of Health and Mental Hygiene*, Index No. 653584/12, 2013 N.Y. Misc. LEXIS 1216 (N.Y. Sup. Ct., March 11, 2013) (permanently enjoining implementation of New York City Health Code, § 81.53), *affirmed*, 2013 N.Y. App. Div. LEXIS 5423 (N.Y. App. Div. 1st Dep't, July 30, 2013), *leave to appeal granted*, 2013 N.Y. LEXIS 2894 (October 17, 2013).

29. See generally T. S. Jost (1995), "Oversight of the Quality of Medical Care: Regulation, Management, or the Market?" *Arizona Law Review*, 37: 825–68, at 859 ("The deficiencies of the market and of management insure the existence of a continuing legitimate role for quality regulation").

30. See L. T. Kohn, J. M. Corrigan, and M. Donaldson (1999), *To Err Is Human: Building a Safer Health System* (Washington, DC: National Academies Press).

31. See, e.g., L. I. Palmer, "Patient Safety, Risk Reduction, and the Law," *Houston Law Review* (1999), 36: 1609–61, at 1638 ("Advocates for patient safety have offered solutions from the airline industry without noting how different health care is from the airline industry in terms of both organization and surrounding legal structure").

32. See, e.g., 40 Pa. Cons. Stat. § 1303.313(a) (duty of medical facilities to report serious events to government officials, but without any information that would identify the individual patient); *id.* at § 1303.311(a) (certain documents are not discoverable or admissible in evidence).

33. See, e.g., proposed Stop All Frequent Errors (SAFE) in Medicare and Medicaid Act of 2000, S. 2378, 106th Cong. (2000) (bipartisan bill would have established mandatory reporting by providers with confidentiality for the reported information).

34. Patient Safety and Quality Improvement Act of 2005, Pub. L. No. 109-41, 119 Stat. 424 (2005).

35. See, e.g., *Michigan v. Rogers*, 641 N.W.2d 595 (Mich. App. 2001) (upholding prosecution of a "natural doctor" who used a machine to

diagnose a child with ear problems as having a tapeworm, a bacterial infection, and a brain aneurysm).

36. Jost, *supra* note 29, at 827.

37. See Health Security Act, H.R. 3600, 103rd Cong. § 1161 (1993).

38. U.S. Department of Health and Human Services, Office of Inspector General, *State Medical Boards and Medical Discipline*, OEI-01-89-00560 (August 1990): 15.

39. *Griffiths v. Superior Court*, 96 Cal. App. 4th 757, 769–72 (Cal. App. 2002), *review denied*, 2002 Cal. LEXIS 3826 (2002).

40. See, e.g., *In re Lustgarten*, 629 S.E.2d 886 (N.C. App. 2006).

41. See Chapter 14 *infra* at notes 30–32 and accompanying text.

42. U.S. Department of Labor, www.dol.gov.

43. U.S. Department of Health and Human Services, Office of Inspector General, *The External Review of Hospital Quality: The Role of Medicare Certification*, OEI-01-97-00052 (July 1999): 1, 6.

44. See 42 U.S.C. § 1395bb (2006).

45. See generally L. H. Wolfson (2001), "State Regulation of Health Facility Planning: The Economic Theory and Political Realities of Certificates of Need," *DePaul Journal of Health Care Law*, 4: 261–314.

46. C. J. Conover and F. A. Sloan (1998). "Does Removing Certificate-of-Need Regulations Lead to a Surge in Health Care Spending?" *Journal of Health Politics, Policy & Law* 23 (3): 455–81.

47. See B.R. Furrow, et al. (2000). *Health Law* 2nd ed., Hornbook Series (St. Paul, MN: West Group): at 29 ("the demand for care will always expand to the limits of the supply").

48. *Id.*

49. See Pub. L. No. 93-641, 42 U.S.C. §§ 300k–300n-6 (repealed 1986).

50. National Conference of State Legislatures, "Certificate of Need: State Health Laws and Programs" (2012). www.ncsl.org/issues-research/health/con-certificate-of-need-state-laws.aspx.

51. See, e.g., K. Greene (1997), "Nonprofit Hospitals Win in Georgia," *Wall Street Journal (Southeast Journal)*, March 19, S3.

52. See *Adventist Healthcare Midatlantic, Inc. v. Suburban Hospital, Inc.*, 711 A.2d 158, 166–68 (Md. 1998).

53. N.C. Admin. Code tit. 10, r. 3R.1700 (2002). Updated regulations located today at N.C. Admin. Code tit. 10A, 14C.1701 and 14C.1703 (2006).

6

PROTECTING THE PRIVACY OF MEDICAL INFORMATION

Most patients do not want providers to disclose their medical information to other people, except as specifically authorized by the patient. Disclosure of personal information could be harmful or embarrassing to the patient, especially if it is disclosed to the patient's employer, insurance company, neighbors, spouse, or former spouse. However, more than merely preventing harm or embarrassment to a person is at stake in confidentiality issues.

Inappropriate disclosure of medical information could harm the public health and reduce the quality of care by making people unwilling to provide necessary information to their healthcare providers. If patients had to worry that personal information would be disclosed to others, they would not provide the candid information that practitioners and facilities need to provide appropriate care. Even worse, people might refrain from seeking necessary treatment out of fear that information about them would be disclosed. Therefore, the underlying goals of medical privacy are to encourage patients to seek appropriate care and to confide fully in their healthcare providers. In these ways, confidentiality should improve the quality of care and promote public health.

From an ethical perspective, the privacy of medical information is based on the ethical principle of autonomy or self-determination. Patients have the right to control the disclosure of their own medical information and the right to condition their consent to treatment on the provider's promise to maintain confidentiality. In addition, improper disclosure of private information could harm the patient and thereby violate the ethical principle of **nonmaleficence**. Finally, to the extent that confidentiality promotes quality of care and public health, it is consistent with the ethical principle of **beneficence**.

Nonmaleficence
The ethical principle of not harming others.

Healthcare professional organizations have recognized these ethical principles and adopted the obligation of confidentiality in their own codes of ethics. In accordance with the traditional Hippocratic Oath, the Principles of Medical Ethics of the American Medical Association (AMA) encourage physicians to "safeguard patient confidences and privacy within the constraints of the law."[1] Similarly, the *Code of Ethics* of the American College of Healthcare Executives provides that healthcare executives have the responsibility to "[w]ork to ensure the existence of procedures that will safeguard the

Beneficence
The ethical principle of helping others.

confidentiality and privacy of patients or others served."[2] Other professional organizations have adopted similar principles for their members.

In some ways, the problem of medical privacy has become more acute now that data are stored on computers and transferred electronically among practitioners, facilities, and third-party payers. As former U.S. Department of Health and Human Services (HHS) Secretary Donna Shalala put it, "Gone are the days when our family doctor kept our records sealed away in an office file cabinet. Patient information is now accessed and exchanged quickly."[3] It is certainly true that electronic storage and transmission of data increase the extent to which information can be disseminated as well as the possibility of improper disclosure.[4] However, keep these technological changes in perspective and avoid undue nostalgia for the supposed good old days, which probably never existed. In fact, the concept of a historical golden age of individual privacy, before the advent of computers, is something of an illusion. In those good old days, when Americans lived in small towns or discrete urban neighborhoods, everyone knew everyone else, and everyone knew everyone else's business. Of course, the family doctor dutifully kept everyone's medical records secure and confidential, but if someone had a medical problem such as mental illness or alcoholism, everyone else in the community would have known about it.[5]

Aside from dealing with changes in information technology and new systems of healthcare financing and delivery, another major problem in protecting privacy is preventing employers from misusing medical information about their employees. This problem arises because, under the U.S. system of health insurance, many people obtain coverage for themselves and their dependents through their place of employment. People with employment-based coverage want their employer or its agent to pay their medical bills but do not want their employer to look at their medical bills. Under this system, the employer or its agent has a legitimate reason to review medical bills and medical records to determine the appropriateness of payment. However, employers should not be allowed to use this personal health information to make other employment-related decisions, such as hiring and promotion. Nevertheless, as others have pointed out, the alternative of a single-payer system of health coverage would pose a different and perhaps more serious threat to privacy by providing the medical bills and medical records of all citizens directly to the government.[6]

Despite the importance of protecting medical privacy, some situations occur in which the public interest requires that information be disclosed, even without the consent of the individual patient.[7] To prevent epidemics, for example, we want physicians to report communicable diseases to public health authorities, even if the individual patient does not want that information to be reported. We also want healthcare providers to report gunshot wounds and suspected cases of child abuse to designated agencies, despite the consequent breach of confidentiality. In addition, the use and disclosure of medical records may be necessary to provide appropriate treatment and to conduct important medical and pharmaceutical research. Therefore, the issue of public policy is not merely how to provide the maximum protection for individual privacy. Rather, it is how to provide sufficient protection for individual privacy without interfering too much with other public needs, such as public safety, communicable disease control, medical treatment, and healthcare research.

State and federal governments have attempted to balance these conflicting policies when developing their laws on the privacy and disclosure of medical information. Historically, the role of the federal government in this area was somewhat limited, and most aspects of patient privacy have been subject to the laws of the states. Since 1996, however, the federal government has played a major role in patient privacy through the enactment of the Health Insurance Portability and Accountability Act (HIPAA) and the adoption of the federal HIPAA privacy rule. Although the federal privacy rule is highly detailed, it does not totally preempt the law of patient confidentiality. Rather, state laws will continue to apply when they impose higher standards than the federal rule. Therefore, considering *both* the federal privacy rule and the laws of the individual states is still necessary.

State Laws on Privacy of Patient Information

Historically, the confidentiality of patient information has been governed by "a patchwork of State laws and regulations that are incomplete and, at times, inconsistent."[8] The laws differ from one state to the next, and some states provide more privacy protection than others. Moreover, even within each specific state, confidentiality laws do not provide comprehensive privacy protection.

Many state privacy laws are provider-specific, in the sense that each law only applies to information in the possession of a specific type of provider. For example, most states have statutes or common law rules of evidence that prevent physicians from having to disclose patient confidences on the witness stand unless the patient waives the physician–patient privilege. Those same states might have separate statutes or regulations that apply to the patient records maintained by hospitals, other healthcare facilities, health departments, pharmacies, insurance companies, and health maintenance organizations (HMOs). Ordinarily, those provider-specific laws do not protect the confidentiality of information once it has been transferred to a different type of entity.

Many state laws are disease-specific as well, in that they only apply to records that indicate a particular diagnosis or treatment for a particular disease. For example, some states have specific statutes or rules that protect the records of patients with AIDS or HIV. States also have laws that require healthcare providers to report communicable diseases and regulate the use of the reported information. However, those state laws are often limited to the specific diseases identified by name in the statutes or regulations.

State laws might also provide a legal remedy for unauthorized disclosure of confidential information. One of the inherent obligations of the provider–patient relationship is to preserve the confidences of the patient. Subject to certain exceptions, healthcare providers have a duty to refrain from disclosing information about their patients. In addition, practitioners and facilities have a duty to exercise reasonable care to prevent disclosure by their employees, and must take reasonable steps to prevent unauthorized access to patients' records by third parties. If these duties are breached, the practitioner or facility could be held liable for damages under the laws of the particular state. As one court explained,

> We repeat here our earlier finding that a doctor who makes an unauthorized divulgence of confidence should respond in damages.
>
> Any time a doctor undertakes the treatment of a patient, and the consensual relationship of physician and patient is established, two jural obligations (of significance here) are simultaneously assumed by the doctor. Doctor and patient enter into a simple contract, the patient hoping that he will be cured and the doctor optimistically assuming that he will be compensated. As an implied condition of that contract, this Court is of the opinion that the doctor warrants that any confidential information gained through the relationship will not be released without the patient's permission. Almost every member of the public is aware of the promise of discretion contained in the Hippocratic Oath, and every patient has a right to rely upon this warranty of silence. The promise of secrecy is as much an express warranty as the advertisement of a commercial entrepreneur. Consequently, when a doctor breaches his duty of secrecy, he is in violation of part of his obligations under the contract.
>
> When a patient seeks out a doctor and retains him, he must admit him to the most private part of the material domain of man. Nothing material is more important or more intimate to man than the health of his mind and body. Since the layman is unfamiliar with the road to recovery, he cannot sift the circumstances of his life and habits to determine what is information pertinent to his health. As a consequence, he must disclose all information in his consultations with his doctor—even that which is embarrassing, disgraceful or incriminating. To promote full disclosure, the medical profession extends the promise of secrecy referred to above. The candor which this promise elicits is necessary to the effective pursuit of health; there can be no reticence, no reservation, no reluctance when patients

discuss their problems with their doctors. But the disclosure is certainly intended to be private. If a doctor should reveal any of these confidences, he surely effects an invasion of the privacy of his patient. We are of the opinion that the preservation of the patient's privacy is no mere ethical duty upon the part of the doctor; there is a legal duty as well. The unauthorized revelation of medical secrets, or any confidential communication given in the course of treatment, is tortious conduct which may be the basis for an action in damages.[9]

In accordance with these principles, patients have filed claims against healthcare providers for unauthorized disclosure to the patient's employer, spouse, and others. In one particularly egregious case, the patient's treating physician allegedly made an unauthorized disclosure about the patient's medical condition and use of prescription drugs to the patient's former spouse, who was also a physician.[10] Then the former spouse used that information against the patient in their pending legal dispute over custody of their children. In that case, the Supreme Court of Washington held that the patient could state a valid claim against the treating physician for unauthorized disclosure under the general state statute for medical malpractice, because the treating physician had made the disclosure in the context of providing healthcare services to the patient.[11]

In other situations, however, healthcare providers may be held legally liable for *failing* to disclose confidential information about a patient who poses a danger to others. For example, in *Tarasoff v. Regents of the University of California*,[12] the patient had told his therapist that he intended to kill a particular person, and subsequently did so. In a suit by the parents of the victim, the court held that the therapist had a duty to take reasonable steps for protection of the intended victim, even though it would have required disclosure of confidential information. As explained by the court in that case,

We recognize the public interest in supporting effective treatment of mental illness and in protecting the rights of patients to privacy . . . and the consequent public importance of safeguarding the confidential character of psychotherapeutic communication. Against this interest, however, we must weigh the public interest in safety from violent assault. . . .

We realize that the open and confidential character of psychotherapeutic dialogue encourages patients to express threats of violence, few of which are ever executed. Certainly a therapist should not be encouraged routinely to reveal such threats; such disclosures could seriously disrupt the patient's relationship with his therapist and with the persons threatened. To the contrary, the therapist's obligations to his patient require that he not disclose a confidence unless such disclosure is necessary to avert danger to others, and even then that he do so discreetly, and in a fashion that would preserve the privacy of his patient to the fullest extent compatible with the prevention of the threatened danger.

> The revelation of a communication under the above circumstances is not a breach of trust or a violation of professional ethics. . . . We conclude that the public policy favoring protection of the confidential character of patient-psychotherapist communications must yield to the extent to which disclosure is essential to avert danger to others. The protective privilege ends where the public peril begins.[13]

In addition to balancing the public policies in that case, the court attempted to establish a standard to guide practitioners in determining when disclosure is required.

> When a therapist determines, or pursuant to the standards of his profession should determine, that his patient presents a serious danger of violence to another, he incurs an obligation to use reasonable care to protect the intended victim against such danger. The discharge of this duty may require the therapist to take one or more of various steps, depending upon the nature of the case. Thus it may call for him to warn the intended victim or others likely to apprise the victim of the danger, to notify the police, or to take whatever other steps are reasonably necessary under the circumstances.[14]

As the court pointed out, disclosure of patient information under these circumstances is consistent with the AMA's Principles of Medical Ethics.[15] In fact, the current version of the AMA's Fundamental Elements of the Patient–Physician Relationship provides that "[t]he physician should not reveal confidential communications or information without the consent of the patient, unless provided for by law or by the need to protect the welfare of the individual or the public interest."[16]

Under these circumstances, healthcare providers may be held liable under state law for improperly disclosing patient information or for improperly failing to disclose patient information. The legal duties to disclose and not to disclose will depend on the specific facts of each case—disclosure of patient information might be prohibited, required, or permitted at the option of the provider. In addition, providers must comply with the requirements of federal law as discussed in the next section of this chapter.

Federal Law and the HIPAA Privacy Rule

Before 1996, federal involvement in patient privacy issues was limited to a few specific areas. Federal law restricts the disclosure of treatment records for alcoholism and substance abuse.[17] In addition, federal law provides rules for conducting research with human subjects in institutions that receive federal support, including a requirement for "adequate provisions to protect the privacy of subjects and to maintain the confidentiality of data."[18] Of course, federal law also regulates the confidentiality and disclosure of records in the possession of federal agencies.[19]

The most significant federal involvement in patient privacy began in 1996 when Congress enacted HIPAA.[20] In that statute, Congress recognized that electronic transmission of health information could improve the efficiency of the healthcare system[21] but also recognized the importance of protecting "the privacy of individually identifiable health information."[22] Therefore, Congress required the secretary of HHS to adopt various standards for electronic exchange of information, such as standards for transactions, data elements, and code sets; a standard unique health identifier; electronic signatures; and the security of health information.[23]

With regard to privacy, however, Congress took a different approach to developing federal standards, and set in motion a process with a series of statutory deadlines.[24] First, Congress directed the secretary of HHS to make recommendations to Congress within one year on the protection of privacy, including consideration of individual rights and the appropriate use and transfer of medical information. In addition, Congress gave itself three years to enact privacy standards by means of additional legislation. Under the HIPAA statute, if Congress failed to enact privacy standards by new legislation within three years, the secretary of HHS would be required to adopt standards for protecting privacy by means of a rule.

The secretary of HHS made her recommendations to Congress on the privacy of medical information, but Congress was unable to enact additional legislation by the end of the three-year period. Congress did consider some proposals for additional legislation,[25] but the issues of privacy and disclosure proved to be too complicated and controversial for further action.

Therefore, on November 3, 1999, the secretary of HHS issued her standards for protecting privacy in the form of a proposed rule.[26] During the public comment period, HHS received 52,000 comments on the proposed rule. After that period, on December 28, 2000, the secretary issued the final rule[27] (actually a long and complicated set of rules). When published in the *Federal Register* with three columns of small print per page, the final rule was 31 pages and was accompanied by 336 additional pages of explanatory material from HHS. Ironically, the HIPAA privacy rule was adopted to implement provisions of the statute entitled "administrative simplification."

Originally, the final rule was supposed to become effective on February 26, 2001. However, because of an administrative error, it did not become effective until April 14, 2001. Most individuals and organizations that were subject to the rule had to be in compliance by April 14, 2003, although small health plans had until April 14, 2004, to comply. Some healthcare organizations challenged the validity of the privacy rule on a variety of constitutional and statutory grounds, but courts have rejected those arguments.[28]

Healthcare providers, payers, researchers, and other organizations devoted substantial attention and resources to making the procedural and technological changes needed to comply with the rule. Not surprisingly, the government and the industry had different perceptions of the burden and different estimates of the cost of compliance. The truth was probably somewhere in the middle of those competing estimates. When the U.S. government adopted its HIPAA privacy rule, it estimated the cost at $18 billion over 10 years.[29] However, the government claimed that its other rules for "administrative simplification" would save the health system $30 billion over 10 years. Thus, the government claimed that the result of all those rules would be a net savings for the U.S. health system.

In addition to raising concerns about the cost and burden of compliance, many industry organizations argued that the privacy rule would have the unintended and undesired effects of interfering with some healthcare treatment and research. For example, providers complained that requirements for prior written consent by patients for using or disclosing information could delay necessary medical care. In addition, medical schools and other research organizations argued that strict requirements for the use of individually identifiable data would prevent important medical, pharmaceutical, and healthcare research.

The federal government responded to some of these concerns by making several changes to the final privacy rule in 2002. After issuing proposed modifications on March 27, 2002,[30] HHS issued a final rule on August 14, 2002, that modified the previous final rule.[31] According to HHS, "The purpose of these modifications is to maintain strong protections for the privacy of individually identifiable health information while clarifying certain of the Privacy Rule's provisions, addressing the unintended negative effects of the Privacy Rule on health care quality or access to health care, and relieving unintended administrative burdens created by the Privacy Rule."[32]

In its August 2002 modifications, HHS made a significant change on the issue of whether to require prior written consent by patients for using or disclosing information for some purposes. As discussed previously, some providers had argued that the original requirements for prior consent would cause delays in providing necessary care. Therefore, in the August 2002 modifications, HHS eliminated the requirement for prior written consent in the context of particular functions, such as medical treatment. However, HHS enhanced the requirement to provide notice of the covered entity's privacy policies by requiring those providers who treat patients directly to try in good faith to have patients acknowledge in writing that the notice was received.

At that time, several organizations of healthcare consumers and providers challenged HHS's elimination of the requirement to obtain a patient's prior consent for using or disclosing information. However, in that case the federal district court upheld HHS's August 2002 modifications to the rule, and the Court of Appeals for the Third Circuit affirmed that decision.[33] Both the district court and the appellate court explicitly recognized that the goal of Congress in enacting HIPAA was not simply to protect privacy but rather to achieve a balance between privacy and efficiency in the health system. Following is an excerpt from the decision of the Court of Appeals in that case.

Citizens for Health v. Leavitt, 428 F.3D 167 (3RD CIR. 2005), *cert. denied*, 127 S. CT. 3 (2006) (CITATIONS, FOOTNOTES, AND SOME PARTS OF TEXT OMITTED)

Appellant Citizens for Health, along with nine other national and state associations and nine individuals (collectively "Citizens"), brought this action against the Secretary of the United States Department of Health and Human Services ("HHS" or "Agency") challenging a rule promulgated by the Agency pursuant to the administrative simplification provisions of the Health Insurance Portability and Accountability Act of 1996 ("HIPAA"). Citizens allege that the "Privacy Rule"—officially titled "Standards for Privacy of Individually Identifiable Health Information"—is invalid because it unlawfully authorizes health plans, health care clearinghouses, and certain health care providers to use and disclose personal health information for so-called "routine uses" without patient consent. . . . Citizens challenge subsection (a) as authorizing disclosures that, they contend, violate individual privacy rights.

The District Court granted summary judgment to the Secretary on all of Citizens' claims based on its conclusions that the promulgation of the Privacy Rule did not violate the Administrative Procedure Act [the "APA"], that the Secretary did not exceed the scope of authority granted to him by HIPAA, and that, insofar as the Privacy Rule is permissive and does not compel any uses or disclosures of personal health information by providers, it does not affirmatively interfere with any right protected by the First or Fifth Amendments. Because we reason to the same conclusions reached by the District Court, albeit under a slightly different analysis, we will affirm.

I. BACKGROUND

The objectionable provision is only one aspect of a complex set of regulations that is the last in a series of attempts by HHS to strike a balance

(continued)

(continued from previous page)

between two competing objectives of HIPAA—improving the efficiency and effectiveness of the national health care system and preserving individual privacy in personal health information.

A. HIPAA

HIPAA was passed by Congress in August 1996 to address a number of issues regarding the national health care and health insurance system. The statutory provisions relevant to the issues in this case are found in Subtitle F of Title II. Aimed at "administrative simplification," HIPAA Sections 261 through 264 provide for "the establishment of standards and requirements for the electronic transmission of certain health information." More specifically, these provisions direct the Secretary to adopt uniform national standards for the secure electronic exchange of health information.

Section 264 prescribes the process by which standards regarding the privacy of individually identifiable health information were to be adopted. This process contemplated that, within a year of HIPAA's enactment, the Secretary would submit detailed recommendations on such privacy standards, including individual rights concerning individually identifiable health information, procedures for exercising such rights, and the "uses and disclosures of such information that should be authorized or required," to Congress. If Congress did not enact further legislation within three years of HIPAA's enactment, the Secretary was directed to promulgate final regulations implementing the standards within 42 months of HIPAA's enactment. The Act specified that any regulation promulgated pursuant to the authority of Section 264 would provide a federal baseline for privacy protection, but that such regulations would "not supersede a contrary provision of State law, if the provision of State law imposes requirements, standards, or implementation specifications that are more stringent than the requirements, standards, or implementation specifications imposed under the regulation."

B. The Privacy Rule

Because Congress did not enact privacy legislation by its self-imposed three-year deadline, the Secretary promulgated the privacy standards contemplated in Section 264 through an administrative rulemaking process. During this process, the Rule went through four iterations: the Proposed Original Rule, the Original Rule, the Proposed Amended Rule, and

(continued)

(continued from previous page)

the Amended Rule. The Original Rule required covered entities to seek individual consent before using or disclosing protected health information for routine uses. Before the Original Rule could take effect, however, the Secretary was inundated with unsolicited criticism, principally from health care insurers and providers, warning that the Original Rule's mandatory consent provisions would significantly impact the ability of the health care industry to operate efficiently. He responded by reopening the rulemaking process. The final result was the Amended Rule—the currently effective, codified version of the Privacy Rule which is the subject of Citizens' challenge here.

The Amended Rule retains most of the Original Rule's privacy protections. It prohibits "covered entities"—defined as health plans, health care clearinghouses, and health care providers who transmit any health information in electronic form in connection with a transaction covered by the regulations—from using or disclosing an individual's "protected health information"—defined as individually identifiable health information maintained in or transmitted in any form or media including electronic media—except as otherwise provided by the Rule. Covered entities must seek authorization from individuals before using or disclosing information unless a specific exception applies. Uses and disclosures that the Amended Rule allows must be limited to the "minimum necessary" to accomplish the intended purpose.

The Amended Rule departs from the Original Rule in one crucial respect. Where the Original Rule required covered entities to seek individual consent to use or disclose health information in all but the narrowest of circumstances, the Amended Rule allows such uses and disclosures without patient consent for "treatment, payment, and health care operations"—so-called "routine uses." "Health care operations," the broadest category under the routine use exception, refers to a range of management functions of covered entities, including quality assessment, practitioner evaluation, student training programs, insurance rating, auditing services, and business planning and development. The Rule allows individuals the right to request restrictions on uses and disclosures of protected health information and to enter into agreements with covered entities regarding such restrictions, but does not require covered entities to abide by such requests or to agree to any restriction.

(continued)

(continued from previous page)

The Rule also permits, but does not require, covered entities to design and implement a consent process for routine uses and disclosures.

Importantly, the Rule contains detailed preemption provisions, which are consistent with HIPAA Sections 1178(a)(2)(B) and 264(c)(2). These provisions establish that the Rule is intended as a "federal floor" for privacy protection, allowing state law to control where a "provision of State law relates to the privacy of individually identifiable health information and is more stringent than a standard, requirement, or implementation specification adopted under [the Privacy Rule]."

II. PROCEDURAL HISTORY

Citizens filed this action on April 10, 2003. In its Amended Complaint, Citizens alleged that the Secretary violated the APA and Sections 261 through 264 of HIPAA in promulgating the Amended Rule, and that, to the extent that the Amended Rule rescinded or eliminated the need for consent for the use and disclosure of individually identifiable health information for "routine uses," the Amended Rule violated privacy rights protected by the Fifth Amendment and free speech rights protected by the First Amendment of the United States Constitution. Both parties moved for summary judgment, and, after a hearing on December 10, 2003, the District Court granted summary judgment in favor of the Secretary.

On Citizens' APA claims, the Court concluded that the Secretary had adequately informed the public regarding the proposed rulemaking, examined the relevant data, responded to public comments, and provided a reasoned analysis that rationally connected the facts with the decision to rescind the consent requirement in the Amended Rule. Regarding Citizens' claims alleging violations of HIPAA, the Court concluded that the changes in the Amended Rule were reasonably related to the legislative purpose of Subtitle F of the Act, and, because the Amended Rule was promulgated before the Original Rule took effect, the Amended Rule did not eliminate any "rights" created under the Original Rule. Finally, regarding Citizens' constitutional claims, the Court concluded that because (1) neither the First Amendment nor the Fifth Amendment places an affirmative obligation on the State to protect individuals' rights from harm by third parties and (2) the Amended Rule is wholly permissive as to whether covered entities seek consent from

(continued)

(continued from previous page)

an individual before using or disclosing personal health information for routine uses, the Amended Rule did not violate individual rights under either Amendment. . . .

On appeal, Citizens reassert the claims they made before the District Court, that the Secretary, by promulgating the Privacy Rule, (1) unlawfully infringed Citizens' fundamental rights to privacy in personal health information under due process principles of the Fifth Amendment of the United States Constitution; (2) unlawfully infringed Citizens' rights to communicate privately with their medical practitioners under the First Amendment of the Constitution; (3) contravened Congress's intent in enacting HIPAA by eliminating Citizens' reasonable expectations of medical privacy; and (4) violated the APA by arbitrarily and capriciously reversing a settled course of behavior and adopting a policy that he had previously rejected. . . .

A. Fifth Amendment Substantive Due Process Claim

. . . We begin our analysis with the premise that the right to medical privacy asserted by Citizens is legally cognizable under the Due Process Clause of the Fifth Amendment, although, as Citizens themselves concede, its "boundaries . . . have not been exhaustively delineated." Whatever those boundaries may be, it is undisputed that a violation of a citizen's right to medical privacy rises to the level of a constitutional claim only when that violation can properly be ascribed to the government. The Constitution protects against state interference with fundamental rights. It only applies to restrict private behavior in limited circumstances. Because such circumstances are not present in this case, and because the "violations" of the right to medical privacy that Citizens have asserted, if they amount to violations of that right at all, occurred at the hands of private entities, the protections of the Due Process Clause of the Fifth Amendment are not implicated in this case. We will accordingly affirm the District Court's finding that the Secretary did not violate Citizens' constitutional rights when he promulgated the Amended Rule. . . .

The fact that covered entities are construing the "may use" language as constituting a new federal seal of approval, and may be ignoring state laws regarding protections to be afforded to such information, is regrettable and disquieting. That routine requests for privacy are apparently

(continued)

(continued from previous page)

being ignored by covered entities is even more unfortunate. But our task here is to determine the constitutionality of the Amended Rule, not the propriety of covered entities' actions under state or common law. Because, for all of the reasons stated above, the covered entities' actions that Citizens challenge do not implicate the federal government, we reject Citizens' Fifth Amendment claim.

B. First Amendment Claim

Citizens' First Amendment claim is that the Amended Rule infringes individuals' right to confidential communications with health care practitioners, i.e., a right to refrain from public speech regarding private personal health information. Citizens argue that the effect of the Amended Rule is to chill speech between individuals and their health care practitioners because the possibility of nonconsensual disclosures makes individuals less likely to participate fully in diagnosis and treatment and more likely to be evasive and withhold important information. . . .

Citizens' First Amendment claim fails on the same grounds as their Fifth Amendment claim: the potential "chilling" of patients' rights to free speech derives not from any action of the government, but from the independent decisions of private parties with respect to the use and disclosure of individual health information. For all of the reasons enumerated above, the decisions of the private parties to use or disclose private health information in reliance on the Amended Rule, which may or may not "chill" expression between health care providers and their patients, does not implicate the government in a way that gives rise to a constitutional claim. We will therefore affirm the District Court's grant of summary judgment to the Secretary on Citizens' First Amendment claim.

C. Claims Alleging Violations of HIPAA

In claims based on HIPAA's statutory language, Citizens argue (1) that the Secretary exceeded the regulatory authority delegated by HIPAA because the Act only authorizes the Secretary to promulgate regulations that enhance privacy and (2) that the Amended Rule impermissibly retroactively rescinded individual rights created by the Original Rule and disturbed Citizens' "settled expectations" in the privacy of their health information. We find the District Court's analysis of these statutory claims to be cogent. Citizens argue that the Secretary has eliminated their reasonable expectations of medical privacy retroactively and

(continued)

(continued from previous page)

prospectively and that such action is inconsistent with Congress's intent in enacting HIPAA. However, Citizens' argument that the controlling policy underlying HIPAA is medical privacy and that the Amended Rule wholly sacrifices this interest to covered entities' interests in efficiency and flexibility ignores the Act's stated goals of "simplifying the administration of health insurance," and "improving the efficiency and effectiveness of the health care system." As the District Court aptly explained, HIPAA requires the Secretary to "balance privacy protection and the efficiency of the health care system—not simply to enhance privacy." We thus conclude that Citizens' first HIPAA claim lacks merit.

We also agree with the District Court's finding that the Amended Rule does not retroactively eliminate rights that Citizens enjoyed under the Original Rule or under various laws or standards of practice that existed before the Amended Rule went into effect. Because the Original Rule was amended before its compliance date, "covered entities were never under a legal obligation to comply with the Original Rule's consent requirement." Citizens, therefore, never enjoyed any rights under the Original Rule at all. Nor does the Amended Rule retroactively eliminate Citizens' reasonable expectations based on state law, standards of medical ethics, and established standards of practice because the Amended Rule does not disturb any preexisting, "more stringent" state law privacy rights. Accordingly, we reject Citizens' second HIPPA [sic] claim as well, and will affirm the grant of summary judgment to the Secretary on these claims.

D. APA Claims

Lastly, Citizens challenge the rulemaking process under the APA, contending that (1) the Secretary's rulemaking was arbitrary and capricious . . . and (2) the Secretary failed to provide adequate notice of the rescission of the consent requirement of the Original Rule. . . . Citizens argue that the Secretary acted arbitrarily and capriciously by failing to adequately explain the rescission of the consent requirement, ignoring earlier findings, and failing to respond to public comments.

We dispose of Citizens' argument that the Secretary did not provide adequate notice to the public of his intention to rescind the consent requirement first. On this point, the District Court correctly pointed out that the APA requires a notice to provide either "the terms or substance of the proposed rule" or "a description of the subjects and issues

(continued)

(continued from previous page)

involved." In this case, the Notice for Proposed Rulemaking did both. We will therefore affirm the District Court's grant of summary judgment to the Secretary on this claim.

We also reject Citizens' claim that the Secretary acted arbitrarily and capriciously in promulgating the Amended Rule. Citizens argue that the Secretary acted arbitrarily and capriciously in promulgating the Amended Rule by improperly reversing a "settled course of behavior" established in the Original Rule and adopting a policy that he had previously rejected. When an agency rejects a "settled course of behavior," however, it need only supply a "reasoned analysis" for the change to overcome any presumption that the settled rule best carries out the policies committed to the agency by Congress. Such an analysis requires the agency to "examine the relevant data and articulate a satisfactory explanation for its action including a "rational connection between the facts found and the choice made.'"

Here, the Secretary examined the relevant data, and gave adequate consideration to the large volume of public comments that HHS received during the rulemaking process. The Secretary considered other alternatives and explained why they were unworkable. The Secretary also considered Congress's dual goals in devising the privacy standards, i.e., protecting the confidentiality of personal health information and improving the efficiency and effectiveness of the national health care system.

In sum, the Secretary's decision to respond to the unintended negative effects and administrative burdens of the Original Rule by rescinding the consent requirement for routine uses and implementing more stringent notice requirements was explained in a detailed analysis that rationally connected the decision to the facts. . . . [W]e agree with the District Court's analysis and conclusion that the Secretary's decision was reasonable given the findings and that the Secretary did not act arbitrarily and capriciously in violation of the APA. Accordingly, we will affirm the grant of summary judgment to the Secretary on these claims.

V. CONCLUSION

For the reasons set forth above, we will AFFIRM the judgment of the District Court.

In *Citizens for Health v. Leavitt*, the appellate court recognized that the federal HIPAA privacy rule does not eliminate any rights to privacy that may exist under state laws that are stricter than the federal HIPAA privacy rule. This was a choice made by Congress between two possible alternatives. Some people think privacy should be governed by a single federal standard to have uniformity throughout the country. Under that approach, a single federal law should preempt or supersede all state laws on the subject of healthcare privacy. Others argue that a federal law should merely establish the minimum standard or floor for privacy protection, and each state government should be permitted to impose more stringent protections within its particular state. In the HIPAA legislation, Congress resolved this issue of federalism in favor of greater flexibility for the states instead of nationwide uniformity. Under HIPAA, the privacy rule adopted by HHS does *not* supersede or preempt state laws that provide a higher level of protection for the privacy of healthcare information.[34]

The federal HIPAA privacy rule is enforced by the HHS Office for Civil Rights. Violating the rule results in significant penalties, including high civil penalties and even some criminal penalties for more serious violations. The HIPAA statute does not explicitly provide a private cause of action for patients to seek damages from those who improperly disclose their records. However, creative lawyers might be able to assert claims for civil liability under existing state laws, by arguing that the federal privacy rule is the "standard of care" for purposes of state law claims.[35]

As a practical matter, the requirements of the privacy rule are complex. Most requirements have exceptions, and often there are exceptions to the exceptions. In general, the privacy rule protects health information that identifies an individual or could be used to identify an individual. In some situations, however, disclosure of patient information is allowed even without the authorization of the patient.

Negative obligations Requirements to refrain from specific conduct or action.

Healthcare providers, health plans, and other entities that are subject to the rule have both **negative obligations** and **affirmative obligations**. First, they have the negative obligation to not use or disclose information except in accordance with the rule. For some purposes, they must limit disclosure to the minimum amount of information necessary to accomplish that purpose. The rule sets forth additional requirements that must be satisfied if the disclosure is made for purposes such as marketing or fundraising. In regard to affirmative obligations, they are required to establish policies, provide notices, conduct employee training, designate a privacy official and a person to receive complaints, put safeguards into place to protect confidentiality, and retain documents as provided by the rule.

Affirmative obligations Requirements to perform specific activities.

When it was first adopted, the HIPAA privacy rule only applied to **covered entities**—health plans, healthcare clearinghouses, and healthcare providers that transmit information by electronic means. These categories include health insurance companies, HMOs, the Medicare and Medicaid programs, healthcare facilities, institutional providers, and most physician practices. However, HHS recognized the need to protect health information

Covered entities Health plans, healthcare clearinghouses, and healthcare providers that transmit information by electronic means.

when covered entities use the services of other organizations, such as accountants, lawyers, computer technicians, and accrediting organizations. In performing certain functions for a covered entity, those business associates might have access to individually identifiable information about the patients or members of the covered entity. Because those other organizations are not included within the definition of covered entity, they were not subject to direct regulation under the privacy rule. To address that problem, the original HIPAA privacy rule protected health information in the hands of those organizations by requiring covered entities to enter into specific written agreements with their business associates.

Later, Congress expanded the scope of privacy protection by extending some requirements of the HIPAA privacy rule to business associates. On February 17, 2009, Congress enacted the Health Information Technology for Economic and Clinical Health (HITECH) Act, as part of the American Recovery and Reinvestment Act of 2009.[36] The HITECH Act required HHS to amend its HIPAA privacy rule in several respects, including direct regulation of business associates. To satisfy the mandate of the HITECH Act, HHS issued a comprehensive ("omnibus") final rule on January 25, 2013, which amends the HIPAA privacy rule as well as other rules about security and enforcement.[37] As HHS explained, the 2013 amendments to the privacy rule "[m]ake business associates of covered entities directly liable for compliance with certain of the HIPAA Privacy and Security Rules' requirements."[38]

The 2013 final rule also made other important changes to the law, such as establishing requirements for notification of breach of unsecured health information, as well as imposing new limits on the sale of health information or the use of health information for marketing and fundraising. The 2013 final rule also modifies the requirements for a "notice of privacy practices" and makes changes to the enforcement provisions and penalties. Disclosure of personal health information is also restricted if a patient pays for healthcare services in full out-of-pocket. The 2013 final rule also implements a requirement of a separate federal statute, the Genetic Information Nondiscrimination Act of 2008 (GINA),[39] by generally preventing the use of genetic information for underwriting.

Individuals have certain rights under the HIPAA privacy rule. In general, and subject to various exceptions, individuals have the right to obtain their own health information, request corrections to statements in their medical records, and obtain an "accounting of disclosures" to find out who has received information from their records. The 2013 final rule expands the right of individuals to receive copies of their records in electronic form.[40]

If the individual patient is a minor, the parent would ordinarily have the right to consent to treatment on behalf of the minor and obtain the minor's medical information. However, some states have laws that permit minors to consent on their own for treatment of specific conditions such as substance abuse or sexually transmitted diseases. If the minor may lawfully give consent to treatment, state law might prohibit disclosure of information to the parent. This issue has led to conflict between some healthcare providers, who believe privacy will encourage adolescents to seek treatment, and some former officials at HHS, who believed that parents should have access to medical information about their children, especially with regard to drug abuse and abortion. Under the statutory scheme set forth in HIPAA, this issue is generally governed by state law.[41]

The following reading is an excerpt from the Federal Register in which HHS summarized the components and purposes of its 2013 final rule. After that excerpt, Activity 6.1 provides an opportunity to consider, from both a legal and an ethical perspective, whether patients should retain their rights to privacy if they disclose selected parts of their medical information to the media as part of a complaint against a healthcare provider.

5566 *Federal Register* / Vol. 78, No. 17 / Friday, January 25, 2013 / Rules and Regulations[42]

Department of Health and Human Services
Office of the Secretary
45 CFR Parts 160 and 164
RIN 0945–AA03

Modifications to the HIPAA Privacy, Security, Enforcement, and Breach Notification Rules Under the Health Information Technology for Economic and Clinical Health Act and the Genetic Information Nondiscrimination Act; Other Modifications to the HIPAA Rules

AGENCY: Office for Civil Rights, Department of Health and Human Services.

ACTION: Final rule.

SUMMARY: The Department of Health and Human Services (HHS or "the Department") is issuing this final rule to: Modify the Health Insurance Portability and Accountability Act (HIPAA) Privacy, Security, and Enforcement Rules to implement

(continued)

(continued from previous page)

statutory amendments under the Health Information Technology for Economic and Clinical Health Act ("the HITECH Act" or "the Act") to strengthen the privacy and security protection for individuals' health information; modify the rule for Breach Notification for Unsecured Protected Health Information (Breach Notification Rule) under the HITECH Act to address public comment received on the interim final rule;

modify the HIPAA Privacy Rule to strengthen the privacy protections for genetic information by implementing section 105 of Title I of the Genetic Information Nondiscrimination Act of 2008 (GINA); and make certain other modifications to the HIPAA Privacy, Security, Breach Notification, and Enforcement Rules (the HIPAA Rules) to improve their workability and effectiveness and to increase flexibility for and decrease burden on the regulated entities.

DATES: Effective date: This final rule is effective on March 26, 2013.

Compliance date: Covered entities and business associates must comply with the applicable requirements of this final rule by September 23, 2013. . . .

I. Executive Summary and Background

A. *Executive Summary*

i.   Purpose of the Regulatory Action Need for the Regulatory Action

This final rule is needed to strengthen the privacy and security protections established under [HIPAA] for individual's health information maintained in electronic health records and other formats. This final rule also makes changes to the HIPAA rules that are designed to increase flexibility for and decrease burden on the regulated entities, as well as to harmonize certain requirements with those under the Department's Human Subjects Protections regulations. These changes are consistent with, and arise in part from, the Department's obligations under Executive Order 13563 to conduct a retrospective review of our existing regulations for the purpose of identifying ways to reduce costs and increase flexibilities under the HIPAA Rules. We discuss our specific burden reduction efforts more fully in the Regulatory Impact Analysis.

(continued)

(continued from previous page)

This final rule is comprised of four final rules, which have been combined to reduce the impact and number of times certain compliance activities need to be undertaken by the regulated entities.

Legal Authority for the Regulatory Action

The final rule implements changes to the HIPAA Rules under a number of authorities. First, the final rule modifies the Privacy, Security, and Enforcement Rules to strengthen privacy and security protections for health information and to improve enforcement as provided for by the [HITECH Act] . . . . The rule also includes final modifications to the Breach Notification Rule, which will replace an interim final rule originally published in 2009 as required by the HITECH Act. Second, the final rule revises the HIPAA Privacy Rule to increase privacy protections for genetic information as required by [GINA]. Finally, the Department uses its general authority under HIPAA to make a number of changes to the Rules that are intended to increase workability and flexibility, decrease burden, and better harmonize the requirements with those under other Departmental regulations.

ii. Summary of Major Provisions

This omnibus final rule is comprised of the following four final rules:

1. Final modifications to the HIPAA Privacy, Security, and Enforcement Rules mandated by the [HITECH Act], and certain other modifications to improve the Rules, which were issued as a proposed rule on July 14, 2010. These modifications:

    • Make business associates of covered entities directly liable for compliance with certain of the HIPAA Privacy and Security Rules' requirements.

    • Strengthen the limitations on the use and disclosure of protected health information for marketing and fundraising purposes, and prohibit the sale of protected health information without individual authorization.

    • Expand individuals' rights to receive electronic copies of their health information and to restrict disclosures to a health plan concerning treatment for which the individual has paid out of pocket in full.

(continued)

(continued from previous page)

- Require modifications to, and redistribution of, a covered entity's notice of privacy practices.
- Modify the individual authorization and other requirements to facilitate research and disclosure of child immunization proof to schools, and to enable access to decedent information by family members or others.
- Adopt the additional HITECH Act enhancements to the Enforcement Rule not previously adopted in the October 30, 2009, interim final rule (referenced immediately below), such as the provisions addressing enforcement of noncompliance with the HIPAA Rules due to willful neglect.

2. Final rule adopting changes to the HIPAA Enforcement Rule to incorporate the increased and tiered civil money penalty structure provided by the HITECH Act, originally published as an interim final rule on October 30, 2009.

3. Final rule on Breach Notification for Unsecured Protected Health Information under the HITECH Act, which replaces the breach notification rule's "harm" threshold with a more objective standard and supplants an interim final rule published on August 24, 2009.

4. Final rule modifying the HIPAA Privacy Rule as required by [GINA] to prohibit most health plans from using or disclosing genetic information for underwriting purposes, which was published as a proposed rule on October 7, 2009. . . .

B. *Statutory and Regulatory Background*

i.   HIPAA and the Privacy, Security, and Enforcement Rules
The HIPAA Privacy, Security, and Enforcement Rules implement certain of the Administrative Simplification provisions of title II, subtitle F, of [HIPAA] . . . . The HIPAA Administrative Simplification provisions provided for the establishment of national standards for the electronic transmission of certain health information, such as standards for certain health care transactions conducted electronically and code sets and unique identifiers for health care providers and employers. The HIPAA Administrative Simplification provisions also required the establishment of national standards to protect the privacy and security of personal health information and established

(continued)

(continued from previous page)

civil money penalties for violations of the Administrative Simplification provisions. The Administrative Simplification provisions of HIPAA apply to three types of entities, which are known as "covered entities": health care providers who conduct covered health care transactions electronically, health plans, and health care clearinghouses.

The HIPAA Privacy Rule, 45 CFR Part 160 and Subparts A and E of Part 164, requires covered entities to have safeguards in place to ensure the privacy of protected health information, sets forth the circumstances under which covered entities may use or disclose an individual's protected health information, and gives individuals rights with respect to their protected health information, including rights to examine and obtain a copy of their health records and to request corrections. Covered entities that engage business associates to work on their behalf must have contracts or other arrangements in place with their business associates to ensure that the business associates safeguard protected health information, and use and disclose the information only as permitted or required by the Privacy Rule.

The HIPAA Security Rule, 45 CFR Part 160 and Subparts A and C of Part 164, applies only to protected health information in electronic form and requires covered entities to implement certain administrative, physical, and technical safeguards to protect this electronic information. Like the Privacy Rule, covered entities must have contracts or other arrangements in place with their business associates that provide satisfactory assurances that the business associates will appropriately safeguard the electronic protected health information they create, receive, maintain, or transmit on behalf of the covered entities.

The HIPAA Enforcement Rule, 45 CFR Part 160, Subparts C–E, establishes rules governing the compliance responsibilities of covered entities with respect to the enforcement process, including the rules governing investigations by the Department, rules governing the process and grounds for establishing the amount of a civil money penalty where a violation of a HIPAA Rule has been found, and rules governing the procedures for hearings and appeals where the covered entity challenges a violation determination.

(continued)

(continued from previous page)

Since the promulgation of the HIPAA Rules, legislation has been enacted requiring modifications to the Rules. In particular, the [HITECH Act] . . . modifies certain provisions of the Social Security Act pertaining to the HIPAA Rules, as well as requires certain modifications to the Rules themselves, to strengthen HIPAA privacy, security, and enforcement. The Act also provides new requirements for notification of breaches of unsecured protected health information by covered entities and business associates. In addition, [GINA] calls for changes to the HIPAA Privacy Rule to strengthen privacy protections for genetic information. This final rule implements the modifications required by GINA, as well as most of the privacy, security, and enforcement provisions of the HITECH Act. This final rule also includes certain other modifications to the HIPAA Rules to improve their workability and effectiveness.

ii.   The Health Information Technology for Economic and Clinical Health Act

The HITECH Act is designed to promote the widespread adoption and interoperability of health information technology. Subtitle D of title XIII, entitled "Privacy," supports this goal by adopting amendments designed to strengthen the privacy and security protections for health information established by HIPAA. These provisions include extending the applicability of certain of the Privacy and Security Rules' requirements to the business associates of covered entities; requiring that Health Information Exchange

Organizations and similar organizations, as well as personal health record vendors that provide services to covered entities, shall be treated as business associates; requiring HIPAA covered entities and business associates to provide for notification of breaches of

"unsecured protected health information"; establishing new limitations on the use and disclosure of protected health information for marketing and fundraising purposes; prohibiting the sale of protected health information; and expanding individuals' rights to access their protected health information, and to obtain restrictions on certain disclosures of protected health information to health plans. In addition, subtitle D adopts provisions designed to strengthen and expand HIPAA's enforcement provisions. . . .

(continued)

(continued from previous page)

iii.   The Genetic Information Nondiscrimination Act

[GINA] prohibits discrimination based on an individual's genetic information in both the health coverage (Title I) and employment (Title II) contexts. In addition to the nondiscrimination provisions, section 105 of Title I of GINA contains new privacy protections for genetic information, which require the Secretary of HHS to revise the Privacy Rule to clarify that genetic information is health information and to prohibit group health plans, health insurance issuers (including HMOs), and issuers of Medicare supplemental policies from using or disclosing genetic information for underwriting purposes.

ACTIVITY 6.1: HILLTOP MEMORIAL HOSPITAL

Hilltop Memorial Hospital (HMH) is an acute care general hospital in Windsor County. It is owned and operated by a private, nonprofit corporation, and it has tax-exempt status under federal and state tax laws. HMH provides a large volume of uncompensated care and service to Medicaid patients, but it receives no public funds from the county government.

Windsor County has no public hospital. The only other hospital in the county is a for-profit facility that provides relatively little uncompensated care. Therefore, HMH is the safety-net hospital for uninsured, underinsured, and Medicaid patients in the region. Under these circumstances, HMH relies heavily on its insured patients to subsidize its indigent care and its losses on Medicaid patients.

On April 6, 2013, George Long went to the outpatient department of HMH for diagnosis and treatment of back pain. Long had made an appointment for that outpatient visit, and he arrived at HMH on schedule. Long had been to HMH many times for his back pain and for treatment of his mental health conditions. As indicated by his medical record at HMH, Long had a history of mental health problems, including episodes of delusion.

On that particular day, Long was escorted to an examining room in HMH's outpatient department and was instructed to wait for the nurse.

(continued)

(continued from previous page)

A few minutes later, the nurse arrived to find Long running around the examining room in an agitated manner. The nurse was unable to calm him and immediately called for the doctor. The doctor and nurse held Long's arms for about one minute until he became calm. After Long assured them that he could remain calm, the doctor completed examination of his back and instructed him to return in two weeks if he was still in pain.

One week later, Long went to the office of a private, nonprofit advocacy organization called Patient Rights of Windsor County (PRWC) to discuss his recent experience at HMH. Long told the president of PRWC that during his visit to HMH on April 6, 2013, the doctor and nurse at HMH had slapped him in the face and hit him in the stomach.

With the help of the president of PRWC, Long called the local newspaper and gave this same account to a reporter. The reporter took detailed notes of the conversation with Long and then called the CEO of HMH to hear her side of the story. However, the CEO replied that, because of privacy laws, she could not comment or provide any information about any individual patient at HMH. The local newspaper published a story about Long's allegations, including the details of his statement and the fact that HMH's CEO had no comment. Long has not filed a complaint with the police or with any government agency about this alleged incident, nor has he filed any legal action against HMH or the individual healthcare professionals.

During the next few weeks, members of PRWC participated in a series of demonstrations on the public sidewalk in front of HMH. Many of the PRWC members carried signs that stated "Stop HMH from beating patients." The local newspaper published three stories about those demonstrations, in which the newspaper repeated Long's allegations and HMH's refusal to comment.

In the three months since the first newspaper report about Long's allegations, HMH has experienced a severe drop in visits by patients who have coverage through commercial health insurance or employer-based health plans. It appears that a substantial majority of those insured patients have chosen to receive care at the for-profit hospital in the county or at hospitals in other counties. HMH relies heavily on those insured patients to subsidize its indigent care and its losses on Medicaid patients. HMH has determined that it will be unable to pay all of its operating expenses if this situation continues for another six months.

(continued)

(continued from previous page)

The CEO of HMH attempted to communicate with Long in an effort to resolve the matter or, at least, obtain his consent to allow HMH to release his medical record to the local newspaper. The CEO even suggested that it might be possible to make a financial settlement with him, in exchange for a neutral press release that would be acceptable to both sides. However, Long refused to discuss any type of settlement and refused to consent to the release of his medical record.

The board of trustees of HMH ("the board") held an emergency meeting to discuss the situation and consider its options. After receiving an update from the management of HMH, members of the board suggested various alternatives. Board member A argued that HMH must continue its current position of refusing to make any comment or provide any information about an individual patient. In contrast, board member B took the position that Long gave up his privacy by giving the mass media information—albeit false information—about his treatment at HMH. Therefore, Long would have no right to complain if HMH were to set the record straight by releasing his medical record, which would show that he has a long history of delusional episodes. Board member C stated that only a stupid law would prevent HMH from defending itself and its staff under these circumstances, and disclosing a small amount of information about Long's medical history would be a technical violation at most. Finally, board member D argued that ethical considerations require disclosing Long's history of delusional episodes, because the potential harm to Long from his loss of privacy is vastly outweighed by the greater good of preserving the community's safety-net hospital, which is at serious risk of insolvency.

Please evaluate HMH's alternatives from both an ethical and a legal perspective, including consideration of the federal HIPAA privacy rule. Also, please decide whether the current law should be clarified or amended. Be prepared to explain the reasons for your conclusions.

Notes

1. American Medical Association, *Code of Medical Ethics, Principles of Medical Ethics, Preamble*, point IV (2001). www.ama-assn.org/ama/pub/physician-resources/medical-ethics/code-medical-ethics/principles-medical-ethics.page.

2. American College of Healthcare Executives (2003). *Code of Ethics.* www.ache.org/ABT_ACHE/code.cfm.

3. U.S. Department of Health and Human Services, "HHS Announces Final Regulation Establishing First-Ever National Standards to Protect Patients' Personal Medical Records" (2000). Press Release, December 20. aspe.hhs.gov/admnsimp/final/press2.htm.

4. See Standards for Privacy of Individually Identifiable Health Information, 65 Fed. Reg. 82462, 82465 (December 28, 2000) ("[T]he disclosure of information may require only the push of a button").

5. *Id.* ("In some ways, this imperfect system of record keeping created a false sense of privacy among patients, providers, and others").

6. D. A. Hyman and M. Hall (2001). "Two Cheers for Employment-Based Health Insurance," *Yale Journal of Health Policy, Law & Ethics,* (II)(1): 23–58, at 33.

7. See generally C. Scott, "Is Too Much Privacy Bad for Your Health? An Introduction to the Law, Ethics, and HIPAA Rule on Medical Privacy." *Georgia State University Law Review* (2000), 17(2): 481–529, at 494–95 ("Maine citizens seem to have concluded that too much privacy could be bad for their health").

8. 65 Fed. Reg. at 82466.

9. *Hammonds v. Aetna Casualty & Surety Co.*, 243 F. Supp. 793, 801–802 (N.D. Ohio 1965) (applying Ohio law where the jurisdiction of the federal court was based on diversity of citizenship).

10. *Berger v. Sonneland*, 26 P.3d 257 (Wash. 2001).

11. *Id.* at 265–67 (rejecting the treating physician's argument that the state medical privacy statute was the exclusive remedy, in which case the patient's claim would have been time-barred by failure to meet the statute of limitations).

12. 551 P.2d 334 (Cal. 1976).

13. 551 P.2d at 346–47 (citations and footnotes omitted).

14. *Id.* at 340.

15. *Id.* at 347.

16. American Medical Association, *Code of Medical Ethics*, 10.01: Fundamental Elements of the Patient-Physician Relationship. www. ama-assn.org/ama/pub/physician-resources/medical-ethics/code-medical-ethics/opinion1001.page.

17. 42 C.F.R. §§ 2.1 *et seq.* (2005).

18. 45 C.F.R. § 46.111(a)(7) (2005) (criteria for IRB approval).

19. See Scott, *supra* note 7, at 508.

20. Health Insurance Portability and Accountability Act of 1996, Pub. L. No. 104-191, 110 Stat. 1936 (1996).

21. *Id.* § 261, 110 Stat. at 2021.

22. *Id.* § 264, 110 Stat. at 2033.

23. *Id.* § 262, 110 Stat. at 2021.

24. *Id.* § 264, 110 Stat. at 2033.

25. See, e.g., proposed Medical Information Privacy and Security Act, S. 573, 106th Cong. (1999) [sponsored by Senators Patrick Leahy (D-VT), Thomas Daschle (D-SD), Byron Dorgan (D-ND), and Edward Kennedy (D-MA)]; proposed Consumer Health and Research Technology Protection Act, H.R. 3900, 105th Cong. (1998) [sponsored by Representatives Christopher Shays (R-CT) and Thomas Barrett (D-WI)].

26. Standards for Privacy of Individually Identifiable Health Information, 64 Fed. Reg. 59918 (Nov. 3, 1999) (proposed rule).

27. Standards for Privacy of Individually Identifiable Health Information, 65 Fed. Reg. 82462 (Dec. 28, 2000) (final rule).

28. See, e.g., *South Carolina Medical Association v. Thompson*, 327 F.3d 346 (4th Cir. 2003); *Association of American Physicians & Surgeons, Inc. v. U.S. Department of Health and Human Services*, 224 F. Supp. 2d 1115 (S.D. Tex. 2002), *aff'd* 67 Fed. Appx. 253 (5th Cir. 2003).

29. 65 Fed. Reg. at 82760.

30. Standards for Privacy of Individually Identifiable Health Information, 67 Fed. Reg. 14776 (March 27, 2002) (proposed rule; modification).

31. Standards for Privacy of Individually Identifiable Health Information, 67 Fed. Reg. 53182 (Aug. 14, 2002) (final rule).

32. *Id.* at 53182.

33. *Citizens for Health v. Leavitt*, 428 F.3d 167 (3rd Cir. 2005), *cert. denied*, 127 S. Ct. 3 (2006).

34. Health Insurance Portability and Accountability Act of 1996, Pub. L. No. 104-191, § 264(c)(2), 110 Stat. 1936, 2033–34 (1996).

35. J. Kulynych and D. Korn (2002). "The Effect of the New Federal Medical-Privacy Rule on Research." *New England Journal of Medicine* 346 (3): 201–204, at 203.

36. American Recovery and Reinvestment Act of 2009, Pub. L. No. 111-5.

37. 78 Fed. Reg. 5566 (January 25, 2013).

38. *Id.* at 5566.

39. Genetic Information Nondiscrimination Act of 2008, Pub. L. No. 110-233.

40. 78 Fed. Reg. at 5702.
41. See generally 67 Fed. Reg. at 53200–201.
42. 78 Fed. Reg. 5566 (January 25, 2013).

MEDICAL STAFF MEMBERSHIP AND CLINICAL PRIVILEGES

7

One of the most important aspects of healthcare law is the relationship between physicians and healthcare facilities or organizations. Under the law of medical malpractice, as discussed in Chapter 10, patients often seek to hold a hospital or other healthcare organization liable for a physician's negligence. Ordinarily, the result in that type of case depends on the precise nature of the relationship between the physician and the institution. This relationship also raises legal issues of Medicare fraud and abuse. As explained in Chapter 8, federal law prohibits certain types of financial arrangements between healthcare facilities and referring physicians. Finally, as discussed in Chapter 9, some cases have antitrust law implications when physicians are prevented from practicing in healthcare institutions.

In the hospital context, this relationship has been based primarily on an individual physician's request for permission to treat patients at a particular hospital. In recent years, physicians have also requested permission to affiliate with other types of healthcare organizations, such as networks, preferred provider organizations, and managed care organizations (MCOs). To be able to treat the patients enrolled in a particular plan, or at least to be able to treat those patients on favorable terms, physicians must ask the MCO for permission to join its network of preferred providers.

Inevitably, disputes arise in connection with these new physician relationships, just as they have in the hospital context. An MCO might refuse to allow a physician to join its network, just as hospitals might refuse to grant permission for certain physicians to practice at their facilities. Moreover, a patient might seek to hold an MCO liable for the negligence of an individual physician, just as patients have sought to hold hospitals liable for the negligence of individual physicians.

It is not surprising that courts attempt to resolve these new disputes between physicians and MCOs by analogy to the preexisting legal principles, which were developed in the context of physicians and hospitals. Although the situations are somewhat different, the issues are essentially the same. The first issue is determining when a healthcare organization may refuse to permit a licensed physician to practice in connection with that organization. In the managed care context, MCOs might have the right to exclude and terminate physicians in the process of selective contracting, as discussed in Chapter 14. In addition, if an organization permits a physician to participate, the separate issue arises of determining when that organization will be held liable for the negligence of that individual physician. The potential liability of MCOs for the negligence of participating physicians is discussed in Chapter 10. First, it is necessary to understand the traditional relationship between physicians and hospitals as well as the legal principles that have been developed in connection with that relationship.

The Relationship Between Physicians and Hospitals

To survive economically and fulfill their respective functions in the healthcare system, physicians and hospitals need each other. Most physicians need to have some access to the facilities of a hospital, even if they see many of their patients in an office setting. In addition to admitting patients to the hospital, physicians might rely on the hospital to perform diagnostic tests on their patients. In many cases, hospitals bear the expense of providing the facilities and equipment physicians need to treat their patients.

At the same time, hospitals need physicians to get patients into the hospital. Except in an emergency, a prospective patient cannot simply walk into a hospital and ask for care. Rather, a patient may be admitted to a hospital only under the authority of a physician or other practitioner who has admitting privileges at that particular facility. Once the patient has been admitted, only a physician or other designated practitioner has the authority to order tests and treatments for that patient.

In establishing a relationship, hospitals and physicians can choose from at least three different types of arrangement:

1. employment;
2. contract; or
3. medical staff membership and clinical privileges.

Employment

The parties could decide to make the individual physician an employee of the hospital. Employees receive compensation from their employer, but they are subject to their employer's control. Historically, only a small percentage of physicians were employees of a hospital. Although teaching hospitals employed many physicians, that practice was not common at most community hospitals.

In recent years, however, the use of employment relationships has increased, as hospitals have purchased physician practices and hired physicians as employees of the hospital or an affiliated organization.[1] Many hospitals also employ **hospitalists**, who specialize in caring for inpatients.

From the perspective of physicians, an employment relationship can reduce the need to spend their time on administrative tasks of practice management and can provide a more flexible lifestyle. "Furthermore, the young doctors being hired today tend to value better work–life balance and are more willing than preceding generations to trade higher incomes for the lifestyle flexibility and administrative simplicity provided by hospital employment."[2] The motivations for hospitals to employ physicians include increasing their market share and bargaining power,[3] increasing referrals, reducing costs, and preparing for the changes of health reform.[4] As O'Malley and colleagues have noted, "Following enactment of national health reform in March 2010, hospital executives also increasingly cited physician–hospital integration through physician employment as key to preparing for expected Medicare payment reforms, including bundled payments, accountable care organizations (ACOs) and penalties for preventable hospital readmissions."[5]

In some states, this type of employment arrangement may violate the traditional doctrine that prohibits the corporate practice of medicine. Under that doctrine, only a licensed *individual* may practice medicine, and a corporation may not own or control the practice of an individual physician. Therefore, physicians in those states could not be employees of a corporation, such as a hospital. However, even in those states that follow the traditional doctrine, the restriction can usually be circumvented by making the physicians employees of a separate entity or by using a contract instead of an employment relationship.[6]

An employment relationship also raises several ethical issues for a physician, including the need to maintain the physician's independent medical judgment. In 2012, the American Medical Association (AMA) adopted its AMA Principles for Physician Employment.[7] Some of these principles deal specifically with conflicts of interest, including the following:

(a) A physician's paramount responsibility is to his or her patients. Additionally, given that an employed physician occupies a position of significant trust, he or she owes a duty of loyalty to his or her employer. This divided loyalty can create conflicts of interest, such as financial incentives to over- or under-treat patients, which employed physicians should strive to recognize and address.

(b) Employed physicians should be free to exercise their personal and professional judgment in voting, speaking, and advocating on any matter regarding patient care interests, the profession, health care in the community, and the independent exercise of medical judgment. Employed physicians should not be deemed in breach of their employment agreements, nor be retaliated against by their employers, for asserting these interests.

Hospitalists
Physicians employed by hospitals and specializing in the care of inpatients.

(c) In any situation where the economic or other interests of the employer are in conflict with patient welfare, patient welfare must take priority.[8]

Contractual Relationship

In this situation, the physician is not an employee but rather is an independent contractor. The hospital cannot tell the contracting physician how to perform the work, as it could with an employee; it can only require that the physician meet the obligations set forth in the contract. Instead of contracting directly with an individual physician, the hospital might contract with a professional corporation or professional association, which will hire individual physicians as employees of the professional corporation or professional association.

Frequently, hospitals use contracts to obtain the services of hospital-based physicians (HBPs). HBPs are responsible for providing all of the necessary medical coverage in a particular department of the hospital, such as radiology, pathology, anesthesiology, or emergency. Ordinarily, those hospital contracts are exclusive, and only the contracting physicians may provide services in that particular department for the duration of the contract. This type of exclusive arrangement has several advantages for the hospital, such as convenience in scheduling; quality control; consistency in the use of procedures, equipment, and supplies; and ensuring full-time medical coverage for all patients, including those who are unable to pay for their care.

Medical Staff Membership and Clinical Privileges

In this category, the physicians are not employees of the hospital, and they have not entered into a contract to operate a particular department of the hospital. Rather, they are physicians in the private practice of medicine who have applied for the privilege of admitting and treating their patients at that particular facility. As discussed here, physicians are not automatically entitled to admit their patients to a particular hospital, even if they are licensed to practice medicine in the state. Rather, they must apply for membership and privileges under the criteria set forth in the bylaws of the hospital's medical staff.

Under these circumstances, many of the physicians practicing in U.S. hospitals are not employees of the hospital. Nevertheless, those non-employee physicians have the power to make decisions and take actions that will significantly affect the quality of care provided by the hospital as well as its financial viability. As discussed in Chapter 8, hospitals may gain or lose money under the Medicare prospective payment system as a result of treatment and discharge decisions made by physicians who are not employees of the hospital. In addition, as discussed in Chapter 10, a hospital may be held liable for the negligence of a physician who is not an employee of the hospital if it reasonably appears to the patient that the physician was an employee or agent of the hospital. Thus, a hospital's legal liability and financial viability, as well as its overall quality of care, will depend to a large extent on the actions of physicians who are not under the direct control of the hospital, but merely are members of the hospital's organized medical staff. A hospital may also be held liable under the doctrine of corporate negligence for failing to adequately screen physicians who apply for clinical privileges and membership on the hospital's medical staff.

The Organized Medical Staff

The medical staff of a hospital is not a separate corporation. Rather, it is an association that has its own members, officers, and bylaws. It is also part of the larger hospital organization.

Although a medical staff has a great deal of influence, it is not the ultimate authority in a hospital. As in any corporation, that authority is the board of directors, which is sometimes referred to as the board of trustees or governing board. The board oversees the operation of the hospital and is responsible for ensuring that it is operated in a lawful, prudent, and fiscally responsible manner.

Most members of hospital boards are neither healthcare professionals nor experts in healthcare management. In a public or nonprofit hospital, trustees are usually civic leaders with experience in business or charitable activities, as well as respected representatives of various constituencies in the community. If the hospital is owned by a for-profit chain, the board is likely to consist of representatives who were designated by the parent company. Of course, the board will usually rely on the administrative staff for matters of day-to-day operation and will usually defer to the medical staff on matters that involve professional expertise.

The roles and responsibilities of the hospital's medical staff are described in the accreditation standards of The Joint Commission.[9] As discussed in Chapter 5 of this text, accreditation by The Joint Commission is voluntary, but most hospitals participating in Medicare are accredited. Thus, most acute care, general hospitals in the United States conform to the organizational structure that is set forth in Joint Commission standards, including the standards for the organized medical staff. As set forth in The Joint Commission's *Comprehensive Accreditation Manual for Hospitals (CAMH)*, "The self-governing organized medical staff provides oversight of the quality of care, treatment, and services delivered by practitioners who are credentialed and privileged through the medical staff process. The organized medical staff is also responsible for the ongoing evaluation of the competency of practitioners who are privileged, delineating the scope of privileges that will be granted to practitioners and providing leadership in performance improvement activities within the organization."[10]

The physicians who treat patients at a hospital might have their own private practices in competition with each other. However, as a group, they are responsible for overseeing the quality of services provided at the hospital by each individual member of the group. "The primary function of the organized medical staff is to approve and amend medical staff bylaws and to provide oversight for the quality of care, treatment, and services provided by practitioners with privileges."[11] Moreover, Joint Commission standards require accountability to the hospital's governing body for performance of those functions.[12]

The medical staff is responsible for developing medical staff bylaws, as well as policies, rules, and regulations.[13] The medical staff bylaws require approval by the hospital's governing body.[14] However, once they are in effect, the bylaws may not be amended unilaterally by either the governing body or the medical staff.[15] The 2012 *CAMH* specifies the requirements which must be included in the bylaws, but it allows other details to be set forth in policies, rules, or regulations.[16] The requirements that *must* be in the bylaws include qualifications for membership, the process for appointment and reappointment, the process for granting and renewing privileges, procedures for recommending adverse action against a practitioner in regard to membership or privileges, and procedures for fair hearings and appeals.[17]

Historically, The Joint Commission required hospitals to limit their medical staffs to licensed doctors and dentists. This requirement enabled hospitals to use Joint Commission standards as a reason to deny applications from other categories of independent practitioners, such as chiropractors and podiatrists, who have a right under state law to practice without supervision. Nonphysician practitioners want the opportunity to use the facilities of hospitals for diagnosing and treating their patients. Some hospitals and physicians have argued that granting membership and privileges to nonphysicians would adversely affect the quality of care provided in hospitals. In response, nonphysicians have argued that medical doctors were merely trying to keep out competition and perpetuate their monopoly of hospital services.

After challenges were made under federal antitrust law, The Joint Commission changed its standards to leave the decision up to each individual hospital, subject only to the limits of state professional licensure laws. The 2012 *CAMH* indicates that a hospital's medical staff is *not* limited to doctors and dentists, but may also include other practitioners who are licensed to provide care independently without supervision and may include other practitioners as well.[18] Moreover, The Joint Commission has broadened the category of practitioners who may be given privileges by separating the concepts of staff membership and clinical privileges. Under the 2012 *CAMH*, "[a]pplicants for privileges need not necessarily be members of the medical staff."[19]

Privileges may be granted for a maximum of two years, with a process to apply for renewal.[20] In addition to the process for periodic renewal of privileges, a separate process exists for "Ongoing Professional Practice Evaluation," which can result in revocation of current privileges before the designated time for renewal.[21]

The *CAMH* requires that decisions about granting, denying, or renewing privileges be made in a process that is objective and based on evidence.[22] Criteria for decisions about privileges must include factors such as licensure and training, which must be verified by primary sources of information.[23] Of course, "[g]ender, race, creed, and national origin are not used in making decisions regarding the granting or denying of clinical privileges."[24]

How should hospitals consider an applicant's physical and mental health? On one hand, ensuring that patients are not harmed by physicians with problems such as substance abuse, mental illness, failing vision, or memory loss is important. However, under some circumstances, a physician's mental or physical problem could constitute a disability, and hospitals may not discriminate on the basis of disability. The *CAMH* explains that criteria for privileges must include "[e]vidence of physical ability to perform the requested privilege."[25] Apart from the disciplinary process, the *CAMH* provides a separate process for handling health issues of practitioners, which is designed to promote rehabilitation as well as protection of others.[26]

For example, if a physician is HIV-positive or has AIDS, the hospital must determine if that is a legitimate reason to deny, revoke, or restrict the physician's membership and privileges. In attempting to balance the interests of the hospital, its patients, and the infected physician, one approach is to rely on the concept of informed consent. Under that approach, the legal issue is whether hospitals may require HIV-positive physicians to give prior notice to their patients about their medical status as a condition of treating patients at the hospital. In one case, a trial court approved the hospital's action in requiring a surgeon who had AIDS to obtain the specific informed consent of his patients before performing surgery as a condition of restoring his surgical privileges.[27]

As discussed, hospitals often make exclusive contracts with HBPs to provide all of the medical coverage in a particular department of the hospital. In those situations, the physician's clinical privileges might terminate on expiration of the contract, without the need to demonstrate good cause for terminating those privileges. Alternatively, the hospital might permit contract physicians to retain their privileges on termination of the contract but effectively prevent them from practicing at the hospital by awarding an exclusive contract to someone else.

Denial or Termination of Membership and Privileges

As discussed in Chapter 10, in malpractice cases hospitals can be held liable for allowing an incompetent physician to provide services in the facility. In that type of case, an injured patient—or the estate of a patient—would sue the physician for alleged negligence in diagnosis or treatment and may also sue the hospital for its own alleged negligence in failing to properly screen applicants for clinical privileges. This legal theory of hospital liability is referred to as **corporate negligence**, and it can also be applied to the decision of a network or an MCO permitting a physician to become a participating provider. Under these circumstances, hospitals and other healthcare organizations have an incentive to be extremely careful in screening and selecting applicants.

Corporate negligence
Liability for breach of a hospital's duty to a patient, such as the duty to exercise reasonable care in allowing a physician to treat patients at the hospital.

However, if the organization denies the application, it may be sued by the disappointed applicant—a no-win situation from the organization's point of view. In effect, the organization has to choose whether it would prefer to be sued by an angry practitioner for allegedly unlawful exclusion or by patients or their estates for allegedly negligent credentialing. From the practitioner's point of view, the denial or termination of privileges would interfere with the ability to earn a living and cause a lifelong injury to professional reputation.

In the past, physicians who had their privileges revoked might be able to get a fresh start by moving to a different part of the country and obtaining privileges at a different hospital. Often, cases of threatened revocation were handled by means of a negotiated settlement. In many of those cases, the physician would voluntarily resign, and the hospital would agree to provide a neutral reference so that the physician could obtain privileges at a different hospital. Although state laws may have required hospitals to report adverse credentialing decisions to the state medical licensing board, those actions were characterized as voluntary resignations, rather than as adverse decisions, to avoid the need to make a report.

Obviously, that system did not address the problem with the physician's abilities but merely transferred the problem to another hospital and to other patients. Therefore, some states have strengthened their requirements for reporting adverse credentialing decisions to include a voluntary resignation under threat of revocation. In addition, the Federation of State Medical Boards established a data bank on physician disciplinary actions, and the federal government established the National Practitioner Data Bank (NPDB) pursuant to a 1986 federal statute.[28] Under that statute, hospitals and MCOs are required to notify the NPDB of adverse credentialing actions against physicians. In addition, insurance payments on behalf of physicians for medical malpractice must also be reported. Information about individual physicians in the NPDB is not available to the public, but hospitals must obtain information from the data bank when physicians apply for clinical privileges and every two years thereafter. In fact, the *CAMH* requires hospitals to request information from the NPDB when considering applications for new privileges or renewal of existing privileges.[29]

Despite some weaknesses in the system of reporting to the NPDB, more publicity surrounds disciplinary matters than in the past. As already discussed, some state governments have strengthened their reporting requirements, and state licensing boards are sharing information about disciplinary actions. In fact, some state boards make information about disciplinary actions available to the public on the Internet.

Under this more intensive system of reporting and publicity, a practitioner has a much more difficult time starting over in a new location, which has resulted in more protection for the public as a whole. At the same time, the new system increases the economic and professional consequences of an adverse credentialing decision for the affected practitioner. Under these circumstances, ensuring that every credentialing decision has a legitimate basis, as well as a realistic way to challenge any decision that is improper, is more important than ever.

In some cases, hospitals have revoked clinical privileges for valid reasons, such as incompetence, unethical behavior, and uncontrolled alcoholism or addiction. However, some hospitals have also excluded or expelled practitioners to prevent them from competing with the hospital or with existing members of the medical staff.

Moreover, in matters of credentialing, the healthcare industry has a long history of discrimination on the basis of race, gender, religion, and national origin. Before the passage of civil rights legislation, membership on some hospital medical staffs was explicitly limited by discriminatory criteria in the medical staff bylaws. Even after the passage of civil rights laws, some discrimination in credentialing has continued, but it is usually hidden under expressions of purported concern for the applicant's qualifications or ability to work with others. As in cases of employment discrimination, it may be difficult to determine whether a credentialing decision was based on a person's qualifications or on discrimination, in which case the supposed concern for the person's qualifications was merely a pretext. Finally, in the world of complex human relationships, some decisions on employment or credentialing involve a mixture of proper and improper motives.

The concern for a physician's ability to work with others has taken on increased significance as part of the ongoing movement to improve patient safety and quality of care. In some cases, claims about a physician's alleged inability to work with others could be a pretext for discrimination or anti-competitive conduct. In other cases, however, an inability to work with others could present a genuine risk to quality of care and the safety of patients. As The Joint Commission explained in a *Sentinel Event Alert*, "Intimidating and disruptive behaviors can foster medical errors, contribute to poor patient satisfaction and to preventable adverse outcomes, increase the cost of care, and cause qualified clinicians, administrators and managers to seek new positions in more professional environments. Safety and quality of patient care is dependent on teamwork, communication, and a collaborative work environment. To assure quality and to promote a culture of safety, health care organizations must address the problem of behaviors that threaten the performance of the health care team."[30] For these reasons, The Joint Commission's *CAMH* includes general competencies of "professionalism" and "interpersonal and communication skills."[31]

As one appellate court explained, a hospital should not terminate a physician's medical staff membership and clinical privileges merely because that physician is annoying to other people.

> The mere fact that a physician is irascible, however, or that he or she generally annoys other physicians, nurses or administrators does not constitute sufficient cause for termination of his or her hospital privileges. Likewise, a physician should not be removed from medical staff membership merely because he or she has criticized hospital practices or other health care personnel at the hospital. On the other hand, a physician may be so disruptive as to throw the hospital, or a segment of it, into turmoil and to prevent it from functioning effectively. So substantial a disruption reasonably could lead the hospital authorities to find that overall patient care may be threatened, thereby constituting good cause for termination of the physician's hospital privileges.[32]

In that case, the court held that hospitals may provide in their medical staff bylaws for denial or revocation of staff membership and clinical privileges on the ground of disruptive behavior when that behavior is sufficiently serious that it might affect patient care.[33] Of course, that standard raises a difficult factual question. Conflicting testimony about whether the behavior is sufficiently serious that it might affect patient care is likely. In the following excerpt, a federal court evaluated the evidence in regard to a particular physician's inability to work with others. After that excerpt, Activity 7.1 will provide an opportunity to consider these issues under a specific set of facts.

Everhart v. Jefferson Parish Hospital District No. 2, 757 F.2D 1567 (5TH CIR. 1985) (CITATIONS AND SOME TEXT OMITTED).[34]

ROBERT MADDEN HILL, Circuit Judge:

Appellant Francis J. Everhart, M.D., (Everhart) applied for and was denied admission to the medical staff of appellee East Jefferson General Hospital, located in Jefferson Parish, Louisiana. Everhart brought this action seeking declaratory and injunctive relief in connection with that denial of admission. Everhart sought declaratory relief from alleged denials of procedural and substantive due process of law in violation of the Fourteenth Amendment to the United States Constitution. In addition, he requested preliminary and permanent injunctive relief requiring that the hospital appoint him to the medical staff.

After conducting hearings on April 1 and April 21, 1981, the district court denied Everhart's request for preliminary injunctive relief. We affirmed the district court's denial in a per curiam opinion entered March 4, 1982. The case was then tried on its merits and the district court entered judgment in favor of defendants, with comprehensive written reasons, dismissing plaintiff's complaint. Everhart then timely appealed from that judgment. For the reasons that follow, we affirm.

I. FACTS

Everhart is a licensed physician, duly authorized to practice medicine in the State of Louisiana. He is board certified and specializes in cardiology. Jefferson Parish Hospital District No. 2, which does business as East Jefferson General Hospital (the hospital), is a political subdivision of the State of Louisiana, having been created by Ordinance No. 4049 of the Jefferson Parish Louisiana Council pursuant to the authority granted it under Louisiana Revised Statute Title 46, Chapter 10. The hospital is governed by the Board of Directors, which is appointed by the Jefferson Parish Louisiana Council.

The medical staff of the hospital is made up of over 400 doctors, is organized separately from the hospital itself, and has its own by-laws. Under the by-laws, an application for medical staff membership is sent

(continued)

(continued from previous page)

to the executive director of the hospital. After the director collects all references and other materials deemed pertinent, the completed application is referred to the credentials committee for its consideration. This committee then transmits the completed application to the medical staff's executive committee which makes a recommendation to the hospital board; the board then makes the final decision to grant or deny staff membership.

On March 24, 1980, Everhart submitted his application for medical staff membership to Mose Ellis, the executive director. At that time he also requested privileges in internal medicine and cardiology. The application form submitted by Everhart reflects that he graduated from medical school in 1962, completed his internal medicine residency in 1965 and was licensed to practice medicine in nine states. In addition, from July 1967, when Everhart first entered the private practice of medicine, until 1980, when he first arrived in Louisiana, he had begun and left six different practices. The application further reflects that his staff privileges had been suspended from Sacred Heart Hospital in Spokane, Washington, from July 1975 to November 1975 for "inappropriate behavior."

Pursuant to the by-laws, Everhart's application was referred to the credentials committee for review. On August 7, 1980, the committee reviewed twelve applications, and voted to recommend to the executive committee that eleven physicians be granted staff privileges. Although it found Everhart's "credentials in order," it made no recommendation to the executive committee as required by the by-laws. On August 12 the executive committee denied Everhart's application for membership to the medical staff.

On August 13 Ellis wrote Everhart, informing him that the executive committee voted not to recommend his appointment; the letter gave no reason for the committee's action. The next day Everhart requested a review of the executive committee's action, reasons for the adverse decision and the data that was reviewed by both the credential and executive committees as well as other materials. Pursuant to this request and in accordance with Art. VIII, Sec. 3, of the by-laws, Dr. Gustavo Colon, president of the medical staff at the hospital and chairman of the executive committee, appointed an ad hoc committee, consisting

(continued)

(continued from previous page)

of Drs. George Welch, chairman, Isadore Yager, chief of medicine, Samuel Leonard, Robert Miller and Irving Rosen.

On August 22 Dr. Colon notified Everhart in writing that the ad hoc committee would meet on August 27 and provided him with a list of the committee members. The notice did not contain the reasons for the adverse decision of the executive committee. Nevertheless, the ad hoc committee conducted hearings on August 27, September 8, and September 25. Everhart was present at each hearing and a record of the hearings was made by an electronic recording unit. On October 7 the ad hoc committee voted to recommend to the executive committee that Everhart not be appointed to the medical staff; on the same date the executive committee accepted the recommendation of the ad hoc committee.

After receiving notice of the committee's decision, on October 15 Everhart requested appellate review by the hospital board as well as a transcript of the committee hearings. On October 31 Ellis notified Everhart that a hearing would be conducted by the hospital board on November 6. On November 6 a duly appointed committee of the governing body, consisting of eight board members held a hearing at which Everhart, represented by counsel, was present. On February 17, 1981, the board found that the executive committee had not acted arbitrarily or capriciously and affirmed its decision denying the application for staff membership. Thereafter, Everhart brought this action before the district court complaining that his constitutional right to procedural and substantive due process had been violated in the denial of his admission to the medical staff of the hospital.

II. Procedural Due Process

Everhart contends that the procedures followed by the defendants which culminated in the denial of his application for staff membership, taken together, deprived him of his right to procedural due process. . . .

Everhart has several specific complaints regarding his procedural due process claim. First, he asserts, correctly, that the credentials committee, in violation of Art. V, Sec. 2(a), of the by-laws, failed to recommend to the executive committee that he be accepted, rejected,

(continued)

(continued from previous page)

or that his application be deferred. While the committee's failure to make such a recommendation to the executive committee does indeed constitute a technical violation of the by-laws, we fail to see how it has harmed Everhart. This technical violation certainly does not rise to the level of a deprivation of a constitutional right.

Everhart also contends that the notice he received of the ad hoc committee hearing stated only the time and place of the hearing and not the reasons for which the executive committee denied him staff membership as required by Art. VIII, Sec. 3(b), of the by-laws. The evidence, however, is clear that Everhart knew the reason he had been rejected was because of his past history of inappropriate behavior and his difficulty with interpersonal relationships at other hospitals. Everhart had ample notice to be apprised of the reasons for the rejection and to prepare his defense. Moreover, after a member of the ad hoc committee at the hearing asked Everhart if he desired written notice of the reasons for his rejections, Everhart expressly waived the requirement. We find no constitutional deprivation here.

Everhart next challenges the timing of the notice and the sufficiency of the materials provided to him for his appeal to the hospital board. Article VIII, Sec. 6(e), of the by-laws required that Everhart have (a) access to the ad hoc committee hearing record and all materials considered in the decision against him, and (b) fifteen days to submit a written statement in his behalf. Defendants concede that Everhart received notice on November 3, 1980, and that pursuant to such notice the board hearing was scheduled three days later for November 6. The evidence reveals, however, and Everhart concedes in his brief on appeal, that he expressly waived the procedural deficiency in the notice in order to proceed immediately with the appeal to the hospital board. In addition, Everhart had access to and in fact reviewed tapes prior to the hearing before the hospital board. The testimony of Drs. Yager and Colon establishes that Everhart received all pertinent, available documents. The appeal to the hospital board was not procedurally defective.

Finally, Everhart contends that two doctors sitting on separate committees were biased because at that time they were members of a corporation that had an exclusive right to practice invasive cardiology at the hospital, and thus had direct economic conflicts of interest with

(continued)

(continued from previous page)

Everhart. There is no evidence to support such a contention. Everhart would have us believe that a letter to the credentials committee, written by one of the doctors, raising a question as to Everhart's prior difficulties is evidence of such bias. We disagree. The doctor testified that he wrote the letter only after reviewing Everhart's application and file and only after becoming familiar with the reference letters that question Everhart's ability to work effectively with a medical staff. Further, Everhart brought forth no evidence to contradict the admittedly self-serving testimony of both doctors—the fact that Everhart sought cardiology privileges had nothing to do with their voting to deny him staff membership.

Everhart's complaint points this Court to several technical violations of the medical staff by-laws; we do not believe, however, that even taken together, these violations rise to the level of a constitutional deprivation of procedural due process. Everhart was fully aware of the reason for his rejection and, further, he had access to all the materials and reports that were relied upon and utilized by the defendants. In addition, he was afforded sufficient notice and an adequate opportunity (several lengthy hearings) and the means by which (calling any witnesses and presenting any evidence) to address and respond to the reason for his rejection. In some respects where the hearings were procedurally defective, Everhart expressly waived those defects. . . . The procedures utilized in reviewing and rejecting Everhart's application for admission to the medical staff were adequate and appropriate under the circumstances and nature of this case.

III. SUBSTANTIVE DUE PROCESS

Everhart contends that the hospital's decision to deny him staff membership was based on grounds having no reasonable relationship to the purpose of providing adequate medical care, i.e., his difficulty in interpersonal hospital relationships. He also contends that there was no evidence that his relationship with the hospital staff would affect patient care. We find both contentions unavailing.

. . . Article III, Sec. 2(a), of the by-laws, the basis for Everhart's rejection, requires that an applicant document his background, experience,

(continued)

(continued from previous page)

training and demonstrated competence, his adherence to professional ethics, his good reputation and his "ability to work with others, with sufficient adequacy to assure the medical staff and the governing body that any patient treated by him in the hospital will be given a high quality of medical care." Everhart contends that one's "ability to work with others" has no reasonable relation to the provision of high quality or even adequate medical care. Even if this consideration is reasonably related to the provision of the appropriate degree of medical care, he contends there was no evidence that had he joined the medical staff, that patient care would then be impacted negatively.

. . . We think Everhart's ability to work with others—his interpersonal relationships at the hospital—is a consideration that is reasonably related to the provision of adequate medical care. Consequently, the board's reliance upon this factor to deny staff membership to Everhart was neither arbitrary nor capricious and did not deprive him of substantive due process. . . .

We do not agree with Everhart's contention that his relationship with hospital personnel and the potential effects of poor interpersonal relationships is not a matter of medical expertise. While we agree that the character of a man is, in essence, a question of human nature, when that character becomes embroiled in the confines of a hospital environment, his character and his ability to work effectively in such an environment is a question uniquely suited to the hospital board. . . .

There was certainly sufficient evidence to indicate that Everhart had a history of difficulties with hospital personnel; he had been suspended for five months from Sacred Heart Hospital in Spokane, Washington, for inappropriate behavior. Further, the defendants received numerous letters from various individuals in hospitals that had been associated with Everhart indicating not only his difficulties with interpersonal relationships but also some emotional problems. Moreover, the high number of hospitals at which he had worked over a relatively short period of time could lead one to infer that Everhart would not have been able to effectively deal with those persons he came in contact with at the hospital. In addition, there was sufficient evidence that quality patient care demands that doctors possess at least a reasonable "ability to work with others." During the hearing process several doctors testified

(continued)

(continued from previous page)

specifically, contrary to Everhart's assertion, to the disruptive and potentially serious effect that poor interpersonal relationships may have on the smooth and efficient operation of the hospital.

Accordingly, we hold that there was sufficient evidence to justify the board's conclusion that Everhart was unable competently to work with others on the hospital staff and that such inability would have endangered the hospital's ability to provide quality medical care. Everhart failed to demonstrate that the decision to reject his application for admission to the medical staff of the hospital violated his right to substantive due process.

AFFIRMED.

ACTIVITY 7.1: DR. MICHAEL HENRY

Please assume the following facts. You are a member of the board of trustees (BOT) of Adams Memorial Hospital (AMH). AMH is an acute care, general hospital owned and operated by a private, nonprofit corporation. It is the only hospital in Adams County, which is in a mountainous region popular with retirees and vacationers.

Dr. Michael Henry is a surgeon. He received his education and training at prestigious institutions, and his technical skills are excellent. Dr. Henry is a perfectionist. He holds himself to very high standards and has little patience with other people who fail to meet similarly high standards. He expects the other healthcare professionals he deals with to do their jobs as well as he does his job.

Last year, Dr. Henry moved to Adams County. He obtained a license from the state medical licensing board and established a private practice in Adams County as a sole practitioner. He applied to AMH for medical staff membership and clinical privileges. Pursuant to the bylaws of the AMH medical staff, his application was reviewed and approved. Aside from Dr. Henry, all of the surgeons who practice at AMH are partners or employees of Adams Surgical Group, P.A.

(continued)

(continued from previous page)

Since his arrival, Dr. Henry has been critical about the level of care provided by doctors and nurses at AMH. He has complained in writing to the chief of surgery and the director of nursing about the equipment and procedures at AMH as well as about the performance of specific individuals. The chief of surgery responded in writing that Dr. Henry should not expect a community hospital in an area like Adams County to have the same equipment and procedures as the prestigious urban hospitals at which Dr. Henry received his education and training. Moreover, the chief of surgery pointed out that there was no evidence to prove that the issues raised by Dr. Henry had resulted in any harm to patients at AMH.

On several occasions, Dr. Henry has yelled at nurses and technicians during surgery. Three nurses and technicians have complained to the director of nursing, who forwarded their complaints to the chief of surgery.

Six months ago, Dr. Henry informed the director of nursing that he would no longer work with Nurse Ross because he considers her to be incompetent. The director of nursing denied Dr. Henry's allegations, and pointed out that Nurse Ross has a B.S. degree in nursing, a license from the state as a registered nurse, and 37 years of experience. Since then, the director of nursing has avoided scheduling Nurse Ross to work in the same operating room as Dr. Henry. However, that has created scheduling difficulties in the operating rooms.

Three months ago, after Dr. Henry yelled at another nurse during surgery, the chief of surgery gave Dr. Henry a written warning about his disruptive behavior. Dr. Henry has continued to yell at nurses and technicians during surgery, despite the written warning.

Subsequently, the medical staff of AMH notified Dr. Henry that, in accordance with the bylaws of the medical staff, it had started proceedings to revoke Dr. Henry's clinical privileges and his membership on the medical staff. The AMH medical staff bylaws provide that clinical privileges and medical staff membership may be revoked for disruptive behavior that might affect the care and safety of patients.

The medical staff followed all of the procedures set forth in the bylaws, including written notice to Dr. Henry and opportunities for hearings by the credentials committee and the executive committee of the medical staff. Dr. Henry participated in both of those hearings and

(continued)

(continued from previous page)

testified on his own behalf. Nevertheless, both the credentials committee and the executive committee recommended that his medical staff membership and clinical privileges be revoked on the ground of disruptive behavior that might affect the care and safety of patients.

As allowed by the bylaws of the medical staff, Dr. Henry requested a hearing before the BOT. That hearing was held one week ago. Dr. Henry participated in that hearing with his attorney and made this statement:

> *I am the best surgeon at this hospital, and everybody knows it. When I arrived, I was shocked at the outdated equipment, inadequate procedures, and poor performance by some of the employees and surgeons at AMH. Now they want to get rid of me because I am shaking up the status quo. In fact, the other surgeons want to drive me out so they can avoid competition and go back to their old monopoly, in which all of the surgeons who practice at AMH were partners or employees of one surgical group practice. Since I arrived at AMH, I have been trying to improve the quality of care provided by this hospital. This hospital is still using old-fashioned procedures rather than the best practices that were developed by evidence-based medicine. Finally, no evidence exists whatsoever that my so-called disruptive behavior has ever caused any harm to a patient.*

After Dr. Henry finished speaking, the director of nursing stated as follows:

> *Dr. Henry keeps yelling at nurses and technicians in surgery. He has been warned to stop doing that, but he just won't stop. His refusal to work with Nurse Ross has caused serious problems in scheduling personnel to work in the operating rooms. Nurse Ross is an employee in good standing at this hospital, and she has a license from the state as a registered nurse. She also has the most seniority on the nursing staff, which is supposed to give her the right under AMH policies to have first choice of shifts. Under the policies of AMH, no surgeon has the right to dictate the staffing schedule by refusing to work with a particular nurse. What would happen if every surgeon at AMH did that? Moreover, Dr. Henry's disruptive behavior poses a risk to the safety of patients. If a nurse observes a dangerous situation during surgery, such as a surgeon preparing to operate on the wrong part of the body or administering the*

(continued)

(continued from previous page)

wrong drug, the nurse is supposed to politely inform the surgeon of the apparent error. However, nurses are afraid to disagree with Dr. Henry in any way, because he always yells at people who disagree with him. Therefore, if a dangerous situation were to arise, the nurses would be afraid to inform Dr. Henry, and the patient might suffer a serious injury or death.

Finally, the chief of surgery made the following statement.

I admit that Dr. Henry has excellent technical skills. But he just cannot work with other people, especially the people here at AMH whom he considers to be beneath his level of performance. We have warned Dr. Henry in the past, including a written warning a few months ago. He just won't stop or can't stop, and we can't go on like this any longer. As the director of nursing explained, Dr. Henry's disruptive behavior poses a serious risk to the patients at this hospital. We simply have no other alternative at this point. For the good of AMH, its patients, and its employees, Dr. Henry's medical staff membership and clinical privileges must be revoked.

At the conclusion of the hearing, the chair of the BOT stated that a decision would be issued in ten days.

Your task, as a member of the BOT, is to decide whether to revoke Dr. Henry's medical staff membership and clinical privileges, under the facts set forth above. Be prepared to explain the reasons for your decision.

Judicial Review of Credentialing Decisions

For the reasons already discussed, a legal remedy must be available by which practitioners can appeal an inappropriate denial or termination of their privileges. However, the extent to which credentialing decisions should be subject to review and reversal by the courts is a complex policy issue.

In fact, tension exists between conflicting public policies in this area of the law. On one hand, we want to ensure that practitioners will have an effective right of appeal in cases of improper exclusion. However, we also want to encourage hospitals and their medical staffs to keep out incompetent or unethical practitioners who would be likely to pose a danger to the public. In almost all cases, those incompetent or unethical practitioners hold licenses from the state, which demonstrates that government regulation alone is not sufficient to protect the public health and ensure the quality of care. Therefore, we need to supplement government regulation with professional self-regulation through the mechanism of peer review. The goal for the legal system is to develop a remedy that will be effective for the aggrieved practitioner without interfering with the important function of medical peer review in the process of credentialing.

Over time, various legal theories have been in and out of favor as possible remedies for allegedly improper credentialing decisions. At first, excluded practitioners argued that they had been deprived of their constitutional right to due process of law. However, that theory has not been effective in this context for several reasons. The constitutional obligation to comply with due process of law only applies to units of government, such as public hospitals, the actions of which are deemed to be the actions of the state. Therefore, a private hospital's denial or revocation of privileges is not subject to the requirement of due process of law. Under current law, a private hospital's receipt of Medicare and Medicaid reimbursement or receipt of funding from the Hill-Burton program does not turn that private hospital's actions into "state action."[35]

Finally, for a public hospital that *is* subject to the requirements of due process, the hospital would only be required to show that it provided notice and an opportunity to be heard, as well as some reasonable basis for its decision.

Apart from the constitutional requirement of due process, some states have statutes or common law precedents that allow courts in those states to review the credentialing decisions of private hospitals. Most state courts would require some evidence that a fair procedure was used and some reasonable basis for the decision, but the court's review of the hospital's decision would be superficial. Courts recognize that the procedure for credentialing hearings may be informal, and a hospital is not required to follow all of the procedural requirements of a civil or criminal trial. Moreover, in reviewing the substantive basis for a credentialing decision, courts will ordinarily defer to the judgment of the hospital. As one court has explained,

> No court should substitute its evaluation of such matters for that of the Hospital Board . . . . Human lives are at stake, and the governing board must be given discretion in its selection so that it can have confidence in the competence and moral commitment of its staff. The evaluation of professional proficiency of doctors is best left to the specialized expertise of their peers, subject only to limited judicial surveillance . . . . In short, so long as staff selections are administered with fairness, geared by a rationale compatible with hospital responsibility, and unencumbered with irrelevant considerations, a court should not interfere. Courts must not attempt to take on the escutcheon of Caduceus.[36]

Under these circumstances, and because of the court's limited standard of judicial review, it is difficult for excluded physicians to prevail in this type of case. Even if they were driven out for discriminatory or anticompetitive reasons, they were probably given a written notice in advance and some apparent opportunity to be heard. The hospital's written decision, which might have been written by the hospital's attorney, is likely to contain some reason that appears to be valid and a recitation of some evidence in support of that decision.

In addition, state and federal governments have provided immunity for most activities in the process of medical peer review. To encourage physicians to express themselves freely in the peer review process, states have enacted statutes that provide some immunity for participants and confidentiality for their statements and documents. Similarly, Congress has provided immunity from damages for good-faith participation in peer-review activities. That immunity applies to claims by excluded physicians under various legal theories, including the antitrust claims which are discussed in Chapter 9.

The theory of these state and federal laws is that quality of care requires an effective system of peer review, and effective peer review requires immunity from damages for the participants. In other words, physicians would not participate in the process or provide candid evaluations of their peers unless they were given significant protection against the possibility of damages and the cost of litigation.

Theoretically, these state and federal immunities have exceptions that preserve the possibility of pursuing legitimate claims. In reality, however, obtaining effective legal relief is difficult for a practitioner, even if the credentialing decision was made for an improper reason. Thus, our society has made the policy decision to promote quality of care by means of professional self-regulation, even though some legitimate grievances by practitioners might not be effectively redressed.

Notes

1. A. S. O'Malley, A. M. Bond, and R. A. Berenson (2011). "Rising Hospital Employment of Physicians: Better Quality, Higher Costs?" Center for Studying Health System Change, Issue Brief No. 136, www.hschange.com/CONTENT/1230/1230.pdf; R. Kocher and N. Sahni (2011). "Hospitals' Race to Employ Physicians—The Logic Behind a Money-Losing Proposition." *New England Journal of Medicine* 364 (19): 1790–93.
2. Kocher and Sahni, *supra* note 1, at 1791.
3. O'Malley, Bond, and Berenson, *supra* note 1, at 1 and 3.

4. Kocher and Sahni, *supra* note 1, at 1790–92.

5. O'Malley, Bond, and Berenson, *supra* note 1, at 2.

6. See, e.g., O'Malley, Bond, and Berenson, *supra* note 1, at 1. ("Exceptions are Orange County, where California law bars hospitals from directly employing physicians, but physicians tend to be tied closely to hospitals through other means. . . .").

7. American Medical Association, "AMA Principles for Physician Employment" (2012). www.ama-assn.org/resources/doc/hod/ ama-principles-for-physician-employment.pdf.

8. *Id.* at 1.

9. The Joint Commission, *Comprehensive Accreditation Manual: CAMH for Hospitals (CAMH)* (2012), MS-1 to MS-46. Oakbrook Terrace, IL: Joint Commission Resources.

10. *Id.* at MS-1.

11. *Id.* at MS-2.

12. *Id.*

13. *Id.* at MS-5 to MS-6.

14. *Id.* at MS-6.

15. *Id.* at MS-13.

16. *Id.* at MS-7.

17. *Id.* at MS-7 to MS-11.

18. *Id.* at MS-1.

19. *Id.* at MS-2.

20. *Id.* at MS-31.

21. *Id.* at MS-23, MS-38 to MS-39.

22. *Id.* at MS-28.

23. *Id.*

24. *Id.* at MS-30.

25. *Id.* at MS-28.

26. *Id.* at MS-40 to MS-42.

27. *Estate of Behringer v. Medical Center at Princeton*, 592 A.2d 1251 (N.J. Super. 1991).

28. See Health Care Quality Improvement Act of 1986, Pub. L. No. 99-660, §§ 421–27, 100 Stat. 3743, 3788–92 (1986), codified as amended at 42 U.S.C. §§ 11131–37 (2005).

29. *CAMH, supra* note 9, at MS-29.

30. The Joint Commission (2008). "Behaviors That Undermine a Culture of Safety," Sentinel Event Alert Issue 40. www.jointcommission.org/ assets/1/18/SEA_40.PDF (endnotes omitted).

31. *CAMH, supra* note 9, at MS-25 and MS-26.

32. *Mahmoodian v. United Hospital Center, Inc.*, 404 S.E. 2d 750, 761 (Supreme Court of Appeals of West Virginia 1991), cert. denied, 502 U.S. 863 (1991).

33. *Id.* at 759–60.

34. *Everhart v. Jefferson Parish Hospital District No. 2*, 757 F.2d 1567 (5th Cir. 1985).

35. See, e.g., *Modaber v. Culpepper Memorial Hospital, Inc.*, 674 F.2d 1023, 1025–26 (4th Cir. 1982).

36. *Sosa v. Val Verde Memorial Hospital*, 437 F.2d 173, 177 (5th Cir. 1971).

THE LAW OF GOVERNMENT PAYMENT PROGRAMS: MEDICARE, MEDICAID, AND FRAUD AND ABUSE

To provide coverage to persons who are elderly, disabled, or indigent, Congress enacted the Medicare and Medicaid laws. The programs created by those laws have caused profound changes in the U.S. healthcare system and have made the federal government the largest buyer of healthcare services. The 2010 federal health reform legislation (the Patient Protection and Affordable Care Act, or ACA) made important changes to the law of government health programs. Those changes include improvements in coverage for beneficiaries, revisions to payment mechanisms, and efforts to reduce costs, improve efficiency, and increase the quality of care. In addition, the ACA made important changes to the law of fraud or abuse.

Since the creation of Medicare and Medicaid in the 1960s, many legal disputes have raised questions about the statutes, regulations, and policies that were adopted to implement the programs. Some of those disputes have involved the legal structure and financing of the programs. Other disputes can be categorized as issues of eligibility, benefits, or payment. *Eligibility* refers to the criteria an individual must meet to qualify as a beneficiary of the program. *Benefits* is a matter of defining the services covered by the program. In other words, assuming that a person has qualified as an eligible beneficiary, what services are covered and to what extent? *Payment* refers to the amount of money the program will pay to the facility or practitioner as compensation for providing covered services to an eligible beneficiary, as well as the methodology by which that compensation is determined. A separate set of issues involves fraud and abuse of the government payment programs, such as false claims, kickbacks, and self-referrals, which are discussed in detail in this chapter.

Medicare

Legal Structure and Financing
The Medicare program was established by federal statute, Title XVIII of the Social Security Act. It is a purely federal program administered by the Centers

for Medicare & Medicaid Services (CMS) and is part of the Department of Health and Human Services (HHS). Because Medicare was created by statute, a fundamental change in the program requires an act of Congress.

To implement the program, CMS has adopted regulations, which are contained in the *Code of Federal Regulations* and the *Federal Register*, and has published numerous policy manuals on various aspects of the program. In addition, the federal government makes contracts with private insurance companies to act as intermediaries or carriers on behalf of the government and with quality improvement organizations in each state to promote quality and efficiency of services.

At the time Medicare was created in 1965, the intent of Congress was merely to provide insurance for elderly persons, not to help the larger community or achieve broader social aims.[1] Over time, Medicare has become a mechanism to support other goals, such as care for the indigent, graduate medical education, and healthcare facilities in rural areas.[2] In addition, Congress uses Medicare participation as a "hook" by imposing various requirements on healthcare providers that choose to participate. In 2000, the U.S. Supreme Court concluded that "[t]he structure and operation of the Medicare program reveal a comprehensive federal assistance enterprise aimed at ensuring the availability of quality health care for the broader community."[3]

Medicare has two inconsistent aspects. In some respects, Medicare resembles an insurance plan, because part of the program is funded by premiums paid by beneficiaries. On the other hand, part of the program is financed by payroll taxes and government revenues. Thus, Medicare also resembles a tax-funded social welfare program, which redistributes wealth among different individuals and groups.

In general, Medicare is not means-tested; therefore, wealthy retirees can qualify for the program. In fact, some of the beneficiaries have much more income and assets than the workers who are taxed to support the program. Of course, wealthy and middle-class beneficiaries view the Medicare program as a type of insurance for which they insist they already have paid. The Medicare Prescription Drug, Improvement, and Modernization Act (MMA)[4] takes a significant step toward means-testing by requiring beneficiaries with high incomes to pay more for Part B coverage.[5] As one commentator has pointed out, the move toward means-testing could erode the level of political support for Medicare as a whole.[6]

As discussed in Chapter 11, the U.S. Constitution does not require Congress to establish and maintain a Medicare program. In other words, Congress had the authority to create Medicare, but it was not constitutionally obligated to do so. In the absence of a constitutional mandate, Congress has considerable flexibility to determine which groups of people to assist and which services to cover. Congress also has the legal authority to change or even eliminate Medicare on a prospective basis, regardless of the expectations of beneficiaries or the financial contributions of employees.[7] As a matter of law, individuals have no vested right to receive the Medicare benefits that existed at the time they paid taxes or at the time they became eligible for the program.

Of course, eliminating Medicare altogether would not be politically feasible and would certainly not be desirable. However, serious concerns have arisen about the long-term solvency of the program and its ability to meet the needs of the aging baby boom generation. To maintain long-term solvency, Congress may find it necessary in the future to reform the program in ways that would be detrimental to the interests of beneficiaries, and Congress certainly has the legal authority to do so.

As one type of fundamental reform, some have argued in favor of changing Medicare to a premium support or voucher system. Under that type of system, the government would not act as an insurer and would not pay the medical bills incurred by beneficiaries. Instead, the government would give beneficiaries a sum of money or a voucher to purchase the coverage of their choice in the private health insurance market. This type of approach would be similar to a defined contribution retirement plan or 401(k) plan, in which the employees make their own investment decisions with the money contributed by their employers. Changing the Medicare program in that manner would have advantages and disadvantages.[8] Advantages include placing a limit or "cap" on federal government spending and the possibility that competition among health plans might reduce costs and improve quality. Disadvantages include the possibility of higher costs for Medicare beneficiaries and the possibility that private health plans would try to contain cost by using techniques, such as prospective utilization review and limited provider panels, that previously caused a backlash when used by managed care organizations. Under these circumstances, proposals for premium support or vouchers have been met with strong opposition as well as support. Compounding this issue are political and philosophical disputes about the appropriate roles of government and the private sector in the healthcare system.

Medicare Eligibility and Benefits

Medicare provides health insurance coverage to more than 50 million people, which makes it the largest health plan in the country. People may qualify for Medicare if they are over the age of 65, are permanently disabled, or have end-stage renal disease. Part A of Medicare primarily covers inpatient hospital services; Part B covers outpatient hospital care, physician services, and some other services and supplies.

Part C, now known as Medicare Advantage, allows each beneficiary to choose from a variety of approved managed care plans. For several years, members of Congress from both political parties had attempted to reform the Medicare program in an effort to use the cost-saving mechanisms of managed care and provide more choices to beneficiaries. Although Medicare had a health maintenance organization program for many years, only a small percentage of Medicare patients were enrolled in those managed care plans. As part of the Balanced Budget Act of 1997 (BBA),[9] Congress added the Medicare+Choice system as Part C. Under the BBA, a beneficiary could remain in the traditional fee-for-service program under Parts A and B or could choose from a variety of qualified Medicare+Choice plans under Part C.

In the 2003 MMA, Congress again revised the Medicare managed care program. Beneficiaries may now choose to join a Medicare Advantage Plan, which is operated by a private company and approved by Medicare. In a Medicare Advantage Plan, the beneficiary's premiums and copayments may be lower than in traditional Medicare, and the Medicare Advantage Plan might provide some additional benefits. However, the Medicare Advantage Plan might impose additional restrictions, such as limiting the choice of physicians and requiring approval to consult a specialist. Each beneficiary has the option to remain in the traditional fee-for-service program under Parts A and B, which is the default option unless she elects to join a Medicare Advantage Plan. In the fee-for-service program, beneficiaries have the right to select the provider of their choice.[10]

Under traditional fee-for-service Medicare, the government acts as an insurer and bears the risk of having to pay for all of the covered services needed. In contrast, Part C operates somewhat like a voucher system. If the beneficiary chooses a Medicare managed care plan, the government will make a specified payment to that plan on behalf of the beneficiary, instead of paying the expenses incurred by the beneficiary under Parts A and B. In that way, the government can shift the risk of unanticipated expenses to the managed care plan. In addition to limiting the government's potential liability, the government could be in the politically advantageous posture of providing desirable benefits to the voters while forcing private managed care plans to make the difficult and unpopular decisions on utilization review and denial of care.

Medicare Part D was created in 2003 to provide coverage for prescription drugs. Historically, one of the most significant limitations on the scope of Medicare benefits was the lack of coverage for prescription drugs on an outpatient basis. Congress responded to these concerns in 2003 by enacting the MMA.[11]

Beneficiaries are not required to enroll in Part D, but they may choose to enroll by joining a Medicare drug plan or a Medicare managed care plan that includes prescription drug coverage. Medicare drug plans are operated by health insurance companies or other private companies that are approved by Medicare. If the beneficiary chooses a Medicare Advantage Plan under Part C, that plan might also include coverage for prescription drugs.

The MMA includes complex rules about alternatives, costs, and coverage. Different plans may have different levels of coverage and different costs. In addition, Medicare prescription drug plans may have a gap in coverage after the beneficiary exhausts the standard amount of coverage and before the beneficiary qualifies for the catastrophic coverage. This gap is known as the "doughnut hole." Subsequently, the 2010 ACA provided for the reduction and eventual elimination of the doughnut hole.

One of the most controversial issues in the Medicare prescription drug program is whether the federal government should negotiate prices directly with pharmaceutical manufacturers or, alternatively, rely on private drug plans to negotiate with manufacturers. Rather than using Medicare's usual system of government-administered pricing, the MMA prohibits HHS from establishing the prices or formularies under Medicare Part D and participating in those negotiations with manufacturers.[12] In a subsection of the law entitled "noninterference," Congress provided that the secretary of HHS "may not interfere with the negotiations" between pharmaceutical manufacturers and the sponsors of private prescription drug plans.[13] Some people support the current system. However, others object to the noninterference provision and argue that the federal government should attempt to negotiate for lower drug prices on behalf of Medicare beneficiaries.

Another significant gap in the scope of Medicare benefits has been the limitation of coverage for long-term care services. Although Medicare pays for some home health services, the program is restrictive about paying the costs for a nursing home. As part of the ACA, Congress established a separate program of voluntary insurance for long-term care services, entitled Community Living Assistance Services and Supports (CLASS). Under that separate program, workers could choose to pay a monthly insurance premium, in exchange for a daily benefit, in the event that they need help with activities of daily living or because of cognitive impairment. However, HHS determined that the CLASS program could not be implemented on a financially solvent basis. Therefore, HHS suspended its implementation, and that part of the ACA was eventually repealed in January 2013.[14] Under these circumstances, Congress has yet to deal effectively with the increasing costs of long-term care or the limitation of coverage for long-term care services under Medicare.

Medicare Payment Issues

Providers are not legally required to participate in Medicare, even though participation may be a financial necessity as a practical matter. Because participation is voluntary, the federal government has broad authority to impose conditions on healthcare facilities and practitioners who choose to

Conditions of participation
Standards developed by the federal government for healthcare organizations in Medicare.

participate. In imposing those **conditions of participation**, the government is acting as a buyer, rather than a regulator. However, the government is a unique type of buyer because it has the power to fine or imprison healthcare providers who violate its rules.

The Medicare statute explicitly prohibits federal control of the practice of medicine or the operation of healthcare facilities.[15] As a practical matter, however, courts have allowed Medicare to influence the practice of medicine and the operation of healthcare facilities, such as by limiting the payment of providers and using mechanisms of cost containment.[16] From the provider's point of view, the relationship with the government may appear to be a contractual arrangement, in which the facility or practitioner performs services for beneficiaries and receives payment from the government for providing those services. However, courts have held that the provider's relationship with the government is more than merely a contract to perform services in exchange for payment. The U.S. Supreme Court has held that providers, as well as patients, are recipients of benefits under the federal Medicare program.[17]

The mere receipt of federal reimbursement does not turn any action of a private hospital into an action of the state; therefore, private hospitals are not subject to the same constitutional obligations as government agencies.[18] However, by receiving Medicare reimbursement, a healthcare facility becomes a recipient of federal financial assistance, and thereby subjects itself to the requirements of additional federal laws.[19]

Almost any licensed provider may choose to participate in Medicare and receive payment for treating Medicare beneficiaries. The methodology for paying each type of provider is set forth by statute and can be quite inflexible. Historically, the program could not pay more to particular providers as compensation for a higher level of quality or efficiency. More recently, the Medicare program developed some pay-for-performance (P4P) initiatives and authorized several demonstration projects to experiment with alternative methods of purchasing services and compensating providers.[20]

In the 2010 ACA, Congress created an innovation center within CMS to use pilot programs and demonstration projects for innovations such as bundled payment.[21] The ACA also makes some adjustments to Medicare payment on the basis of quality, by reducing the level of payment to hospitals that have a high rate of hospital-acquired conditions or an excessive rate of readmissions. Finally, the ACA promotes the development of accountable care organizations (ACOs) under the Shared Savings Program, in which groups of healthcare providers deliver quality care to Medicare patients in a coordinated manner and share the cost savings resulting from those efforts.

Originally, Medicare paid hospitals for services rendered to Medicare patients on the basis of retrospectively determined costs. In effect, the government looked at all of the costs that the hospital had incurred during the previous year and then paid the hospital the portion of the costs that was attributable to the treatment of Medicare beneficiaries. This payment methodology required each hospital to prepare detailed cost reports listing each item of cost in each department of the hospital and allocate various overhead costs to particular allowable and nonallowable cost centers. Of course, the government or its intermediaries had to audit those cost reports, and frequent disputes occurred over the amount of reimbursement to which the hospital was entitled.

In addition to being incredibly complex, this system of retrospective, cost-based reimbursement was inherently inflationary, and it provided perverse incentives for hospital managers. For those reasons, the Medicare program eliminated retrospective, cost-based reimbursement of hospitals and replaced it with a **prospective payment system** (PPS). Under a PPS, a hospital that treats a Medicare patient will receive an amount of money that is determined prospectively (i.e., in advance of treating the patient). The amount of that payment will depend on the patient's diagnosis, which will be placed in one of the hundreds of **diagnosis-related groups** (DRGs). Because the payment to the hospital is *not* based on the hospital's costs, the hospital would not increase its reimbursement merely by increasing its costs.

In fact, the incentive under PPS is just the opposite. If an inpatient remains in the hospital for a long time and receives a lot of expensive tests and treatments, the cost for treating him will probably exceed the prospectively determined amount for that DRG, and the hospital could lose money on treating him. However, if the hospital can treat the patient for less than the DRG amount, the hospital essentially makes a profit on that patient. Thus, some people say hospitals now have an incentive to discharge patients "quicker and sicker."

Significantly, a hospital has only a limited ability to control its costs for treating a particular patient. As discussed in Chapter 7, decisions on when to discharge a patient and what services to provide are made by the physician, who is often not an employee of the hospital. Under these circumstances, some hospitals have tried to encourage their physicians to discharge Medicare patients as soon as possible and to consider how their decisions regarding tests and treatments affect the hospital financially. Some hospitals have even tried to give their physicians financial incentives to reduce the cost of treatment. However, Congress has prohibited hospitals from paying physicians to reduce the level of services for Medicare and Medicaid patients.[22]

When the Medicare program was enacted, physicians were paid on the basis of "reasonable charges," which were similar to the charge screens used by commercial insurers. Subsequently, Medicare adopted the Resource-Based Relative Value Scale (RBRVS), under which the program pays more

Prospective payment system
The federal government's method of paying hospitals for treatment of Medicare patients on the basis of prices determined before treatment regardless of the hospital's costs.

Diagnosis-related groups
The federal government's categories of medical conditions that Medicare uses to determine the amount of payment for each patient.

for physician services that require a higher level of training and resources. In addition, the Medicare program limits the amounts that physicians may charge for services rendered to Medicare patients.

In an effort to control Medicare costs, a formula called the sustainable growth rate (SGR) in the federal statute uses specific economic criteria to raise or lower Medicare payments to physicians. For many years, that formula would have required significant reductions in Medicare payments to physicians. However, Congress has repeatedly stopped those reductions, in what is commonly called the "doc fix." Congress has been unwilling to repeal the SGR on a permanent basis, in part because repeal would require the official cost projections of Congress to recognize a severe budgetary impact over a long period of time. Instead, Congress acts as if each failure to reduce costs is merely temporary, and assumes that all future reductions in physician payments under the SGR will be made as scheduled. In addition to being unrealistic, this situation distorts the official projections of Medicare costs.

Another controversial issue is whether a willing patient may make a private contract with a willing physician to pay more than the limit for services that are covered by Medicare. For example, if a private insurance company would pay $200 for a particular physician service, and if Medicare would pay only $100 for that service, a physician might decide to not accept any more Medicare patients and instead devote more time to treating privately insured patients. To obtain the services of that particular physician, some Medicare patients might be willing to pay the $200 out of their own pocket, or at least the incremental difference of $100, assuming they can afford to do so. However, the law severely restricts the ability of Medicare patients and their physicians to do that. Supporters of private contracting argue that Medicare should not interfere with the free-enterprise system. Moreover, they argue that the prohibition against private contracts denies access to the services of desirable physicians and prevents those who are willing from purchasing services of higher quality. Opponents respond that private contracting would force patients to pay higher fees for physician services, would put elderly patients at a disadvantage in bargaining with their physicians, and would effectively create one Medicare program for the rich and one for the poor.

Many healthcare providers complain that Medicare does not adequately pay for services rendered to patients and that the government has refused to provide appropriate increases in rates of payment. As a political matter, Congress may find it easier to cut payments to providers or reduce the rate of increase in payments to providers, rather than cutting Medicare benefits or increasing taxes and premiums. However, at some point, there is a danger that reductions in provider payments may have adverse effects on quality and access to care, especially if providers are unable to shift their costs to other payers.

Medicaid

Legal Structure and Financing

Medicaid is a means-tested, social welfare program that uses tax revenues to provide health coverage for persons who cannot afford private health insurance. Unlike Medicare, which is a purely federal program, Medicaid is operated and funded by both state and federal governments. This situation gives rise to complex issues of federalism, as well as occasional disputes over the powers and duties of each level of government.

The federal Medicaid statute, known as Title XIX of the Social Security Act, was enacted by Congress pursuant to its conditional spending power. In effect, Congress makes an offer to the government of each state. If a state establishes a medical assistance program that meets all of the federal standards, the federal government will provide a large share of the cost of that program in the form of federal financial participation (FFP). States have the option of establishing a medical assistance program, but they are not required to do so. Even though the program is voluntary, every state has established a Medicaid program to obtain its share of FFP.

If a state decides to participate, it is required to comply with the federal statutes and regulations, and states are required to submit their Medicaid plan to HHS for approval. As a general rule, the secretary of HHS has the ability to compel state Medicaid agencies to comply with federal laws by threatening to reduce or terminate their federal Medicaid funds. States do have flexibility in some aspects of their programs, and the federal government may grant waivers of specific requirements at the state's request.

Nevertheless, some people think the federal government should give even more flexibility to states to design and operate their own medical assistance programs without having to meet federal requirements or request a federal waiver. This issue has been debated for many years. In 1995, the Republican-dominated House of Representatives passed a bill to change Medicaid to a block-grant system, under which the federal government would provide funding for the individual states to operate their own medical assistance programs.[23] However, the Democratic minority in Congress argued that eliminating federal standards would have an adverse effect on Medicaid beneficiaries. Eventually, the bill containing the Republican block-grant proposal was vetoed by President Clinton, but the debate continues about the appropriate roles for federal and state governments in the Medicaid program.

More recently, the limits of federal authority under the conditional spending power were tested by the expansion of Medicaid in the 2010 ACA. The ACA provides that, beginning January 1, 2014, Medicaid would provide coverage for individuals who have income up to 133 percent of the poverty level, provided those individuals are under age 65 and are not eligible for Medicare. Significantly, this expansion would provide coverage for poor adults under age 65 who have no dependent children and who had been unable to qualify for Medicare or Medicaid. As explained by the CMS Office of the Actuary,

> The Patient Protection and Affordable Care Act, as amended by the Health Care and Education Reconciliation Act of 2010, will substantially reduce the number of people in the U.S. without health insurance. Much of this reduction will occur as a result of expanded eligibility criteria for Medicaid, which we estimate will increase the number of Medicaid enrollees by about 20 million in 2019. Medicaid provides a relatively low-cost way to increase the number of people with health coverage, since its payment rates for health care services and health plans are low compared to other forms of health insurance. Even so, aggregate Medicaid costs will increase significantly as a result of the Affordable Care Act, due to the very large number of additional enrollees starting in 2014.[24]

The federal government will bear most of the cost for the expansion of Medicaid, at least in the early years. Nevertheless, some states have expressed concerned about their share of the costs. Although they objected to the expansion, those states wanted to continue to participate and receive FFP for the pre-ACA Medicaid program. The federal government took the position that states must participate in the Medicaid expansion under the ACA or withdraw entirely from Medicaid. Under these circumstances, some states challenged the Medicaid expansion in federal courts on the grounds that it constituted federal coercion of state governments and exceeded the authority of Congress.

The U.S. Supreme Court agreed with the states.[25] Its ruling on this issue was part of its June 28, 2012, decision on the constitutionality of the ACA. The court held that the federal government cannot withdraw existing Medicaid funds from states that decline to participate in the expansion. Thus, expansion of Medicaid is optional for the states, and some state governments have refused to participate.

The Supreme Court acknowledged that Congress has the power to impose conditions on spending but clarified the constitutional limits of that power. Under its conditional spending power, Congress may impose conditions on states that go beyond what it could otherwise require states to do. Congress may use financial incentives to persuade or encourage the states, but it may not coerce the states. However, distinguishing between permissible persuasion and impermissible coercion is difficult.

Rather than attempting to distinguish between persuasion and coercion, the Supreme Court resolved this case by focusing on a different limitation on the conditional spending power, which provides that Congress may impose conditions on the use of specific federal funds, but may not impose conditions that relate to the use of other federal funds. For example, if a state refuses to comply with the conditions on a federal grant for an education program, the federal government may withhold funding for that education program but not for transportation or healthcare programs.

In this case, the Supreme Court resolved the challenge to the Medicaid expansion by treating it as a different federal program from the preexisting Medicaid program, distinguishing between "new" Medicaid funds and "existing" Medicaid funds. As the court explained, "[w]hat Congress is not free to do is to penalize States that choose not to participate in that new program by taking away their existing Medicaid funding. Section 1396c gives the Secretary of Health and Human Services the authority to do just that . . . . In light of the Court's holding, the Secretary cannot apply § 1396c to withdraw existing Medicaid funds for failure to comply with the requirements set out in the expansion."[26]

Medicaid Eligibility and Benefits

As a social welfare program, Medicaid eligibility is restricted to persons with limited income and assets. Some people are considered to be categorically eligible for Medicaid because they fit within certain categories of persons on public assistance. In the past, persons receiving cash payments under the Aid to Families with Dependent Children program were categorically eligible for Medicaid, as were disabled persons who received payments under the Supplemental Security Income program. However, the 1996 welfare reform legislation abolished the Aid to Families with Dependent Children program, substituted the new Temporary Assistance for Needy Families program, and made categorical eligibility for Medicaid more complicated.

Medicaid eligibility is limited to U.S. citizens and to those immigrants who fit within the category of "qualified aliens." Thus, undocumented immigrants are generally not eligible for Medicaid. However, there is an exception for emergency treatment, including labor and delivery. Every individual who is born in the United States is a U.S. citizen, regardless of the citizenship or visa status of that individual's parents. Therefore, infants who are born in the United States are eligible for Medicaid benefits if they meet the usual criteria on income and assets.

In addition to qualification for Medicaid as "categorically needy," some people may qualify for Medicaid as "medically needy" if they have high medical expenses. For example, people with chronic conditions may spend so much money on medical care that they spend down to the poverty level, in which case they may qualify for Medicaid. Similarly, many residents of nursing homes will exhaust all of their resources and thereby qualify for

Medicaid. Most Americans do not have long-term care insurance, and most health insurance policies will not pay for room and board in a nursing home, which can be extremely expensive. In addition, Medicare is restrictive about paying for nursing home care. Therefore, even if people enter nursing homes as private, paying residents, they may quickly exhaust their remaining funds, at which time Medicaid may become responsible for their expenses. For this reason, Medicaid is not merely a program for recipients of public assistance. It is also a way of paying the nursing home costs for many middle-class retirees instead of imposing those costs on their own adult children.

Some people go so far as to transfer their remaining assets to other family members as a way to qualify for Medicaid, a practice that raises several legal and ethical issues. Some people believe it is unethical for wealthy retirees to give substantial assets to their adult children and then apply for Medicaid when they have no more resources. However, others respond that people who worked hard and paid taxes for 40 or 50 years ought to be able to leave some of their money or property to their families, without having every penny dissipated for nursing home care. As a legal matter, people who transfer assets for less than fair market value within a certain number of years before entering a nursing home and applying for Medicaid may be disqualified for nursing home benefits for several years.[27]

States have some flexibility on which Medicaid benefits to cover, provided that the states meet the basic federal requirements. In fact, federal law specifies services all states *must* cover, services states *may* cover, and services states *may not* cover at all with Medicaid funds. The minimum federal requirements are different for the categorically needy and the medically needy.[28] If a state chooses to do so, it may offer certain optional services, such as eyeglasses, and the state will receive FFP for those costs.

The federal regulation at 42 C.F.R. § 440.230(c) provides that a state "may not arbitrarily deny or reduce the amount, duration, or scope of a required service . . . to an otherwise eligible beneficiary solely because of the diagnosis, type of illness, or condition." In other words, a state Medicaid agency may limit a service on the basis of medical necessity, but it may not provide less coverage on the basis of the particular type of illness. For example, the Iowa Medicaid agency decided that it would not use its limited funds to pay for sex reassignment surgery, on the grounds that it is never a medically necessary treatment for the condition of transsexualism. However, the surgery is the only available treatment for that condition. Therefore, a federal court of appeals ruled that Iowa was arbitrarily denying services to Medicaid beneficiaries solely because of the diagnosis, type of illness, or condition.[29]

That type of case is one example of the difficult policy issue about how to use limited Medicaid resources. Similar issues have arisen in cases seeking Medicaid funding for expensive organ transplants.[30] In those cases, a state's refusal to pay for the transplant might cause the death of an identifiable child or adult. Instead of paying for the transplant, however, the state could use that money to provide healthcare services to hundreds of unidentifiable people who might go without care if the federal government forces the state to use its Medicaid funds to pay for the transplant. Aside from the ethical issue of determining the right thing to do, separate issues exist of determining who should make the decision and how the decision should be made.

In the 1990s, the state of Oregon squarely addressed these difficult questions by requesting a federal waiver as a demonstration project for its state Medicaid program.[31] Oregon wanted to avoid the federal requirements on the broad scope of covered services and procedures. First, Oregon used a public process to prioritize different procedures in terms of their cost and benefit, and then decided to cover only those procedures that ranked above a particular cutoff point on the list. With the money Oregon would save by not covering low-ranking procedures, it would expand Medicaid eligibility to many more people in the state. That proposal required a waiver from the federal government, which eventually was granted. In granting that waiver, the federal government took an important step toward state flexibility in the Medicaid program and allowed an important experiment in the use of limited resources.

In addition to specifying services which a state *must* cover or *may* cover, federal law specifies a particular service which state Medicaid programs *may not* cover. The federal law known as the Hyde Amendment generally prohibits the states from using Medicaid funds, which include a large percentage of FFP, to pay for abortions.[32] States have the option of using their own non-Medicaid funds to pay for abortions.

As discussed in Chapter 13, abortion at an early stage of pregnancy is a lawful procedure, which state governments may not prohibit. Therefore, some people have argued that the government is required to pay for that lawful procedure for persons the government recognizes to be unable to pay for their medical care. However, the U.S. Supreme Court rejected that argument and held that the government may prohibit the use of Medicaid funds to pay for abortions.[33] In other words, the government cannot stop a woman from choosing to have an abortion at an early stage of pregnancy, but the government is not obligated to pay for the procedure. As the Supreme Court explained in that case:

> [I]t simply does not follow that a woman's freedom of choice carries with it a constitutional entitlement to the financial resources to avail herself of the full range of protected choices . . . although government may not place obstacles in the path of a woman's exercise of her freedom of choice, it need not remove those not of its own creation. Indigency falls in the latter category. The financial constraints

that restrict an indigent woman's ability to enjoy the full range of constitutionally protected freedom of choice are the product not of governmental restrictions on access to abortions, but rather of her indigency.[34]

In addition, the Supreme Court reasoned that Congress has a legitimate interest in protecting potential life; therefore, Congress may give financial incentives to women on Medicaid to encourage them to choose childbirth over abortion.[35] Under these circumstances, Medicaid may pay the costs of childbirth but not the costs of abortion. Although many people would disagree with the Supreme Court's reasoning, it is currently the law of the land. Nevertheless, some state supreme courts have held that a right to public funding of abortion exists under their state constitutions.[36]

Medicaid Payment Issues

Because of increasing costs and budgetary problems, states have tried to reduce Medicaid payments to healthcare facilities and practitioners, or at least reduce the rate of increases in those payments. As discussed previously with Medicare, there is a danger that reducing payments to providers may cause problems in quality and access to care. In 1998, one of the largest nursing home chains in the country threatened to withdraw from Medicaid at many of its facilities because of the company's dissatisfaction with Medicaid payment rates.[37] Although that company subsequently changed its plans, the problems of low Medicaid rates and provider dissatisfaction continue.

For individual practitioners, such as physicians and dentists, low payment rates might discourage participation in the program and thereby create serious problems in access to care. According to the federal statute, state Medicaid plans must ensure that payment is "sufficient to enlist enough providers so that care and services are available under the plan at least to the extent that such care and services are available to the general population in the geographic area."[38] In practice, however, Medicaid payment rates are often too low to satisfy this federal mandate. For example, at one time only 16 percent of dentists in North Carolina participated in Medicaid, which led beneficiaries to file suit against state officials on the ground that they had been denied the equal access required by federal law.[39]

However, a legal dispute has simmered for many years about whether Medicaid providers and beneficiaries have the right to sue state Medicaid agencies in federal court to require a state to comply with federal statutes and regulations.[40] The mere fact that a federal law exists on a subject does not necessarily mean individuals have a private right of action as a means of enforcing that law. Some people argue that only the federal government may require states to comply with the law about the sufficiency of Medicaid rates.

For example, when the state of California tried to reduce some Medicaid rates, providers and beneficiaries sued state officials. The providers and beneficiaries argued that the state Medicaid law that reduced payment rates conflicted with the federal Medicaid law that required sufficient payment rates. Plaintiffs argued that the state law was preempted by federal law under the U.S. Constitution's Supremacy Clause. The U.S. Court of Appeals for the Ninth Circuit agreed with plaintiffs and stopped the state from reducing the rates. Subsequently, the U.S. Supreme Court made a ruling in that case that failed to resolve the underlying legal issue but raised doubts about this type of legal challenge.[41]

In the California case, the U.S. Supreme Court did not decide the legal issue of whether providers or beneficiaries may sue state officials under the Supremacy Clause to enforce the federal Medicaid law. Instead, the court **remanded** the case to the Ninth Circuit to consider the effect of the recent approval of California's rates by the federal government.[42] Four of the nine justices simply would have held that, in the absence of a statutory right to enforce a federal law, private parties may not enforce it under the Supremacy Clause. In contrast, the five justices in the majority did not go that far, but they recognized the problems inherent in allowing private parties to sue in federal court under the Supremacy Clause. Private parties already have the right to pursue administrative appeals and judicial review against CMS, in regard to CMS's approval of reduced state Medicaid rates. Allowing a parallel action under the Supremacy Clause could lead to multiple results, which could be either inconsistent or redundant.

Remand
To send a case back to a lower court for further action.

As a practical matter, the decision of the Supreme Court raises potential problems for providers and beneficiaries. If providers and beneficiaries may not challenge state Medicaid rates under the Supremacy Clause, they would need to challenge CMS's approval of the reduced state Medicaid rates by means of administrative appeal and judicial review. As discussed in Chapter 2, the processes of administrative appeal and judicial review can be difficult and frustrating for parties that are challenging the action of an administrative agency. Parties must exhaust all administrative remedies before they have a right to seek judicial review of an agency's action. Then, in judicial review, courts ordinarily give deference to the decision of the agency. Under these circumstances, challenging reductions in state Medicaid rates will be difficult for providers and beneficiaries.

The State Children's Health Insurance Program

In the BBA of 1997, Congress created the State Children's Health Insurance Program (SCHIP) as Title XXI of the Social Security Act.[43] The purpose of the new law was to provide federal funding to the states to provide health insurance coverage for targeted low-income children who do not have access to other forms of coverage. In essence, these children fall through the cracks in the system because their families have too much money to qualify for Medicaid and not enough money to purchase health insurance in the private market. Under Title XXI, states have the option of using the federal funds to expand their state Medicaid program, create a separate program, or do some combination of both. In 2010, the ACA preserved the program—now known simply as the Children's Health Insurance Program (CHIP)—by extending program funding for several years with the same income-based eligibility levels.

CHIP is similar to Medicaid in that each state operates its own program pursuant to a federally approved plan, with funding from both federal and state governments. However, important differences exist between CHIP and Medicaid, as explained in a 2002 report by the U.S. General Accounting Office (now called the Government Accountability Office, or GAO).

> Medicaid is an open-ended entitlement, meaning the federal government will pay its share of state expenditures for people covered under a state's approved Medicaid plan, and enrollment for those eligible cannot be limited. . . .
>
> In contrast to Medicaid, SCHIP is not an open-ended entitlement. The Congress in 1997 appropriated a fixed amount for the program. . . . In certain circumstances states may restrict enrollment if their allotment of federal funds has been expended, but to date, SCHIP spending for most states has fallen well below allotment levels for a variety of reasons.[44]

In fact, the federal CHIP statute explicitly provides that "[n]othing in this title shall be construed as providing an individual with an entitlement to child health assistance under a State child health plan."[45] However, the statute does provide a state entitlement to the allotment of federal funds, and thereby obligates the federal government to pay those amounts to the states.[46] As some commentators have explained, "The legislation entitles states, not children."[47]

Fraud and Abuse of Medicare and Medicaid

Fraud and abuse of government payment programs have been among the top enforcement priorities of the federal Department of Justice and U.S. attorneys. In addition, many states are devoting substantial resources to fighting Medicaid fraud. The priority given to healthcare fraud and abuse should not be surprising in light of the amount of money involved. For example, in 2012 a chain of healthcare facilities agreed to pay more than $42 million to settle claims of overbilling Medicare.[48]

In addition to fines and other monetary penalties, some types of healthcare fraud and abuse are punishable by imprisonment in the federal penitentiary. Moreover, one of the most severe penalties for a healthcare provider is exclusion from Medicare and Medicaid because that could effectively put that provider out of business.

Suits can also be brought by whistle-blowers, who claim that particular healthcare providers have cheated the federal government.[49] Under the federal False Claims Act (FCA), the whistle-blower may receive a share of any money that the provider is forced to pay to the government, and that might amount to millions of dollars for the whistle-blower. Under these circumstances, disgruntled employees or former employees, from executives to billing clerks, have a tremendous incentive to turn in their employers.

As will be discussed, some healthcare providers and provider associations have argued that the government is inappropriately using fraud and abuse laws to challenge honest mistakes and good-faith differences of opinion. Government officials, however, insist that there are no penalties for honest mistakes, other than promptly returning the money that was erroneously claimed. Moreover, commentators have found providers' complaints to be somewhat exaggerated.[50]

Some cases of alleged fraud and abuse have involved differences of opinion over the proper interpretation of complex reimbursement rules. Other cases have involved providers that were clearly dishonest, such as those that billed for services they never provided at all. Even if only a small percentage of Medicare and Medicaid claims are improper, that could represent millions or even billions of dollars in government funds.

As described in Exhibit 8.1, false or fraudulent claims are only one of three categories in the substantive law of healthcare fraud and abuse. In addition, laws prohibit kickbacks in exchange for referrals and certain types of self-referral arrangements. Each of these three categories is analyzed in detail in the sections that follow. Then, the chapter addresses compliance programs and corporate integrity agreements, including the link between quality of care and fraud or abuse. The chapter concludes by analyzing the application of laws about fraud and abuse to ACOs and their participants.

False Claims

Healthcare facilities and practitioners provide services to individual Medicare and Medicaid beneficiaries, and then rely on the government or its agents to pay the bills for services that already have been rendered. From the perspective of the government and its taxpayers, this situation presents a difficult practical problem. When the government purchases tangible goods, such as computer equipment or battleships, agents of the government can inspect the goods to ensure that they have been delivered and meet all applicable specifications. When the government purchases services, however, verifying that the tasks were really performed and appropriately completed may be

EXHIBIT 8.1

The Substantive
Law of Fraud
and Abuse

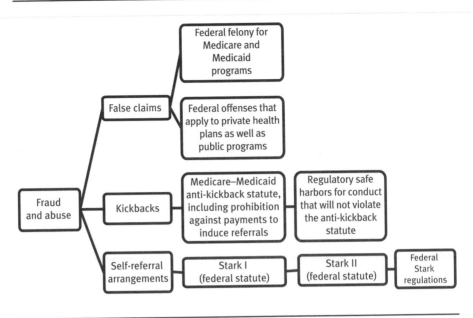

more difficult, especially when the services are not provided at a government facility or are not provided to agents of the government.

That problem is precisely the one presented by the Medicare and Medicaid programs. Specifically, these programs contend with the following issues:

1. The government is usually purchasing services rather than tangible goods.
2. The services are provided to beneficiaries of the programs rather than to agents of the government.
3. The services are usually provided at thousands of remote locations rather than at an office of a payment program.
4. The complexity of professional services makes questioning their quality and appropriateness difficult.
5. The personal and confidential nature of medical care makes it impossible for agents of the government to observe the services at the time they are performed.

Under these circumstances, the government ordinarily has to rely on the word of the provider that is asking to be paid or on written documentation created by that provider. Government payment programs have various mechanisms to audit claims, and most healthcare providers are both honest and careful. However, the payment system necessarily operates in large part on good faith and trust. When that trust is abused, the government can rely on the law of false or fraudulent claims.

In requesting payment from government programs, healthcare facilities and practitioners submit claims and make certain representations with regard to the nature and appropriateness of their services. If they knowingly and intentionally misrepresent the facts to obtain payments to which they are not entitled, that would constitute fraud. One type of fraud is submitting claims to be paid for services that were never rendered. Another type is knowingly and intentionally submitting a claim under an inappropriate diagnostic or procedural code to obtain a higher rate of reimbursement, which is known as **upcoding**. Like a dishonest salesperson who lies to a customer by claiming that a cubic zirconium is really a valuable diamond, healthcare providers who knowingly and intentionally give false statements to government programs have made fraudulent claims.

As indicated by empirical research, some physicians think making false statements about a patient's condition to third-party payers, such as managed care organizations, may be justifiable as a way to obtain services that patients need and could not otherwise afford.[51] In addition to raising serious issues of personal and professional ethics, lying to the Medicare or Medicaid programs in that manner could subject a provider to civil and criminal liability.

Aside from misrepresenting a patient's condition or the nature of the services rendered, some providers have billed Medicare or Medicaid for services to patients they never treated at all. As described in the following excerpt from a Special Fraud Alert by the HHS Office of Inspector General (OIG), some providers have even attempted to defraud the government by billing for services to patients who were already dead at the time of the alleged services.[52]

Upcoding
Submitting a claim under an inappropriate diagnostic or procedural code to obtain a higher rate of reimbursement.

DEPARTMENT OF HEALTH AND HUMAN SERVICES
Office of Inspector General

PUBLICATION OF OIG SPECIAL FRAUD ALERT: FRAUD AND ABUSE IN THE PROVISION OF SERVICES IN NURSING FACILITIES
. . . Nursing facilities and their residents have become common targets for fraudulent schemes. Nursing facilities represent convenient resident "pools" and make it lucrative for unscrupulous persons to carry out fraudulent schemes. The OIG has become aware of a number

(continued)

(continued from previous page)

of fraudulent arrangements by which health care providers, including medical professionals, inappropriately bill Medicare and Medicaid for the provision of unnecessary services and services which were not provided at all. Sometimes, nursing facility management and staff also are involved in these schemes . . .

Claims for Services Not Rendered or Not Provided as Claimed

Common schemes entail falsifying bills and medical records to misrepresent the services, or extent of services, provided at nursing facilities. Some examples follow:

- One physician improperly billed $350,000 over a 2-year period for comprehensive physical examinations of residents without ever seeing a single resident. The physician went so far as to falsify medical records to indicate that nonexistent services were rendered.
- A psychotherapist working in nursing facilities manipulated Medicare billing codes to charge for 3 hours of therapy for each resident when, in fact, he spent only a few minutes with each resident. In a nursing facility, 3 hours of psychotherapy is highly unusual and often clinically inappropriate.
- An investigation of a speech specialist uncovered documentation showing that he overstated the time spent on each session claimed. Claims analysis showed that the speech specialist actually claimed to spend 20 hours with residents every day, far more time than possible. Further investigation revealed that some residents had never met the specialist, and some were dead at the time when the specialist claimed to have provided speech services to them.
- A company providing mobile X-ray services made visits to nursing facilities, and billed for taking two X-rays when only one was actually taken. The case also presented serious concerns about quality of care when the investigation revealed that company personnel were not certified to take X-rays.

Claims Falsified to Circumvent Coverage Limitations on Medical Specialties

Practitioners of medical specialties have been found to misrepresent the nature of services provided to Medicare and Medicaid beneficiaries

(continued)

(continued from previous page)

because the Federally funded programs have stringent coverage limitations for some specialties, including podiatry, audiology, and optometry. For instance:

- The OIG has learned about podiatrists whose entire practices consisted of visits to nursing facilities. Non-covered routine care is provided, e.g., toenail clipping, but Medicare is billed for covered services which were not provided or needed. In one case, an investigator discovered suspicious billing for foot care when it was reported that a podiatrist was performing an excessive number of toenail removals, a service that is covered but not frequently or routinely needed. This podiatrist billed Medicare as much as $100,000 in one year for toenail removals. Investigators discovered one resident for whom bills were submitted claiming a total of 11 toenail removals.

- An optometrist claimed reimbursement for covered eye care consultations when he, in fact, performed routine exams and other non-covered services. His billing history indicated that he claimed to have performed as many as 25 consultations in one day at a nursing home. This is an unreasonably high number, given the nature of a Medicare-covered consultation.

- An audiologist made arrangements with a nursing facility and affiliated physicians to get orders for hearing exams that were not medically necessary. The audiologist used this access to residents exclusively to market hearing aids. In this case, the facility and physicians, in addition to the audiologist, could be held liable for false or fraudulent claims if they acted with knowledge of the claims for unnecessary service.

What to Look for in the Provision of Services to Nursing Facilities
The following situations may suggest fraudulent or abusive activities:

- "Gang visits" by one or more medical professionals where large numbers of residents are seen in a single day. The practitioner may be providing medically unnecessary services, or the level of service provided may not be of a sufficient duration or scope consistent with the service billed to Medicare or Medicaid.

(continued)

(continued from previous page)

- Frequent and recurring "routine visits" by the same medical professional. Seeing residents too often may indicate that the provider is billing for services that are not medically necessary.
- Unusually active presence in nursing facilities by health care practitioners who are given or request unlimited access to resident medical records. These individuals may be collecting information used in the submission of false claims.
- Questionable documentation for medical necessity of professional services. Practitioners who are billing inappropriately may also enter, or fail to enter, important information on medical charts . . .

To Report Suspected Fraud, Call or Write

1-800-HHS-TIPS, Department of Health and Human Services, Office of Inspector General, P.O. Box 23489, L'Enfant Plaza Station, Washington, D.C. 20026-3489.

Dated: May 29, 1996.
June Gibbs Brown,
Inspector General.

As a legal matter, the consequences of submitting an incorrect claim usually depend on the provider's knowledge and intent at the time it was submitted. For example, did the provider know the claim was improper, or was the claim so obviously improper that the provider should have known it was unlawful? Did the provider act with intent to defraud the government? Alternatively, was this just an honest mistake or carelessness on the part of the provider? In addition to affecting issues of liability and penalties, the answers to these questions can determine whether the case will be governed by civil or criminal law, as set forth in Exhibit 8.2.

In some cases, healthcare providers have submitted improper claims as a result of a mistake or simple negligence. The usual remedy in those cases is merely to give back the overpayment. What if a healthcare provider thought the claim was proper at the time it was submitted, but later discovered it was improper and should not have been submitted in that manner? Although legal consequences usually depend on knowledge or intent at the time a claim was submitted, recent changes in the law have made it clear that failing to repay an overpayment in a timely manner constitutes a false claim to the government payment program. The federal Fraud Enforcement and Recovery Act of 2009 (FERA)[53] made it a false claim to not pay an obligation that

Category	Legal Standard	Penalties
Mistake	Honest mistake or mere negligence.	None—just give back the money. However, failing to repay an overpayment in a timely manner after discovery is a false claim. Moreover, the 2010 ACA provides that a violation of the anti-kickback statute is also a basis for liability as a false claim under the False Claims Act.
Criminal fraud (with intent to defraud)	Knowingly and willfully made a false statement of material fact in an application for payment. (The government must prove its case beyond a reasonable doubt.)	Felony (up to five years in prison), plus fines and exclusion from Medicare and Medicaid.
Civil False Claims Act	Knowingly presented a false claim. However, *knowingly* means actual knowledge of the information *or* deliberate ignorance of the truth or falsity of the information *or* reckless disregard of the truth or falsity of information. (The government does not need to prove a specific intent to defraud or prove its case beyond a reasonable doubt.)	Civil penalties and treble damages. (Statistical sampling might be used to calculate the number of false claims.)

EXHIBIT 8.2
False Claims to Medicare or Medicaid

is owed to the government. Subsequently, the ACA provided that overpayments must be reported and repaid by a deadline, which is usually 60 days from the date of discovery. The combined effect of these laws is that failing to repay an overpayment in a timely manner is a false claim, with more serious legal consequences.

Federal statutes make it a crime to defraud any branch of the federal government, and a specific statute relates to fraud in federally supported healthcare programs. As described in Exhibit 8.2, federal law imposes criminal penalties on any person who "*knowingly and willfully* makes or causes to be made any false statement or representation of a material fact in any application for any benefit or payment under a Federal health care program" (emphasis added).[54] Under that statute, fraudulent claims in connection with

Medicare or Medicaid are felonies and are punishable by fines and imprisonment for up to five years.[55]

In a criminal prosecution for Medicare or Medicaid fraud under that
statute, the government bears the heavy burden of proving that the defendant made the false statement or representation "knowingly and willfully."
In addition, because it is a criminal proceeding, the government must prove
its case beyond a reasonable doubt. If the defendant's request for payment
from the government was based on a reasonable interpretation of complex
reimbursement rules, the government would not be able to meet its burden
of proof in a criminal case. For example, in *U.S. v. Whiteside*, two hospital
executives allegedly made a false statement on cost reports by claiming that
all of the interest on a loan was capital related.[56] The government obtained
criminal convictions against the two executives, but those convictions were
reversed on appeal because no clear regulation exists on how interest must
be classified, and reasonable people could differ on the issue. As the appellate
court explained, "In a case where the truth or falsity of a statement centers on
an interpretive question of law, the government bears the burden of proving
beyond a reasonable doubt that the defendant's statement is not true under
a reasonable interpretation of the law."[57]

In contrast, the government's burden of proof is lower in a *civil* case
under the federal False Claims Act (FCA),[58] as described in Exhibit 8.2. The
FCA imposes civil penalties and damages on anyone who "knowingly presents, or causes to be presented, a false or fraudulent claim for payment or
approval."[59] Thus, in an FCA case, the government does not have to prove
that the defendant made a false statement or representation knowingly and
willfully, as required under the criminal statute. In a civil case under the
FCA, the government is only required to prove that the defendant acted
knowingly. The statute provides that the term *knowingly* does not require
actual knowledge. Instead, that term is defined broadly to include not only
actual knowledge but also deliberate ignorance or reckless disregard of the
truth. The FCA also provides explicitly that the government is not required
to prove "specific intent to defraud."[60] However, the government must do
more than merely prove that the claim was submitted by mistake, even if the
mistake was caused by negligence or carelessness.[61]

To prevail in a civil FCA case, moreover, the government is not
required to prove that the defendant healthcare provider had actual knowledge of the Medicare or Medicaid reimbursement regulations. For example,
in *U.S. v. Mackby*, the Court of Appeals for the Ninth Circuit upheld the trial
court's finding that the owner of a physical therapy clinic violated the FCA
by knowingly causing false claims to be submitted, even though he claimed
not to have known about the Medicare rules.[62] In that case, the owner of the
clinic had told the office manager and a billing company to use the provider

identification number of his father, a physician, on claims submitted to Medicare for physical therapy services, although his father had provided no services for the physical therapy clinic or its patients. As the appellate court explained,

> [t]he evidence established that Mackby was the managing director of the clinic. He was responsible for day-to-day operations, long-term planning, lease and build-out negotiations, personnel, and legal and accounting oversight. It was his obligation to be familiar with the legal requirements for obtaining reimbursement from Medicare for physical therapy services, and to ensure that the clinic was run in accordance with all laws. His claim that he did not know of the Medicare requirements does not shield him from liability. By failing to inform himself of those requirements, particularly when twenty percent of Asher Clinic's patients were Medicare beneficiaries, he acted in reckless disregard or in deliberate ignorance of those requirements, either of which was sufficient to charge him with knowledge of the falsity of the claims in question.[63]

Thus, the court affirmed the civil judgment against Mackby under the FCA. The court also noted that, in a civil suit under the FCA, the government only has to prove its case by a preponderance of the evidence, rather than having to prove its case beyond a reasonable doubt.

The civil penalty under the FCA is stated in the statute as $5,000 to $10,000 for each improper claim, plus three times the amount of actual damage incurred by the government, but the civil penalty is subject to adjustment for inflation. Moreover, other financial penalties can be imposed under different laws. The penalty for each violation might seem relatively small, but the total penalty can amount to a huge sum of money when the penalty is multiplied by the number of individual claims that are determined to be improper. As others have pointed out, healthcare providers may file thousands of small claims, and the government can extrapolate from a sample of false claims to derive a much larger number of claims that it alleges to be false.[64] The amount of money sought by the government might be so high that agreeing to a settlement is the provider's only practical alternative.[65] In fact, if the amount of money sought by the government under the FCA were so large that it would bankrupt or severely damage a healthcare organization, the trustees or directors of that organization might be required by their fiduciary duty to reach a settlement, even if they dispute the government's allegations. As stewards of the organization's resources, the trustees or directors simply cannot take the risk of losing the case at trial.

Although most of the laws on fraud and abuse relate to government-funded programs such as Medicare and Medicaid, defrauding private health plans is also against the law. In 1996, Congress established new federal crimes that relate to private and public healthcare benefit plans.[66] Under those criminal laws, any person who knowingly defrauds any public or private healthcare benefit program may be imprisoned for up to ten years.[67]

Kickbacks

Under the federal anti-kickback statute, it is unlawful to knowingly and willfully give or receive anything of value to induce someone to refer a Medicare or Medicaid patient or to induce someone to purchase something for which payment may be made under those programs.[68] The statute is broadly worded and applies to any remuneration, whether direct or indirect, overt or covert, in cash or in kind. In addition, it applies to both the party that offers or pays the illegal remuneration and the party that solicits or receives it, but it does not apply to payments to bona fide employees of the organization that is making the payment. Violating the act is a felony punishable by a $25,000 fine and up to five years in prison as well as exclusion from government payment programs. In addition, the OIG may bring administrative proceedings for the purpose of imposing civil monetary penalties and exclusion from government programs. Some states have their own laws about kickbacks, and those state laws might extend beyond government payment programs.

As a matter of policy, the concern is that payment for referrals could increase Medicare and Medicaid costs by giving physicians and other providers an incentive to provide unnecessary treatment. In addition, compensation for referrals could interfere with a provider's independent judgment as to when and where to refer a particular patient. For example, it would be unlawful as well as unethical for a hospital to pay physicians for patient referrals or for a pharmaceutical manufacturer to pay physicians or pharmacists to prescribe or dispense a particular drug.[69] Similarly, it would be unlawful and unethical for a skilled nursing facility or home health agency to give anything of value, in cash or in kind, to the discharge planners at a hospital for the purpose of inducing them to refer patients for postdischarge services. For similar reasons, giving particular types of incentives to Medicare or Medicaid beneficiaries for the purpose of inducing them to choose a particular healthcare provider is unlawful, although exceptions exist that permit other types of incentives to beneficiaries. These beneficiary incentives are discussed in detail in the final part of this chapter regarding waivers for participation in ACOs.

As a legal matter, the primary issue under this federal statute is the intent of the parties. In other words, payment or other consideration is unlawful if it was made with the intent of inducing referrals or purchases. In some cases, ascertaining the intent of the parties is fairly easy. For example, if a hospital made a monthly payment to each physician on its medical staff and if the amount of each payment was based on the number of patients referred to the hospital by each physician during the previous month, the intent to induce referrals would be obvious. Similarly, if a clinical laboratory paid physicians for each sample they sent to that laboratory, the intent of the parties to pay for referrals and encourage more referrals in the future would be obvious.

However, many situations in the healthcare system are not that clear. Some arrangements are more subtle but have the same intent to induce referrals. Therefore, healthcare professionals and managers must develop the ability to recognize situations in which money or something else of value is flowing from someone who would benefit from referrals to someone who is in a position to refer.

Moreover, a business relationship with a potential source of referrals might be motivated by a combination of different factors. Some of those motivating factors might be appropriate while others are not. How should the law deal with these cases of mixed motivation?

In trying to develop a reasonable rule of law, one approach would be to consider the payment to be unlawful if the *sole* purpose of the payment was to induce referrals. However, from the perspective of prosecutors and enforcement agencies, a "sole purpose" test would be too difficult for them to meet and would allow dishonest people to evade the anti-kickback statute by merely pointing to *some* legitimate motivation for their payments. Another alternative would be to consider the payment to be unlawful if its *primary* purpose was to induce referrals, but that type of standard might be difficult to apply as a practical matter and might lead to arbitrary and inconsistent results.

Therefore, courts have developed a different legal standard for evaluating conduct under the anti-kickback statute, and that standard is favorable to prosecutors and enforcement agencies. Under the prevailing legal standard, giving or receiving a payment is unlawful if *any part* of the motivation for that payment is to induce referrals. In other words, it is unlawful if *one purpose* of the payment is to induce referrals.[70] This standard has been referred to as the "lust in your heart test," because any subjective motivation for referrals would make an arrangement unlawful, even if the primary motivation is completely appropriate. For example, if a hospital pays a physician at fair-market value for legitimate services that actually were rendered, the payment is nevertheless unlawful if a small part of the motivation was to encourage referrals of Medicare or Medicaid patients.

Despite the objections of some healthcare providers, most federal courts that have considered the issue have upheld the one-purpose standard in applying the anti-kickback statute. As the Tenth Circuit held, "a person who offers or pays remuneration to another person violates the Act so long as one purpose of the offer or payment is to induce Medicare or Medicaid patient referrals."[71] In a related case, defendants argued that use of the one-purpose test would make almost every relationship between a physician and a hospital illegal, because the hospital executive would always be thinking about referrals to some extent.[72] However, the Tenth Circuit disagreed with the defendants in that case and explained that merely hoping for or expecting referrals as a result of payments that were made entirely for legitimate purposes is not against the law. Similarly, a physician referring patients to a hospital that also pays the physician for services rendered is not unlawful, provided that the payment is made entirely for the performance of those services. In approving the jury instructions that were given by the district court in that case, the Tenth Circuit explained that "[t]his application of the Act by the district court clearly allows business relationships between a hospital and physician where the motivation to enter into the relationship is for legal reasons entirely distinct from the collateral hope for or decision to make referrals. Accordingly, contrary to defendants' assertion, the Act, as applied in this case, does not make all conduct illegal when a hospital executive or physician has referrals in mind."[73]

Despite such attempts at clarification, the prevailing interpretation of the law causes substantial uncertainty for healthcare providers. Is distinguishing between a partial motivation, on one hand, and a mere hope or expectation, on the other hand really possible? Under these circumstances, it may be difficult to determine whether a particular arrangement is lawful.

As always, the goal of the legal system is to develop a set of understandable rules that will prohibit undesirable conduct without interfering with desirable conduct. In other words, the task is to tailor the rules to stop the "bad guys" without making criminals out of the "good guys." However, with regard to the anti-kickback statute, whether our legal system has achieved that delicate balance is not at all clear. Moreover, the uncertainty about what conduct is lawful has resulted in widespread cynicism and disrespect for the law.

Safe harbor
Laws that provide a safety zone from liability if all of the requirements are satisfied.

To give some additional guidance to providers, Congress required HHS to issue regulations that set forth **safe harbors** from the anti-kickback statute.[74] Those regulations are called safe harbors because they provide a zone of safety from legal liability if all of the requirements in the regulations are satisfied. However, the fact that an arrangement does not fit within a safe harbor does not mean the arrangement is illegal. Rather, arrangements that do not satisfy all of the requirements of a safe harbor would have to be evaluated under the terms of the anti-kickback statute itself.

In 1991, the OIG issued final safe harbor regulations that describe payment practices that will not be subject to criminal prosecution and will not provide a basis for exclusion from Medicare or Medicaid.[75] The OIG clarified and expanded those regulations in 1999.[76] Since then, the OIG has issued additional safe harbors from time to time on specific issues, such as arrangements to provide technology for electronic prescription information and electronic health records.[77]

Some people think the safe harbor regulations are too restrictive and still leave uncertainty about what conduct the government is likely to challenge. Therefore, in the 1996 Health Insurance Portability and Accountability Act (HIPAA), Congress required the OIG to issue advisory opinions with regard to proposed conduct under the anti-kickback statute.[78] Previously, the OIG had expressed concern that issuing advisory opinions would inhibit its law enforcement functions and argued that issuing advisory opinions about conduct under a statute that was based on subjective intent would be impractical. However, Congress enacted the requirement, and the OIG has been issuing advisory opinions that are available to the public on its website.[79]

The 2010 ACA makes some important changes to the anti-kickback statute. First, the ACA makes it easier to prove a violation because proving actual knowledge of that law or a specific intent to violate it will not be necessary.[80] In addition, the ACA provides that a violation of the anti-kickback statute is also a basis for liability as a false claim under the FCA.[81]

The ACA also requires greater disclosure of financial relationships, such as expanded disclosure by nursing homes regarding their ownership, control, or management. Moreover, section 6002 of the ACA generally requires manufacturers of drugs, devices, or supplies to report to HHS the details of their payments or other valuable consideration to doctors and teaching hospitals for publication on a website. This part of the ACA is commonly known as the Sunshine Act. Final Sunshine Act regulations were issued on February 8, 2013.[82]

The federal anti-kickback statute deals with financial incentives to make more referrals and provide more care. However, PPS and some cost-containment strategies create incentives to provide less care in particular cases. The legal and policy issues that arise in connection with those financial incentives are addressed in more detail in Chapter 14. For example, some hospitals tried to give financial incentives to physicians to reduce the cost of treating patients to maximize hospital revenues under PPS. However, Congress has prohibited hospitals from paying physicians to reduce the level of services for Medicare and Medicaid patients, as discussed previously in regard to Medicare payment issues.[83] This type of arrangement, which is known as **gainsharing**, can be a basis for imposing civil monetary penalties. Nevertheless, as discussed in Chapter 14, the federal government has indicated that *some* gainsharing arrangements could be permitted under specific circumstances.

Gainsharing
An agreement by a hospital to give physicians part of the hospital's savings on patient care costs, thereby creating a risk that physicians might reduce the level of services for patients.

Self-Referrals

Even if physicians do not receive kickbacks in exchange for referrals, they may have financial incentives to refer patients to facilities that they own in whole or in part. As with kickbacks, incentives for self-referral have a tendency to increase costs and interfere with a physician's independent medical judgment. In fact, several studies have documented that physicians with financial interests in healthcare facilities tend to make more referrals for tests and treatments than physicians without those financial interests.[84]

To address this problem of self-referral, Congress enacted the Ethics in Patient Referrals Act, which is § 1877 of the Social Security Act.[85] This statute is commonly called the Stark Law because its primary sponsor was Congressman Pete Stark. As originally enacted in 1989, the Stark Law only applied to clinical laboratory services. However, in 1993, Congress expanded the prohibition to cover many types of "designated health services" under a revised statute that is commonly called Stark II,[86] and Congress has made further statutory changes since that date.[87] Aside from its comprehensive regulations to implement the Stark Law, CMS issued a specific final regulation in 2006 to create a new exception for certain arrangements involving electronic prescriptions and electronic health records, which was designed to complement the OIG's new safe harbor under the anti-kickback statute.[88]

In addressing the problem of self-referral, Congress might have taken several possible approaches. One alternative was to permit self-referral but require the physician to disclose her ownership interests and compensation arrangements to the patient. These financial arrangements can provide incentives for physicians to make referrals and can influence the decisions that patients make about their treatment. Therefore, these financial incentives arguably ought to be disclosed to the patient. However, when it enacted the Stark Law, Congress did not choose to require full disclosure as a means of dealing with physician self-referral but instead prevented physicians as a practical matter from engaging in certain types of arrangements.

Under this federal law, physicians are not prohibited from owning an interest in a healthcare facility. However, the law makes it impractical to do so in many situations by prohibiting certain referrals as well as reimbursement for services that were rendered as a result of a prohibited referral. Specifically, if a physician or immediate family member has an ownership interest or compensation arrangement with an entity, the physician may not refer a patient to the entity, and the entity may not bill the government program for services that were rendered as a result of the referral. Under these circumstances, many healthcare organizations do not want—or will not permit—referring physicians to have ownership interests or compensation arrangements, because they do not want to lose the opportunity to bill for their referrals.

In effect, the Stark self-referral law uses a transactional approach in which certain arrangements are lawful or unlawful depending on their structure, rather than focusing on the intent of the parties. In that respect, the Stark Law is different from the anti-kickback statute, which is based on the parties' intent in making a particular payment. However, the safe harbor regulations under the anti-kickback statute also use a transactional approach that is similar in some respects to the approach of the Stark self-referral law. Most important, healthcare providers must meet the requirements of *both* the anti-kickback statute *and* the Stark self-referral law. In addition, some state governments have adopted self-referral laws that might not be limited to patients of government payment programs.

The Stark Law applies to many types of designated health services, such as radiology, clinical laboratory, physical and occupational therapy, home health, outpatient drugs, certain types of supplies, and both inpatient and outpatient hospital services. However, the statute and regulations are extremely complex. They contain numerous exceptions and definitions, each of which must be considered in evaluating whether a particular arrangement is lawful.

The complexity of the Stark Law demonstrates the difficulty of prohibiting undesirable conduct without inhibiting activities that are beneficial to society. We want to prohibit those self-referral arrangements that have a tendency to increase cost and interfere with a physician's independent medical judgment. Moreover, we want to make the prohibition sufficiently broad that people will not be able to circumvent the law by merely changing the outward structure of their business relationships. However, we do not want to prohibit the ordinary and necessary patterns of medical practice, such as referring a patient for ancillary services in a physician's office or referring a patient to another physician in the same group practice. Therefore, the Stark Law provides exceptions for legitimate group practices, as defined in the statute and regulations.[89] In addition, an exception exists for those in-office ancillary services that meet all of the requirements set forth in the law.[90]

The Stark Law also provides an exception that allows physicians to refer patients to a hospital if they have an ownership interest in the hospital as a whole or in the chain or network that owns the hospital.[91] However, the ACA limited the exception for ownership interests in hospitals. The ACA does not require physicians to divest their preexisting ownership interests in hospitals, but it imposes limitations on future expansion of physician-owned hospitals.

In addition, the ACA authorized CMS to develop a self-referral disclosure protocol (SRDP) for potential or actual violations of the Stark Law and gave authority to the secretary of HHS to reduce the penalties for violations. CMS published its SRDP on September 23, 2010, and made revisions on May 6, 2011.[92]

Although the Stark Law and regulations are complex, providers can obtain clarification by asking CMS to issue an advisory opinion on a particular arrangement. In the BBA of 1997, Congress required CMS to issue advisory opinions on most self-referral arrangements.[93] These advisory opinions are available at www.cms.gov.[94]

Compliance Programs for Healthcare Providers

Many healthcare organizations have recognized the importance of instituting a comprehensive compliance program. A compliance program is an in-house system of policymaking, education, information gathering, reporting, and accountability. The purpose of this type of program is to prevent illegal and unethical conduct, such as Medicare and Medicaid fraud. Significantly, the ACA has made compliance programs mandatory for some types of healthcare providers and suppliers, including but not limited to physicians.

An effective compliance program benefits an organization in several ways. First, a compliance program will help to prevent some problems from occurring. Second, when problems do occur, despite the organization's best efforts, an effective compliance program will help to limit the extent of the problem and reduce the amount of the penalties assessed by the government. An organization is likely to receive a much lighter penalty if it already had an effective compliance program in effect at the time the problem occurred. Moreover, as discussed in Chapter 4, the directors of a healthcare corporation might be held legally liable if they fail to ensure that the corporation has an effective compliance program.[95] Finally, a compliance program will help to ensure that the officers, directors, and employees meet the standards of ethical conduct that are established by the organization.

An effective compliance program requires a genuine commitment by an organization's top management and board. Everyone in the organization needs to understand that the management and board take compliance seriously. To communicate that message, compliance should be part of each individual's periodic salary and performance review.

For many years, the OIG has published compliance program guidance for various types of healthcare organizations. These guidance documents are not model compliance programs but rather guidelines on how to develop an effective program in various segments of the healthcare industry.[96] As indicated by the OIG, programs should not be limited to merely ensuring compliance with the law; they should also be designed to encourage ethical business behavior.[97] Thus, a compliance program is more than a system of risk management and damage control. Merely complying with legal requirements and avoiding fines or imprisonment should be viewed as the minimum acceptable effort and not something of which an organization or its leaders should be particularly proud. Rather, in developing and implementing a compliance program, each organization should strive for a standard of ethical behavior that exceeds the requirements of law.

Like the self-referral disclosure protocol for violations of the Stark Law, the OIG encourages healthcare providers and suppliers to disclose violations of other laws about fraud and abuse. The OIG also issues advisory opinions, which are available on its website.[98]

In the meantime, the federal government is continuing to link compliance and quality of care. In some situations, the federal government has taken the position that providing poor quality of care may constitute fraud and abuse.[99] The OIG expressed its hope that compliance programs will not only prevent fraud and reduce healthcare costs, but will also enable organizations to improve the quality of care.[100]

In fraud and abuse cases, the OIG often settles with the healthcare provider. If the OIG permits the organization to continue participating in federal programs, the OIG will ordinarily require the organization to operate under the terms of a **Corporate Integrity Agreement**. In addition to requiring organizations to make improvements in their financial controls, the OIG has used Corporate Integrity Agreements to require providers to establish mechanisms to promote quality of care. Some settlements involve arrangements that are explicitly labeled Quality of Care Corporate Integrity Agreements, and these require the appointment of an independent quality monitor.[101] Under these circumstances, quality of care is part of the law of fraud and abuse, and compliance is inextricably linked with efforts to reduce medical errors and promote the quality of care.

Corporate Integrity Agreement
A contract between the OIG and a healthcare organization in the context of settlement, in which the OIG agrees to permit the organization to continue participating in federal programs and the organization agrees to take specific actions to promote compliance.

Fraud and Abuse Issues for Accountable Care Organizations

As discussed previously, the 2010 ACA promotes the development of ACOs under the Shared Savings Program, in which groups of healthcare providers deliver care to Medicare beneficiaries in a coordinated manner. Healthcare providers who participate in an ACO may share cost savings that result from delivering high-quality care more efficiently.

However, ACOs raise potential problems under the law of fraud and abuse. For example, Congress recognized that creation and operation of an ACO might require healthcare providers to share financial resources in ways that could violate existing fraud and abuse laws. Therefore, Congress authorized the secretary of HHS to provide waivers from particular laws as needed to implement the Shared Savings Program.[102]

On November 2, 2011, CMS and OIG issued an Interim Final Rule with Comment Period (IFC).[103] The IFC sets forth waivers from the application of fraud and abuse laws for ACO arrangements under specific conditions. The ACO waivers apply to four laws, and there are five separate ACO waivers from application of those laws. The four laws are:

1. the Stark Law (the physician self-referral law);
2. the anti-kickback statute;

3. the gainsharing civil monetary penalty (CMP); and

4. the beneficiary inducements CMP.

The gainsharing CMP[104] prohibits hospitals from paying physicians to limit or reduce services to Medicare or Medicaid patients, as discussed previously. The beneficiary inducements CMP[105] prohibits offering or giving something of value to Medicare or Medicaid patients that would be likely to influence their choice of provider, subject to some exceptions.

To cover the variety of potential problems under fraud and abuse laws, CMS and OIG established five separate ACO waivers. These five waivers cover:

1. ACO preparticipation;

2. ACO participation;

3. shared savings distributions;

4. ACO arrangements that raise issues under the Stark Law; and

5. patient incentives.

The IFC sets forth the specific conditions that must be satisfied for each of these waivers to apply.[106]

To qualify for a waiver, ACOs and their participants need to meet all of the conditions for that particular waiver. However, failing to qualify for a waiver does not necessarily make an activity unlawful.

Activity 8.1 provides an opportunity to consider the application of the November 2, 2011, IFC to a specific set of facts about an ACO and its participants. As discussed in this activity, the ACO and its participating providers intend to rely solely on the waiver for patient incentives. Activity 8.1 includes an excerpt from the IFC that should be useful in answering the problem. In addition to some introductory material, the excerpt contains the requirements of the waiver for patient incentives, together with additional explanation of those waiver requirements by CMS and OIG.

ACTIVITY 8.1: THE FRAUD AND ABUSE WAIVER FOR ACO PATIENT INCENTIVES

Please assume the following facts. An accountable care organization (ACO) has entered into a participation agreement with the secretary of the U.S. Department of Health and Human Services (HHS) to participate

(continued)

(continued from previous page)

in the Medicare Shared Savings Program. The ACO remains in good standing under its participation agreement. The healthcare providers participating in the ACO include one hospital and approximately 100 physicians.

The ACO is proposing to give all of its Medicare patients a free electronic tablet device. In addition, the ACO will pay all of the costs for installation and monthly service, in order to connect the tablets by satellite. The tablet will contain an app that will remind Medicare patients to take each dose of medication as prescribed or directed by the physician. Moreover, by touching a box on the screen of the tablet, the app will enable patients to record the fact that they have taken the dose, and that information will be transmitted electronically to the offices of their physicians. The medications that will be tracked by the tablet may include some preventive care but will not be limited to preventive care.

The cost of this type of tablet is $600. The cost of installation and monthly service for a one-year contract is $400. Therefore, the total cost for each Medicare patient during the first year will be $1,000. As a practical matter, Medicare beneficiaries might be able to use the tablet for personal purposes and not merely for purposes related to their medical care. For convenience, all of the foregoing information may be referred to simply as "the proposal."

Your task is to answer all of the following questions under the assumed set of facts. If you think you need any additional facts, please state the facts that you think are needed and explain how those facts would affect your analysis.

Your answers should be based on the November 2, 2011, IFC. An excerpt from the IFC follows the questions. Please note that, in this case, the ACO and its participating providers intend to rely solely on the waiver for patient incentives.

1. Identify the federal law (or laws) that would be waived by the specific waiver on which the ACO and its participants intend to rely. Explain what is prohibited by that law (or laws), and explain how the proposal could violate that law (or laws) in the absence of a waiver.

2. Summarize the requirements that must be met to qualify for the specific waiver.

(continued)

(continued from previous page)

3. Analyze whether the proposal meets all of the requirements for the specific waiver. State the arguments (if any) for concluding that the proposal meets all of those requirements, as well as the arguments (if any) for concluding that the proposal does not meet them. Be sure to state your conclusion and explain the basis for it.

4. As a matter of policy, explain whether you think that the requirements for that specific waiver should be changed by the secretary of HHS. Specifically, should the secretary amend the requirements for that specific waiver to balance the goal of beneficiary compliance with care management programs against the risk that ACOs could use extravagant incentives to steer beneficiaries? Be sure to state your conclusion and explain your reasoning for amending or not amending those requirements.

67992 Federal Register / Vol. 76, No. 212 / Wednesday, November 2, 2011. . . .

Medicare Program; Final Waivers in Connection with the Shared Savings Program

AGENCY: Centers for Medicare & Medicaid Services (CMS) and Office of Inspector General (OIG), HHS.

ACTION: Interim final rule with comment period.

SUMMARY: This interim final rule with comment period establishes waivers of the application of the Physician Self-Referral Law, the Federal anti-kickback statute, and certain civil monetary penalties (CMP) law provisions to specified arrangements involving accountable care organizations (ACOs) under section 1899 of the Social Security Act (the Act) (the Shared Savings Program), including ACOs participating in the Advance Payment Initiative. Section 1899(f) of the Act, as added by the Affordable Care Act, authorizes the Secretary to waive certain fraud and abuse laws as necessary to carry out the provisions of section 1899 of the Act.

DATES: *Effective date:* These regulations are effective on November 2, 2011. . . .

I. Introduction and Overview. . . .

A. Connection Between Shared Savings Program and Fraud and Abuse Waivers

[S]takeholders have expressed concern that the restrictions these laws place on certain arrangements between physicians, hospitals, and

(continued)

(continued from previous page)

other individuals and entities may impede development of some of the innovative integrated-care models envisioned by the Shared Savings Program. . . . Based on stakeholder input and other factors, the Secretary has found that it is necessary to waive these fraud and abuse laws in order to carry out the Shared Savings Program.

Accordingly, this IFC sets forth waivers of certain provisions of the Physician Self-Referral Law, the Federal anti-kickback statute, the CMP law prohibiting hospital payments to physicians to reduce or limit services (the Gainsharing CMP), and the CMP law prohibiting inducements to beneficiaries (the Beneficiary Inducements CMP) as necessary to carry out the provisions of section 1899 of the Act. We seek to waive application of these fraud and abuse laws to ACOs formed in connection with the Shared Savings Program so that the laws do not unduly impede development of beneficial ACOs, while also ensuring that ACO arrangements are not misused for fraudulent or abusive purposes that harm patients or Federal health care programs. . . .

B. Overview of Final Waivers

There are five waivers addressing different circumstances—

- An "ACO pre-participation" waiver of the Physician Self-Referral Law, the Federal anti-kickback statute, and the Gainsharing CMP that applies to ACO related start-up arrangements in anticipation of participating in the Shared Savings Program, subject to certain limitations, including limits on the duration of the waiver and the types of parties covered;
- An "ACO participation" waiver of the Physician Self-Referral Law, the Federal anti-kickback statute, and the Gainsharing CMP that applies broadly to ACO-related arrangements during the term of the ACO's participation agreement under the Shared Savings Program and for a specified time thereafter;
- A "shared savings distributions" waiver of the Physician Self-Referral Law, Federal anti-kickback statute, and Gainsharing CMP that applies to distributions and uses of shared savings payments earned under the Shared Savings Program;
- A "compliance with the Physician Self-Referral Law" waiver of the Gainsharing CMP and the Federal anti-kickback statute for ACO arrangements that implicate the Physician Self-Referral Law and meet an existing exception; and

(continued)

(continued from previous page)

- A "patient incentive" waiver of the Beneficiary Inducements CMP and the Federal anti-kickback statute for medically related incentives offered by ACOs under the Shared Savings Program to beneficiaries to encourage preventive care and compliance with treatment regimes.

. . . . An arrangement need only fit in one waiver to be protected; parties seeking to ensure that an arrangement is covered by a waiver for a particular law may look to any waiver that applies to that law. In some cases, an arrangement may meet the criteria of more than one waiver.

II. Shared Savings Program: Background . . . .

IV. Provisions of the Interim Final Rule With Comment Period: Waiver Requirements

A. Overview

. . . .The waivers are intended to be self-implementing. Apart from meeting applicable waiver conditions, no special action (such as the submission of a separate application for a waiver) is required by parties in order to be covered by a waiver. Parties need not apply for an individualized waiver.

This IFC includes five waivers. . . . Because the waivers cover multiple legal authorities and to ensure that the waivers, if modified, remain consistent over time and across relevant laws, we are not codifying the waivers in the Code of Federal Regulations. . . . .

B. The Waivers and Applicable Requirements . . . .

5. Waiver for Patient Incentives

. . . [S]ection 1128A(a)(5) of the Act (relating to the beneficiary inducements CMP) and sections 1128B(b)(1) and (2) of the Act (relating to the Federal anti-kickback statute) are waived with respect to items or services provided by an ACO, its ACO participants, or its ACO providers/suppliers to beneficiaries for free or below fair-market-value if all four of the following conditions are met:

1. The ACO has entered into a participation agreement and remains in good standing under its participation agreement.

(continued)

(continued from previous page)

2. There is a reasonable connection between the items or services and the medical care of the beneficiary.

3. The items or services are in-kind.

4. The items or services—

    a. Are preventive care items or services; or

    b. Advance one or more of the following clinical goals:

        i. Adherence to a treatment regime.

        ii. Adherence to a drug regime.

        iii. Adherence to a follow-up care plan.

        iv. Management of a chronic disease or condition. . . .

V. Provisions of the Interim Final Rule With Comment Period: Explanation of Waiver Requirements . . . .

F. Waiver for Patient Incentives

. . .[S]everal public commenters indicated that, in carrying out the quality and cost reduction goals of the Shared Savings Program, ACOs would need to engage patients in better managing their own health care, including obtaining preventive care and complying with treatment plans for chronic conditions. Therefore, in light of this need, this IFC promulgates a waiver of the Federal anti-kickback statute and Beneficiary Inducements CMP to address arrangements pursuant to which ACOs, ACO participants, and ACO providers/suppliers provide beneficiaries with free or below-fair market value items and services that advance the goals of preventive care, adherence to treatment, drug, or follow-up care regimes, or management of a chronic disease or condition. . . .

In order to balance the goal of beneficiary compliance with care management programs against the risk that ACOs could use extravagant incentives to steer beneficiaries, we are requiring that there be a reasonable connection between the incentives and the medical care of the individual. By way of example, the waiver would cover blood pressure cuffs for hypertensive patients, but not beauty products or theatre tickets. The waiver will protect incentives that are in-kind items or services, but not financial incentives, such as waiving or reducing patient cost sharing amounts (that is, copayment or deductible), which we believe are prone to greater abuse. . . .

(continued)

(continued from previous page)

This waiver does not protect the provision of free or below fair market value items or services by manufacturers or other vendors to beneficiaries, the ACO, ACO participants, or ACO providers/suppliers. The patient incentives waiver would cover ACOs, ACO participants, and ACO provider/suppliers that give beneficiaries items or services that they have received from manufacturers at discounted rates. However, the waiver would not cover the discount arrangement (or any arrangement for free items and services) between the manufacturer and the ACO, ACO participant, or ACO provider/supplier.

. . . Nothing precludes ACOs, ACO participants, or ACO providers/suppliers from offering patient incentives to promote their clinical care if the incentives fit in an applicable safe harbor or exception or do not otherwise violate the Federal anti-kickback statute and Beneficiary Inducements CMP. For example, many such arrangements may fit in the exception to the Beneficiary Inducements CMP for incentives given to individuals to promote the delivery of preventive care . . . .

Notes

1. D. M. Harris (2003). "Beyond Beneficiaries: Using the Medicare Program to Accomplish Broader Public Goals." *Washington & Lee Law Review* 60 (4): 1251–1314, at 1252, 1312.
2. *Id.*
3. *Fischer v. United States*, 529 U.S. 667, 680 (2000).
4. Medicare Prescription Drug, Improvement, and Modernization Act of 2003, Pub. L. No. 108-173, 117 Stat. 2066.
5. T. S. Jost (2005). "The Most Important Health Care Legislation of the Millennium (So Far): The Medicare Modernization Act." *Yale Journal of Health Policy, Law & Ethics* 5: 437–49, at 445 ("The MMA for the first time means-tests part of the Medicare program").
6. *Id.* at 445–46.
7. See R. A. Berenson and D. M. Harris, "Using Managed Care Tools in Traditional Medicare: Should We? Could We?" *Law & Contemporary Problems* (2002), 65: 139–67.
8. Health Affairs/Robert Wood Johnson Foundation (2012). "Health Policy Brief: Premium Support in Medicare." March 22, www.rwjf.org/content/dam/farm/articles/journal_articles/2012/rwjf72492.

9. Balanced Budget Act of 1997, Pub. L. No. 105-33, 111 Stat. 251 (1997).

10. 42 U.S.C. § 1395a(a) (2006).

11. Medicare Prescription Drug, Improvement, and Modernization Act of 2003, Pub. L. No. 108-173, 117 Stat. 2066. See note 4 *supra*.

12. See Jost, *supra* note 5, at 446.

13. 42 U.S.C. § 1395w–111(i) (2006).

14. American Taxpayer Relief Act of 2012, Pub. L. No. 112-240 (2013), § 642.

15. 42 U.S.C. § 1395 (2006).

16. See, e.g., *Home Health Care, Inc. v. Heckler*, 717 F.2d 587, 590–91 (D.C. Cir. 1983).

17. *Fischer v. United States*, 529 U.S. 667, 680 (2000).

18. See *Modaber v. Culpepper Memorial Hospital, Inc.*, 674 F.2d 1023, 1025–26 (4th Cir. 1982).

19. See *United States v. Baylor University Medical Center*, 736 F.2d 1039, 1946 (5th Cir. 1984).

20. Centers for Medicare & Medicaid Services (2005). "Press Release: Medicare 'Pay For Performance (P4P)' Initiatives," January 31, www.cms.hhs.gov/apps/media/press/release.asp?Counter=1343.

21. See S. Guterman and H. Drake, "Developing Innovative Payment Approaches: Finding the Path to High Performance," *Commonwealth Fund* (June 2010), www.commonwealthfund.org/~/media/Files/Publications/Issue%20Brief/2010/Jun/1401_Guterman_developing_innovative_payment_approaches_ib.pdf.

22. See 42 U.S.C. § 1320a–7a(b) (2006).

23. See Medicare Preservation Act of 1995, H.R. 2425, 104th Cong. (1995) (passed by the House of Representatives).

24. Department of Health & Human Services, Centers for Medicare & Medicaid Services, Office of the Actuary, "2010 Actuarial Report on the Financial Outlook for Medicaid" (2010). www.cms.gov/ActuarialStudies/downloads/MedicaidReport2010.pdf.

25. *National Federation of Independent Business v. Sebelius*, 132 S. Ct. 2566 (2012).

26. *Id.* at 2607 (Opinion of Chief Justice Roberts).

27. See 42 U.S.C. § 1396p(c) (2006).

28. See 42 C.F.R. §§ 440.210, 440.220 (2006).

29. See *Pinneke v. Priesser*, 623 F.2d 546, 549 (8th Cir. 1980).

30. See, e.g., *Pereira v. Kozlowski*, 996 F.2d 723 (4th Cir. 1993) (three-year-old child needing heart transplant).

31. See, e.g., New and Pending Demonstration Project Proposals Submitted Pursuant to Section 1115(a) of the Social Security Act: November and December 1994, 60 Fed. Reg. 4418, 4420 (Jan. 23, 1995).

32. The Hyde Amendment was originally enacted in 1976. Departments of Labor and Health, Education, and Welfare Appropriation Act of 1977, Pub. L. No. 94-439, § 209, 90 Stat. 1418, 1434 (1976).

33. *Harris v. McRae*, 448 U.S. 297 (1980)

34. *Id.* at 316.

35. See *id.* at 324–25.

36. See, e.g., *Committee to Defend Reproductive Rights v. Myers*, 625 P.2d 779 (Cal. 1981).

37. See M. Michael and C. Adams, "For Medicaid Patients, Doors Slam Closed: Citing Finances, Nursing Home Evicts the Needy," *Wall Street Journal*, April 7, 1998, B1.

38. 42 U.S.C. § 1396a(a)(30)(A) (2006).

39. *Antrican v. Buell*, 290 F.3d 178 (4th Cir. 2002).

40. See, e.g., *Mandy R. v. Owens*, 464 F.3d 1139 (10th Cir. 2006); *Westside Mothers v. Olszewski*, 454 F.3d 532 (6th Cir. 2006).

41. *Douglas v. Independent Living Center of Southern California, Inc.*, 132 S.Ct. 1204 (2012).

42. *Id.*

43. Balanced Budget Act of 1997, Pub. L. No. 105-33, §§ 4901(a) *et seq.*, 111 Stat. 251, 552 (1997) (codified at 42 U.S.C. §§ 1397aa *et seq.*).

44. U.S. General Accounting Office, *Medicaid and SCHIP: Recent HHS Approvals of Demonstration Waiver Projects Raise Concerns*, GAO-02-817 (July 2002) (footnotes omitted).

45. 42 U.S.C. § 1397bb(b)(4) (2006).

46. 42 U.S.C. § 1397aa(c) (2006).

47. S. Rosenbaum, et al. (1998). "The Children's Hour: The State Children's Health Insurance Program," *Health Affairs* 17: 75, 77.

48. U.S. Department of Justice, Office of Public Affairs (2012). "Dallas-based Tenet Healthcare Pays More Than $42 Million to Settle Allegations of Improperly Billing Medicare," April 10, www.justice. gov/opa/pr/2012/April/12-civ-446.html.

49. See 31 U.S.C. §§ 3729 *et seq.* (2006).

50. See T. S. Jost and S. L. Davies, "The Empire Strikes Back: A Critique of the Backlash Against Fraud and Abuse Enforcement," *Alabama Law Review* (1999), 51: 239–309.

51. V. G. Freeman, et al. (1999). "Lying for Patients: Physician Deception of Third-Party Payers," *Archives of Internal Medicine*, 159: 2263–70.

52. Publication of OIG Special Fraud Alert: "Fraud and Abuse in the Provision of Services in Nursing Facilities," 61 Fed. Reg. 30623 (June 17, 1996).

53. Fraud Enforcement and Recovery Act of 2009 (FERA), 111 Pub. L. No. 21, 123 Stat. 1617 (2009).

54. 42 U.S.C. § 1320a–7b(a) (2006).

55. See *id.*

56. 285 F.3d 1345 (11th Cir. 2002).

57. *Id.* at 1351.

58. 31 U.S.C. § 3729 (2006).

59. *Id.*

60. *Id.*

61. *United States ex rel. Hochman v. Nackman*, 145 F.3d 1069, 1073 (9th Cir. 1998).

62. 261 F.3d 821 (9th Cir. 2001).

63. *Id.* at 828.

64. Jost and Davies, *supra* note 50, at 247–48, 305.

65. See generally T. H. Stanton, "Fraud-and-Abuse Enforcement in Medicare: Finding Middle Ground," *Health Affairs* (2001), 20(4): 28–42, at 32.

66. See Health Insurance Portability and Accountability Act of 1996, Pub. L. No. 104-191, §§ 241–250, 110 Stat. 1936, 2016–21 (codified in scattered sections of 18 U.S.C.).

67. *Id.* at § 242 (codified at 18 U.S.C. § 1347).

68. See 42 U.S.C. § 1320a–7b(b)(1)–(2) (2006).

69. See Publication of OIG Special Fraud Alerts, 59 Fed. Reg. 65372 (December 19, 1994).

70. See, e.g., *United States v. Greber*, 760 F.2d 68, 72 (3rd Cir. 1985).

71. *United States v. McClatchey*, 217 F.3d 823, 835 (10th Cir. 2000).

72. *United States v. LaHue*, 261 F.3d 993 (10th Cir. 2001).

73. *Id.* (citation omitted).

74. Medicare and Medicaid Patient and Program Protection Act of 1987, Pub. L. No. 100-93, § 14, 101 Stat. 680, 697 (1987) (codified at 42 U.S.C. § 1320a–7b).

75. See Medicare and State Health Care Programs: Fraud and Abuse; OIG Anti-Kickback Provisions, 56 Fed. Reg. 35952, 35984–87 (July 29, 1991) (codified at 42 C.F.R. pt. 1001).

76. Medicare and State Health Care Programs: Fraud and Abuse; Clarification of the Initial OIG Safe Harbor Provisions and Establishment of Additional Safe Harbor Provisions Under the Anti-Kickback Statute, 64 Fed. Reg. 63518 (November 19, 1999).

77. Medicare and State Health Care Programs: Fraud and Abuse; Safe Harbors for Certain Electronic Prescribing and Electronic Health Records Arrangements Under the Anti-Kickback Statute; Final Rule, 71 Fed. Reg. 45110 (August 8, 2006). See also 78 Fed. Reg. 21314 (April 10, 2013) (proposed rule to amend and extend the safe harbor).

78. Health Insurance Portability and Accountability Act of 1996, Pub. L. No. 104-191, § 205, 110 Stat. 1936, 2000 (codified at 42 U.S.C. § 1320a–7d).

79. Office of Inspector General, Department of Health and Human Services, "Advisory Opinions." oig.hhs.gov/compliance/advisory-opinions/index.asp.

80. Patient Protection and Affordable Care Act, Pub. L. No. 111-148, § 6402(f)(2) (2010).

81. *Id.* at § 6402(f)(1).

82. 78 Fed. Reg. 9458 (February 8, 2013).

83. See note 22 *supra* and accompanying text.

84. See Medicare and Medicaid Programs: Physicians' Referrals to Health Care Entities with Which They Have Financial Relationships, 63 Fed. Reg. 1659, 1661 (January 9, 1998) (explanatory information for proposed Stark II regulations).

85. Ethics in Patient Referrals Act, Pub. L. No. 101-239, § 6204, 103 Stat. 2106, 2236 (1989) (codified at 42 U.S.C. § 1395nn).

86. Omnibus Budget Reconciliation Act of 1993, Pub. L. No. 103-66, § 13562, 107 Stat. 312, 596 (1993) (codified at 42 U.S.C. § 1395nn).

87. See, e.g., Social Security Act Amendments of 1994, Pub. L. No. 103-432, § 152, 108 Stat. 4398, 4436 (1994) (codified at 42 U.S.C. § 1395nn).

88. 71 Fed. Reg. 45140 (August 8, 2006) (final rule).

89. See, e.g., 42 U.S.C. § 1395nn(b)(1) (2006); 63 Fed. Reg. at 1687–91, 1721.

90. See 42 U.S.C. § 1395nn(b)(2) (2006); 63 Fed. Reg. at 1684–85, 1723.

91. See 63 Fed. Reg. at 1713 (introduction to proposed regulations).

92. Centers for Medicare & Medicaid Services, "Self-Referral Disclosure Protocol" (2013). www.cms.gov/Medicare/Fraud-and-Abuse/PhysicianSelfReferral/Self_Referral_Disclosure_Protocol.html.

93. Balanced Budget Act of 1997, Pub. L. No. 105-33, § 4314, 111 Stat. 251, 389 (1997) (codified at 42 U.S.C. § 1395nn).

94. Centers for Medicare & Medicaid Services, "Advisory Opinions (AOs)" (2013). www.cms.gov/Medicare/Fraud-and-Abuse/ PhysicianSelfReferral/advisory_opinions.html.

95. See *In re Caremark International, Inc.*, 698 A.2d 959, 970 (Del. Ch. 1996).

96. See, e.g., OIG Supplemental Compliance Program Guidance for Hospitals, 70 Fed. Reg. 4858 (January 31, 2005).

97. See Publication of the OIG Compliance Program Guidance for Hospitals, 63 Fed. Reg. 8987 (February 23, 1998) at 8988, 8990, 8998.

98. Office of Inspector General, Department of Health and Human Services, "Advisory Opinions" (2013). oig.hhs.gov/compliance/ advisory-opinions/index.asp. See note 79 *supra*.

99. See K. A. Peterson, Note, "First Nursing Homes, Next Managed Care? Limiting Liability in Quality of Care Cases Under the False Claims Act," *American Journal of Law & Medicine* (2000), 26: 69–88, n. at 72; J. R. Munich and E. W. Lane, "When Neglect Becomes Fraud: Quality of Care and False Claims," *St. Louis University Law Journal* (1999), 43: 27–52, at 36. See generally *U.S. ex rel. Mikes v. Strauss*, 274 F.3d 687 (2nd Cir. 2001).

100. 63 Fed. Reg. at 8998.

101. Office of Inspector General, Department of Health and Human Services, "Quality of Care Corporate Integrity Agreements" (2013). oig.hhs.gov/compliance/corporate-integrity-agreements/quality-of-care.asp.

102. Section 1899(f) of the Social Security Act, as added by section 3022 of the Affordable Care Act.

103. 76 Fed. Reg. 67992 (November 2, 2011).

104. 42 U.S.C. § 1320a–7a(b)(1) and (2).

105. 42 U.S.C. § 1320a–7a(a)(5).

106. 76 Fed. Reg. at 67999–68001.

ANTITRUST LAW IN HEALTHCARE

The U.S. economic system is based on free enterprise and market competition. The competitive market promotes the welfare of consumers by
reducing price, increasing quality, and providing freedom of choice. To
protect the competitive market and the free-enterprise system, Congress
enacted antitrust laws more than a century ago. As the U.S. Supreme Court
has explained, "Antitrust laws in general, and the Sherman Act in particular,
are the Magna Carta of free enterprise. They are as important to the preservation of economic freedom and our free-enterprise system as the Bill of Rights
is to the protection of our fundamental personal freedoms."[1]

Applying antitrust laws to the healthcare field involves unique and
fascinating problems of law and public policy because of the peculiarities of
healthcare economics and the pervasiveness of government regulation. First, a
significant dispute is ongoing as to whether market competition in healthcare
actually promotes or inhibits the welfare of consumers. As discussed in Chapter 5 with regard to certificate-of-need (CON) regulation, a serious question
exists as to whether competition among healthcare providers reduces the cost
of services, as it does in other industries. In fact, the economic theory of the
CON laws is that consumers are better served by less competition, greater
cooperation, and more intensive government regulation.

In addition, healthcare providers and payers operate under a complex
mixture of market competition and government regulation, which significantly affects the application of antitrust law in this context. As a practical
matter, we know how to apply antitrust laws to ordinary competitive markets,
by applying standard antitrust doctrines. We also know that we would not
apply antitrust laws to sectors of the economy that are completely regulated,
such as public utilities or other natural monopolies, in which market competition has been replaced by government regulation. What makes the application of antitrust law to healthcare so interesting is determining how to apply
antitrust principles to a unique market that is neither fully competitive nor
fully regulated but rather somewhere in the middle.

Some people argue that the healthcare industry should be exempt
from antitrust law, or at least that antitrust laws should be applied differently
in the healthcare context. Others argue that antitrust law should be strictly
applied to healthcare providers to encourage competition on price and quality. Predictably, this debate has not been resolved at one extreme or the other

but rather on an issue-by-issue basis. Thus, the healthcare industry is subject to standard antitrust principles in some ways, but healthcare is treated somewhat differently from most other industries in other ways.

These issues are not merely theoretical—they present real choices of law and policy. For example:

1. Should Congress grant statutory exemptions or immunities from antitrust liability for particular activities by healthcare providers, such as joint negotiation with third-party payers?
2. Should state legislatures enact statutes to replace competition with regulatory supervision of healthcare providers in their respective states, and thereby displace the operation of federal antitrust laws?

The healthcare industry has a long history of resistance to competition by some providers and third-party payers. In an effort to preserve the status quo, some physicians have resisted competition from nonphysician practitioners and have opposed expanding new methods of healthcare financing and delivery, such as prepaid group practice and managed care. Healthcare professionals have often tried to justify their actions as necessary to ensure quality of care[2] and have tried to preserve the status quo by means of ethical rules that have the effect of restricting competition.

However, the U.S. Supreme Court has made it clear that the goals of ensuring quality and maintaining ethical standards do not justify interference with free-market competition. Arguing that restraining competition was justified by the need to preserve quality or protect the public interest is no defense.

In an analogous situation involving professional engineering services, a professional organization's ethical code prohibited competitive bidding by members of the organization.[3] When the federal government challenged the ethical rule under the antitrust laws, the organization tried to justify its rule by arguing that price competition by professional engineers would reduce the quality of services and thereby endanger public health and safety. The Supreme Court flatly rejected the organization's defense and characterized it as "nothing less than a frontal assault on the basic policy of the Sherman Act."[4] In a subsequent case involving an organization of dentists, the Supreme Court reasoned that a professional organization "is not entitled to pre-empt the working of the market by deciding for itself that its customers do not need that which they demand."[5]

Even if they are trying to meet other important societal goals, healthcare professionals and organizations may not take matters into their own hands in ways that violate the antitrust laws. Under the economic policy adopted by Congress, we rely on competition to ensure quality and reduce prices.[6] This exclusive focus on competition as the only relevant value under antitrust law is different from many other areas of healthcare law, in which multiple values are balanced to achieve the best public policy. For example, the law of privacy recognizes that the important value of protecting privacy of health information must be balanced in some situations against the equally important value of protecting the public against an epidemic of communicable disease, as discussed in Chapter 6. The antitrust laws, in contrast, recognize only one value because that is the one value that was established by Congress as national economic policy. If competition does not adequately protect the public interest in a particular industry, then the solution is to ask Congress to grant a legislative exemption from the antitrust laws or to ask state legislatures to regulate that industry in particular ways. However, healthcare professionals and organizations may not take matters into their own hands and interfere with competition on the grounds of quality, consumer protection, or cost containment.

The Federal Antitrust Laws

Organizations and individuals face severe civil and criminal penalties for violating federal antitrust laws. In criminal cases for price fixing, individuals have been sent to prison and corporations have been required to pay significant fines. In addition, federal and state governments may enforce antitrust laws in civil cases.

Private parties who are injured by antitrust violations may file their own civil actions in federal district court. In that type of case, a successful plaintiff would recover an amount of money equal to three times its actual damages, which is called treble damages, as well as the attorney's fees the plaintiff incurred in bringing the case. Under these circumstances, antitrust cases usually involve large sums of money, and even a successful defense can be extremely time consuming and expensive.

Federal antitrust laws are applicable to individual healthcare professionals as well as to healthcare facilities and organizations. These laws apply to tax-exempt, nonprofit organizations as well as for-profit businesses. Federal antitrust laws even apply to public healthcare facilities that are owned by units of local government, although antitrust laws apply somewhat differently to those agencies.

At the federal level, antitrust laws are enforced by the U.S. Department of Justice (DOJ) and the Federal Trade Commission (FTC). The FTC provides information on its website about its antitrust actions in the healthcare industry, including the facts and results of specific cases.[7] In addition, the FTC and DOJ have provided guidance to the healthcare industry by issuing

"Statements of Antitrust Enforcement Policy in Health Care."[8] Those statements address specific activities, such as mergers and joint ventures, and they provide safety zones of conduct that the agencies will generally not challenge. As the FTC and DOJ explained, "Most of the nine statements give health care providers guidance in the form of antitrust safety zones, which describe conduct that the Agencies will not challenge under the antitrust laws, absent extraordinary circumstances."[9] To provide guidance on antitrust issues for healthcare providers participating in accountable care organizations (ACOs), in 2011 the FTC and DOJ issued their "Statement of Antitrust Enforcement Policy Regarding Accountable Care Organizations Participating in the Medicare Shared Savings Program."[10] This policy statement about antitrust issues in ACOs is discussed later in this chapter.

The next part of this chapter analyzes the provisions of the most important antitrust statutes and explains the elements that must be proven to establish a violation of each statute. Note that defendants might be able to raise one or more defenses in response to a legal challenge. Some of these defenses provide immunity from liability in antitrust cases, while other defenses merely provide immunity from monetary damages. These defenses are discussed in more detail at various parts of this chapter.

Section 1 of the Sherman Act

Section 1 of the Sherman Act[11] prohibits every contract, combination, or conspiracy in restraint of interstate commerce. As indicated in Exhibit 9.1, the plaintiff or prosecutor must prove three elements under § 1.

First, there must be a contract, combination, or conspiracy, which requires at least two independent parties that can agree, combine, or conspire with each other. This requirement would be satisfied in any activity by an industry or professional organization, such as a medical society or hospital association, because by definition that type of organization is a combination of independent parties. Ordinarily, officers and employees of the same corporation cannot conspire with each other or with their corporation. Similarly, two parts of the same organization cannot conspire with each other. Some courts have held that a hospital's medical staff is part of the hospital organization or is an agent of the hospital for the purpose of credentialing, which is the process of reviewing and making decisions about medical staff membership and clinical privileges. In those jurisdictions, a physician complaining about an adverse credentialing decision by the hospital and its medical staff could not establish that there are two parties capable of conspiring and would not be able to satisfy that element of a § 1 claim.[12]

As indicated in Exhibit 9.1, the second element under § 1 is an effect on interstate commerce. Usually this is easy to prove in a federal antitrust case because the concept of interstate commerce in this context is interpreted

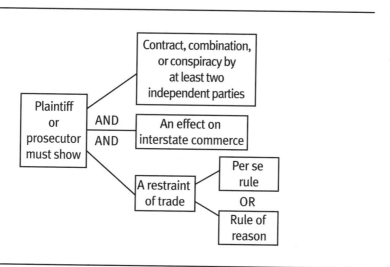

EXHIBIT 9.1
Section 1 of the
Sherman Act

broadly. For example, the Supreme Court held that an alleged conspiracy to block the construction of a local hospital, if proven, would demonstrate a sufficient effect on interstate commerce to invoke the federal antitrust laws.[13] In that case, the Supreme Court reasoned that preventing the construction of a hospital would reduce the flow of money and equipment across state lines. Subsequently, the Supreme Court held that even an individual physician whose clinical privileges had been revoked by a hospital had alleged a sufficient connection with interstate commerce to apply the federal antitrust laws.[14]

The final element of a § 1 claim is the need to demonstrate a restraint of trade. Taken literally, every contract or agreement is a restraint of trade. For example, if Person A makes a contract with Person B to paint A's house for $1,000, that contract restrains A from accepting a subsequent offer from Person C to do the same job for less money. Therefore, the courts have held that, despite its unlimited language, § 1 of the Sherman Act really only prohibits "unreasonable" restraints of trade. However, as discussed below, the term *unreasonable* as used in antitrust law is a technical term of art and does not have its ordinary, common-sense meaning.

As indicated in Exhibit 9.1, whether a restraint is unreasonable for purposes of § 1 may generally be determined in two ways: the **per se rule** and the **rule of reason**. Some types of restraint, such as price fixing among competing sellers, almost always have an adverse effect on competition. Therefore, rather than engage in a lengthy trial about the actual effect on competition in a particular case, courts will simply hold that the agreement is unlawful per se. Under those circumstances, the plaintiff will not need to prove that an adverse effect on competition exists, and the defendant will not be allowed to argue that its activities really promoted competition on the

Per se rule
The rule in antitrust cases that some types of restraint have an adverse effect on competition without the need for any evidence.

Rule of reason
The rule in antitrust cases of determining the effect on competition on the basis of evidence in each case.

facts of that particular case. Traditionally, courts have used per se analysis in cases of price fixing, boycott, and market allocation.

Price Fixing

Price fixing
An unlawful agreement between competitors on prices, such as an agreement on raising, lowering, or maintaining prices.

Price fixing is one of the most serious types of antitrust violation. Under antitrust laws, each seller of goods or services must decide on its own price and may not agree with other competing sellers on the prices that each of them will charge. In the healthcare field, it would be unlawful for competing hospitals or other providers to agree on their prices or agree not to grant discounts to third-party payers.[15] An agreement on price between competitors would be unlawful even if they had agreed to reduce their prices or not increase their prices. Cost containment is not a defense to a claim of violating federal antitrust laws. Thus, the Supreme Court held that it was unlawful per se for a group of competing physicians to agree among themselves on the maximum fees they would charge to certain third-party payers.[16]

However, price fixing is not limited to an explicit agreement on price, which is reached in the proverbial smoke-filled back room. Rather, price fixing may include other methods of collectively affecting prices. For example, using the same sales agent to handle each competitor's goods or services would have the same practical effect as an explicit agreement on price among the competing sellers. In some cases, even the exchange of price information among competitors may violate antitrust laws by making it easier to avoid competing on the basis of price.

Boycotts

Boycott
An unlawful agreement to refuse to deal with another party.

Boycotts are joint, collective, or concerted refusals to deal with another party. Each person or firm may decide on its own not to do business with a particular person or corporation. However, competitors agreeing among themselves that none of them will do business with that person or corporation would be unlawful. For example, physicians in the Michigan State Medical Society had unlawfully agreed among themselves that none of them would participate in the Medicaid program until the state increased the rates of payment for physician services.[17] Although a single healthcare provider or facility may decide not to participate in Medicaid or any other payment program, competing providers may not agree as a group to refuse to participate as a way of pressuring a payer to increase its rates.

When members of a labor union go on strike, they are engaging in a collective refusal to deal with their employer. They are jointly refusing to sell their services as workers until their employer increases their compensation or improves their conditions of employment. That type of collective action, however, is not an illegal boycott because Congress provided an exemption from federal antitrust laws by enacting federal labor laws. Those laws protect the right of employees to collectively bargain and collectively refuse to work. In contrast, labor laws do not provide an antitrust exemption for physicians or other healthcare professionals in private practice who negotiate with third-party payers because healthcare professionals are not employees of those third-party payers.

Market Allocation

Finally, antitrust laws prohibit **market allocation**, or agreements among competitors to assign particular products and services or particular territories to each of the competing sellers. Thus, two hospitals agreeing that one would have the only magnetic resonance imaging scanner in the region and the other would have the only lithotripter in the region would be unlawful. Although that type of decision may be made by a state CON agency, competing providers may not make that type of decision on their own.

Market allocation
An unlawful agreement among competitors to assign particular products and services or particular territories to each of the competing sellers.

 If a restraint does not fit within the category of per se illegal conduct, it will be evaluated under the so-called rule of reason. The rule of reason is really a misnomer. It has nothing to do with whether a challenged practice is reasonable. It has nothing to do with whether it is reasonable to promote competition over other societal values in the circumstances of that case. As the Supreme Court has explained, "the Rule of Reason does not support a defense based on the assumption that competition itself is unreasonable."[18] Rather, the rule of reason merely balances the positive and negative effects on competition as a result of the challenged conduct. As a practical matter, most business practices will increase competition in some ways and reduce competition in other ways. Under the rule of reason, the court will balance the positive effects on competition against the negative effects. If the net effect is that the challenged conduct reduces the level of competition in the marketplace, the conduct will be unlawful under § 1 because it is an unreasonable restraint under the rule of reason. For convenience, the rule of reason could be described as "the rule of determining the effect on competition on the basis of evidence in this particular case," while the per se rule could be described as "the rule of assuming the effect on competition in this type of case without the need for any evidence."

 In recent years, however, several factors have combined to make it less likely that a court would apply the per se rule in a federal antitrust case. First, with regard to boycotts, the Supreme Court has limited its use of the per se rule to those classic situations in which firms try to prevent suppliers or customers from dealing with their competitors, as opposed to other activities that might also be characterized as boycotts. For example, when a group of competing dentists agreed among themselves to not cooperate with utilization review procedures of dental insurers, the Supreme Court stated, "we decline to resolve this case by forcing the Federation's policy into the 'boycott' pigeonhole and invoking the *per se* rule."[19]

Quick look analysis
An intermediate standard for evaluating the effect on competition in an antitrust case, rather than categorizing the conduct as per se unlawful or subject to the rule of reason.

Second, the Supreme Court has taken a more complicated approach to the methods of determining whether a restraint is unreasonable. Rather than categorizing all conduct as either per se unlawful or subject to the rule of reason, the court has recognized a new category called **quick look analysis** and has acknowledged that the different categories of analysis can be somewhat blurred. "The truth is that our categories of analysis of anticompetitive effect are less fixed than terms like '*per se*,' 'quick look,' and 'rule of reason' tend to make them appear. We have recognized, for example, that 'there is often no bright line separating *per se* from Rule of Reason analysis.' . . . As the circumstances here demonstrate, there is generally no categorical line to be drawn between restraints that give rise to an intuitively obvious inference of anticompetitive effect and those that call for more detailed treatment."[20]

Finally, the Supreme Court has emphasized that *some* activities in industries such as healthcare should be analyzed under the more flexible rule of reason. The Supreme Court rejected the idea that healthcare is unique and that *all* activities in healthcare should be treated differently under antitrust law. Some healthcare providers argued that price fixing in healthcare should be evaluated under the rule of reason rather than the per se rule. However, in 1982 the Supreme Court held that, despite the peculiarities of healthcare economics, federal courts should apply the same rules to price fixing in the healthcare field as in any other industry.[21]

Nevertheless, the Supreme Court has indicated that *some* practices in the healthcare industry should be treated differently because they involve the services of professionals, such as medical doctors.[22] In the 1975 case of *Goldfarb v. Virginia State Bar*, the court held that members of "learned professions" are not exempt from federal antitrust laws, but some activities by professionals will be viewed differently from activities by nonprofessionals.[23] If healthcare professionals attempt to excuse their anticompetitive conduct on the grounds of "public service or ethical norms," their conduct will be evaluated under the rule of reason rather than the per se rule.[24] Thus, healthcare professionals are not immune from antitrust liability, but some conduct in the professional context might be viewed under more flexible standards.

In 1999, the Supreme Court reaffirmed the *Goldfarb* principle of special consideration for restraints that are imposed by professionals or professional organizations. In *California Dental Association v. FTC*,[25] the court reasoned that a professional association's ethical rules, which prohibited certain types of advertising, required a detailed analysis by the court to determine their effect on competition. In other industries, restrictions on advertising may be viewed as obviously anticompetitive because they are agreements by competing sellers to refrain from competing with each other. In the context of professional services, however, advertising restrictions might be procompetitive by preventing deceptive or misleading advertising in a market with informational disparities between provider and patient.[26]

Under these circumstances, healthcare professionals and their professional societies will have broader latitude to argue that their restrictions will promote competition and should not be declared per se unlawful under federal antitrust laws. In addition, the court's recognition of informational disparities in the healthcare market might provide a similar opportunity for healthcare facilities to demonstrate that their restraints are procompetitive. Nevertheless, cases that involve price fixing among competing healthcare providers might continue to be treated as per se unlawful. Remember that qualification for the rule of reason does not mean that the conduct was lawful, and it does not allow the providers to argue that it was reasonable to reduce competition. It merely allows the providers to attempt to demonstrate that their challenged conduct had a positive net effect on the level of competition in the marketplace.

Section 2 of the Sherman Act

Another important statute is § 2 of the Sherman Act, which prohibits **monopolization**.[27] Showing that two parties are involved who can agree, combine, or conspire is not necessary to prove monopolization under § 2 of the Sherman Act. A single entity acting alone may commit the offense of monopolization, and a § 2 claim for monopolization might be used as a fallback position by the plaintiff in an antitrust case.

Monopolization
The unlawful possession of monopoly power that was willfully acquired or maintained.

Note that monopolization is not the same as merely having a monopoly or having monopoly power to control a market. Some monopolies are perfectly lawful. For example, having monopoly power because of a better product or greater skill in business or because of historical circumstances is lawful. Similarly, having a monopoly because of a government franchise, such as a patent or CON, is lawful. As indicated in Exhibit 9.2, the plaintiff or prosecutor in a monopolization case under § 2 must demonstrate (1) the possession of monopoly power in a relevant market *and* (2) the willful acquisition or maintenance of that monopoly power. *Willful* is a term of art as used in this context. For the plaintiff in a § 2 case to prove a *willful* acquisition or maintenance of monopoly power, merely showing that the defendant acted intentionally or voluntarily to make as much money as possible is not sufficient. Rather, the plaintiff must prove that the defendant did something coercive or inappropriate to obtain or keep its monopoly power. One example of a coercive tactic is **predatory pricing**, which refers to pricing below cost to drive out a competitor with the intention of raising prices after the competitor is gone.

Predatory pricing
Setting prices below cost to drive out a competitor with a plan to raise prices after the competitor is gone.

What if a hospital has a monopoly as a result of holding the only CON for a particular service and then opposes another hospital's application for a CON to establish a competing service? As stated earlier, the initial acquisition of the monopoly would not constitute monopolization under § 2 because it was lawfully acquired by means of a franchise from the government.

EXHIBIT 9.2
Section 2 of the
Sherman Act
(Monopolization)

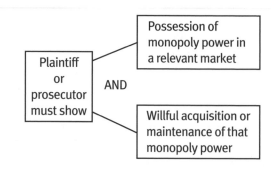

Noerr-Pennington immunity
A defense from antitrust liability that is based on the First Amendment to the U.S. Constitution and protects parties in requesting action from an agency of government.

Moreover, the CON-holder's opposition to another hospital's CON application would not constitute willful maintenance of monopoly power because opposing a competitor through the legal processes of government is lawful. In fact, a specific defense from antitrust liability protects parties in requesting action from an agency of government, as described in Exhibit 9.3. This defense is referred to as the **Noerr-Pennington immunity**, because of the cases in which this doctrine was originally developed.[28]

Under this doctrine, which is based on the First Amendment to the U.S. Constitution, individuals and organizations have the right to petition any agency of government for a legislative, judicial, or administrative action, even if their goal in obtaining governmental action is to harm their competitors. For example, one category of licensed healthcare professionals may request state legislation to restrict the scope of practice by other types of practitioners, thereby limiting competition from those other practitioners. Similarly, healthcare facilities may request a state CON agency to deny applications filed by their competitors. However, the Noerr-Pennington immunity would be forfeit if the alleged petitioning conduct was merely a "sham."[29]

Section 7 of the Clayton Act

Finally, § 7 of the Clayton Act prohibits mergers and acquisitions that might reduce the level of competition in the marketplace. Specifically, § 7 prohibits acquisitions in any relevant geographic market and relevant product market if the effect of the acquisition "*may be* substantially to lessen competition, or to *tend* to create a monopoly."[30] The language used by Congress enables enforcement agencies to prove a violation of § 7 more easily because they do not need to prove that a merger or acquisition will definitely reduce competition or create a monopoly. However, the government's advantage under the language of § 7 is reduced somewhat by the fact that the government bears the burden of proof in seeking a preliminary and permanent injunction.

Defense	Who can raise it?	What does the defendant need to prove?	What is the effect of prevailing on that defense?
State Action Immunity	Any defendant	Clearly articulated state policy to displace competition and active state supervision (but municipalities do not need to prove active state supervision)	Immunity from antitrust liability
Local Government Antitrust Act	Only units of local government	That it is a unit of local government	Immunity from antitrust damages
Health Care Quality Improvement Act	Any defendant in the peer-review or credentialing process involving an individual physician's membership or privileges	Fairness standards in § 11112(a), with a rebuttable presumption in favor of the defendant. Also, must have reported the results to state authorities	Immunity from antitrust damages
Noerr–Pennington Immunity	Any defendant	A genuine attempt to secure governmental action (but the immunity may be lost if the petitioning activity was a sham)	Immunity from antitrust liability

EXHIBIT 9.3
Antitrust
Defenses

Specific Areas of Antitrust Concern in Healthcare

Mergers and Acquisitions

As discussed in Chapter 4, a significant trend toward consolidation of hospitals and other healthcare providers by means of merger, acquisition, and other types of affiliation continues in the healthcare industry. The motivations for this trend include the pressures of healthcare cost containment, the effects of the economic downturn, and the needs of healthcare providers to position themselves for anticipated changes from health reform legislation. In particular, an increase in the number of hospital mergers has been observed.[31]

However, mergers and acquisitions in the healthcare industry raise important public policy concerns. Once they become parts of a single organization, former competitors will no longer compete with each other on price or quality. From the point of view of a large-scale buyer of healthcare services, such as a third-party payer, a merger or acquisition may prevent the buyer from forcing providers to bargain against each other for preferred provider contracts at a discount. Moreover, from the perspective of an individual consumer of healthcare services, a merger may eliminate nonprice competition, by which the merging parties formerly competed for the consumer's business by offering the most attractive package of quality, service, convenience, amenities, and choices. Concerns have also been raised about the elimination of some women's reproductive health services when a secular hospital merges with a religious hospital that opposes provision of those services.[32]

In one sense, a merger poses more of a threat to competition than temporary price fixing. The merged entities will never again compete with each other on price or quality, whereas price fixing may be temporary. However, a merger may have procompetitive effects, such as efficiencies and economies of scale, and it may create a more effective competitor that has the ability to challenge other providers in the market. Therefore, under federal antitrust law, a merger is not unlawful per se. Rather, a merger is evaluated on its specific facts to determine—or at least attempt to predict—the likely effect of that particular merger on competition.

In predicting those effects, we assume that organizations will act in an economically rational manner to maximize their profits. Some people have argued that nonprofit healthcare organizations do not have the same motivation as business enterprises to maximize their profits. However, nonprofits might need to increase their revenues to pay their rising labor and supply costs, subsidize their indigent care, and implement their strategic plans. Therefore, antitrust enforcement agencies usually assume that nonprofit healthcare providers as well as for-profit providers will raise their prices above the levels that would exist in a competitive market, if they can obtain the market power to do so. The underlying principle of merger analysis is to not allow a merger that would enable the combined entity to raise its prices above the competitive level.

To have that market power, a merged entity would probably need to have a large market share and few significant competitors. Therefore, we should not permit a merger that would give the combined entity a large market share in a concentrated market. This usually requires a factual determination of the product market and geographic market in which the merging parties do business. We cannot measure market shares in a vacuum, only as parts of a specific product and geographic market. Ordinarily, government agencies argue that the merging parties operate in a small market, of which they would have a large share after the merger. However, the merging parties respond that they really operate in a huge market, of which they would have only a small share.

For example, hospitals desiring to merge will often argue that they compete with other hospitals outside of their immediate area, but government agencies may view hospital markets as being local. Note that merging firms may sell more than one product or service and may have a different geographic market for each. Patients may be willing to travel farther for some services than for others. Thus, hospitals would have different geographic markets for their routine inpatient care, such as labor and delivery, as opposed to their tertiary care, such as open-heart surgery.

Once we define the relevant market, we can determine whether the merged entity would still face sufficient competition in that market to restrain its ability to raise prices, reduce quality, or limit output. However, antitrust enforcement agencies would also consider other factors, such as the likelihood of entry into the market by potential competitors, efficiencies that would be likely to result from the merger and could not be achieved otherwise, and whether one of the merging parties would go out of business and fail to survive as a competitor in the absence of a merger. Most important, the enforcement agencies would consider actual and potential adverse effects on competition as a result of the merger.

Initially, the government agencies were successful in challenging hospital mergers and won most of their cases.[33] However, between 1994 and 2000, federal and state agencies lost all of the seven cases they tried in federal courts.[34] In some of those cases, the government attempted to define the relevant product and geographic markets in an arbitrary and unrealistic manner, and the courts correctly rejected the government's challenge to those mergers.[35] However, the courts also seem to have been improperly influenced by their overt hostility to managed care organizations and by their desire to protect hospitals, especially nonprofit hospitals, from the cost-cutting process of managed care.[36] In light of those cases, many hospitals concluded that they had greater flexibility to engage in mergers and acquisitions, and that trend of consolidation may have contributed to an increase in the price of hospital services in the United States.

More recently, the antitrust enforcement agencies have changed their strategy for analyzing and challenging mergers, in healthcare and in other industries as well. The agencies have moved away from focusing so extensively on market definition, which is factually complex and easy to dispute. As discussed earlier, problems in defining the relevant market were among the difficulties that enforcement agencies experienced in challenging hospital mergers.

The new strategy focuses primarily on actual anticompetitive effects. In 2010, the agencies issued new "Horizontal Merger Guidelines" to replace

Horizontal merger
A combination of entities at the same level of production or distribution, such as a merger of competing sellers of the same product or service.

Vertical merger
A combination of entities at different levels of production or distribution, such as a manufacturer and a retailer.

their previous guidelines, which had not been revised since 1997.[37] These guidelines apply to **horizontal mergers** in all industries and not merely to mergers of healthcare providers. A horizontal merger is a combination of entities at the same level of production or distribution, such as a merger of competing sellers of the same product or service. In contrast, a **vertical merger** is a combination of entities at different levels, such as a manufacturer and a retailer. As stated in the new 2010 guidelines, "The Agencies' analysis need not start with market definition. Some of the analytical tools used by the Agencies to assess competitive effects do not rely on market definition."[38]

The agencies' new approach is consistent with established legal doctrine. In *FTC v. Indiana Federation of Dentists*, which involved an agreement by dentists not to cooperate with insurance company procedures for utilization review, the U.S. Supreme Court explained that the purpose of market analysis is to predict the effect on competition, and, therefore, evidence of an actual effect on competition makes it unnecessary to conduct a detailed market analysis.[39] As the Court stated, "Since the purpose of the inquiries into market definition and market power is to determine whether an arrangement has the potential for genuine adverse effects on competition, 'proof of actual detrimental effects, such as a reduction of output,' can obviate the need for an inquiry into market power, which is but a 'surrogate for detrimental effects.'"[40]

The FTC used this new type of approach in the hospital industry by challenging a merger in Evanston, Illinois, more than four years after it was completed.[41] As discussed earlier, a postmerger challenge provides some significant advantages to government agencies. Rather than attempting to predict the likely effect of a proposed merger in a battle of competing expert witnesses, the government might be able to introduce evidence of an actual adverse effect on competition as a result of the consummated merger. In addition, the FTC can pursue the case through its own internal process of administrative review, rather than bearing the burden of proving its case in federal court. If the FTC's administrative decision is later appealed to federal court, the appellate court should defer to it.

However, a postmerger challenge presents a significant problem in fashioning an appropriate remedy. Requiring merged hospitals to separate, after operating as a single organization for several years, is somewhat like trying to unscramble eggs. In 2005 the FTC's chief administrative law judge ordered Evanston Hospital to fully divest Highland Park Hospital, with which it had merged in 2000. Ultimately, the FTC agreed that the merger was unlawful but did not order divestiture. Instead, the FTC required the use of separate teams for the hospitals to negotiate their contracts with third-party payers.[42]

In addition to its postmerger challenges, the FTC has continued its previous practice of challenging some proposed hospital mergers. In some cases, the merging parties decided to abandon their challenged transaction. The FTC challenged proposed hospital mergers in Rockford, Illinois, and in northern Virginia, for example, which resulted in abandonment of both transactions.[43] Note that certain large mergers require prior notice to the federal government under the Hart-Scott-Rodino Antitrust Improvements Act.[44]

Nevertheless, the FTC and DOJ have established an antitrust safety zone to indicate that some types of mergers involving small hospitals are unlikely to be challenged.[45] Specifically, the FTC and DOJ stated that they will not challenge a merger of acute care hospitals if one of the two hospitals had fewer than 100 beds and an average daily census of fewer than 40 patients per day during the previous three years. According to the federal agencies, a merger with such a small hospital would probably not reduce competition: First, it may be a rural hospital with no local competitors. Second, a small hospital has few economies of scale and is probably not an effective competitor. Therefore, eliminating that small hospital as an independent competitor would probably not have an adverse effect on competition.

State Action Immunity

Even if a proposed merger does not fit within the requirements of that safety zone, the merging parties might be able to raise a defense in response to a legal challenge. The most important defense in the merger context is the doctrine of **state action immunity**, as shown in Exhibit 9.3. According to the U.S. Supreme Court, Congress did not intend the federal antitrust laws to apply to the acts of a state.[46] In light of the usual relationship between federal and state authority, this doctrine is somewhat counterintuitive. In effect, state action immunity is the opposite of federal preemption because state governments have the authority to negate federal antitrust law by deciding that the state does not want free-market competition in a particular sector of its economy. If the state elects to displace competition and substitute state government regulation, the federal antitrust laws will not apply in that sector of the state's economy.

Moreover, under some circumstances, federal antitrust laws do not apply to private parties that are acting under the authority of a state. For private parties to be protected by state action immunity, they must show two things.[47] First, the state must have adopted a clearly articulated policy to replace competition with regulation. Second, the private conduct must be actively supervised by the government of the state.

In some states, healthcare providers have obtained legislation in an attempt to extend state action immunity to certain cooperative activities such as mergers. State legislatures in at least 18 states have enacted statutes, known as **hospital cooperation acts**, that establish a process for regulatory approval

State action immunity
The rule that federal antitrust laws do not apply to the acts of a state or under some circumstances the conduct of private parties acting under the authority and supervision of a state.

Hospital cooperation act
A state statute that establishes a process for regulatory approval and supervision of particular activities by healthcare providers in an attempt to obtain state action immunity.

and supervision of particular activities by healthcare providers. The statutes express a clearly articulated state policy to replace competition with regulation and create a process for active state supervision of the private conduct. In those states, healthcare providers are not required to submit their activities to state government review. If the providers decide to do so, however, they might be immune from antitrust liability under the state action doctrine. Nevertheless, whether a state regulatory scheme will be sufficient, in its statutory authority or its practical application, to provide the active state supervision required for immunity from federal antitrust law is unclear.[48] In addition to questions about their legal effectiveness, state hospital cooperation acts raise important issues of public policy. As discussed earlier, a long-standing debate argues whether consumers of healthcare services are better served by government regulation or market competition. Even if government regulation is preferable, a serious question exists as to whether all state governments have the resources and expertise to properly evaluate hospital mergers and supervise postmerger conduct on an ongoing basis. Furthermore, whether state government decisions are sufficiently insulated from political influence by hospitals and members of their governing boards is unclear.

Finally, a problem has existed in applying the state action doctrine to mergers or acquisitions by public hospitals because different legal rules apply to the actions of municipal governments.[49] If a public hospital is owned by a municipality, it would not need to demonstrate active state supervision to qualify for state action immunity. Therefore, a merger or acquisition by a public hospital would be immune from federal antitrust law merely by showing a clearly articulated state policy to displace competition. Historically, federal courts made it easy for public hospitals to qualify for state action immunity by applying a low standard for showing a clearly articulated state policy to displace competition.

However, in 2013, the U.S. Supreme Court issued a decision in *FTC v. Phoebe Putney Health System, Inc.*, that set a higher standard and made it more difficult for public hospitals to qualify for state action immunity.[50] The Supreme Court explained that a clearly articulated state policy to displace competition cannot be demonstrated by a mere grant of authority from the state legislature to permit public hospitals to acquire other healthcare facilities or perform other ordinary powers of any public or private entity. Nor does enactment of a state CON law, which limits competition in some ways, demonstrate that the state had intended to displace competition in other ways. In a unanimous opinion, Justice Sonia Sotomayor wrote, "[W]e conclude that respondents' claim for state-action immunity fails because there is no evidence the State affirmatively contemplated that hospital authorities would displace competition by consolidating hospital ownership."[51]

Even if the local public hospital cannot obtain immunity from antitrust *liability* under the state action doctrine, it would still have immunity from antitrust *damages* under the Local Government Antitrust Act of 1984.[52] This federal statute provides that units of local government cannot be held liable for damages in antitrust cases. Therefore, in a suit under federal antitrust law, hospitals that are owned by units of local government are subject only to injunctive relief.

Medical Staff Membership and Clinical Privileges

As discussed in Chapter 7, medical peer review and credentialing are important parts of the system of quality control in healthcare organizations. However, peer review has an inherent danger of anticompetitive conduct, because individual physicians and other practitioners are being evaluated and possibly excluded by their direct competitors. Although the ultimate decisions on membership and privileges are made by the governing body, the competing providers on the medical staff wield substantial influence over those decisions. Therefore, it is not only important to preserve the system of medical peer review but also to ensure that a viable legal remedy is available to correct decisions that are biased or anticompetitive.

Most legal theories are ineffective in challenging an improper denial or termination of privileges, as explained in Chapter 7. In many cases, the record will contain evidence of both anticompetitive motives on the part of the peer reviewers and professional deficiencies on the part of the applicant. When a decision is made to deny or revoke a practitioner's privileges, the written decision is usually prepared by the organization or its lawyer. Therefore, it would not be surprising for the decision to contain some self-serving evidence of the applicant's inadequate performance. If the aggrieved practitioner appeals to a state court, the court will use a limited standard of judicial review. Under those circumstances, the state court is likely to uphold the decision of the organization because some evidence will support it.

In a federal antitrust case, the court should not be limited by that superficial standard of review. Instead, the federal court should permit the aggrieved practitioner to argue and produce evidence to show that the allegedly inadequate performance was merely a pretext to cover up the anticompetitive conduct.

In responding to an antitrust claim by an excluded physician, some healthcare providers tried to use the defense of state action immunity, as shown in Figure 9.3. However, the U.S. Supreme Court held that peer review activities are not protected by state action immunity, because those activities are not supervised by—or subject to reversal by—officials of the state government.[53]

Although the peer review process is not immune from antitrust law under the state action doctrine, the effectiveness of the antitrust remedy in this type of case has been severely curtailed. For an excluded physician to prevail on an antitrust claim is extremely difficult. First, some federal circuit courts have held that a hospital is not legally capable of conspiring with its medical staff or with the individual peer reviewers because those courts consider the medical staff to be part of the hospital organization or an agent of the hospital for purposes of peer review. As discussed previously, a physician whose privileges were improperly denied or revoked could not satisfy the conspiracy element of a § 1 claim in circuits that follow such reasoning. In addition, some courts have held that excluding a single physician from a medical staff or managed care network ordinarily does not give rise to an antitrust claim because it only harms an individual competitor and does not reduce the overall level of competition in the market. Finally, Congress has created a statutory defense for good-faith peer-review activities, by enacting the Health Care Quality Improvement Act (HCQIA) of 1986.[54] The purpose of the HCQIA is to encourage peer review by providing immunity from damages in physician-credentialing cases that meet the requirements of the statute. Although the aggrieved physician might be able to obtain an injunction to require the organization to grant or restore clinical privileges, the physician cannot obtain monetary damages, as shown in Exhibit 9.3.

To qualify for HCQIA immunity, the organization must have provided adequate notice and a hearing and must have reported the results to the state authorities. Moreover, the peer reviewers must meet the fairness standards set forth in the statute, such as acting with a reasonable belief that the action was in furtherance of quality care. However, the statute provides that a professional review action is presumed to have met those fairness standards, unless the plaintiff physician can rebut that presumption by a preponderance of the evidence. Moreover, courts have interpreted the HCQIA in a manner that is favorable to hospitals and peer reviewers by focusing on what reasonable peer reviewers would have done and by ignoring evidence of actual bad faith on the part of the peer reviewers.[55] Under these circumstances, the HCQIA makes prevailing in a credentialing case much more difficult for a physician, and it provides significant protection for participants in the peer-review process.

ACTIVITY 9.1: NORTH FLORIDA WOMEN'S CENTER

The North Florida Women's Center (the "Center") is a nonprofit organization that provides counseling and assistance to women in Tallahassee and nearby areas of Florida and Georgia. Last year, the Center's board of directors decided to expand its services by providing healthcare services to women, including obstetric and gynecological (OB/GYN)

(continued)

(continued from previous page)

services, family planning, contraception, and abortion. The Center will provide these services on a sliding-fee scale, depending on the patient's income and health insurance.

The Center has a written contract with Mary Ellen Stuart, M.D., who is licensed to practice medicine in the state of Florida and is board certified in OB/GYN. Dr. Stuart will care for a large number of patients, some of whom will have no health insurance and limited financial resources. Therefore, both the Center and Dr. Stuart intend to make extensive use of nonphysician providers, such as physician assistants, family nurse practitioners, and midwives. They also want their patients to have a choice in childbirth. Therefore, patients will be able to choose between home birth with only a midwife or hospital birth with Dr. Stuart. Dr. Stuart does not intend to use midwives at the hospital.

In October 2012, Dr. Stuart applied for medical staff membership and clinical privileges at Tallahassee General Hospital ("General"), which is owned and operated by the county and is one of seven hospitals in the county. Because General is close to the Georgia state line, General and its physicians treat a substantial number of patients from Georgia and Florida.

On November 15, 2012, while her application was pending, the 50 current members of General's OB/GYN staff held a meeting, which was called for the purpose of reviewing Dr. Stuart's application. At the meeting, several doctors expressed their concerns about Dr. Stuart, the Center's new healthcare program, the issue of home birth, and the use of midwives. They were worried about having to take care of the Center's home-birth patients in an emergency. For example, if a home-birth patient had a medical emergency during home delivery, the patient would be rushed to General, where she would be cared for by the OB/GYN physician on call, even though she was not the patient of that physician and that physician had never seen the patient before the emergency. The physicians indicated that the potential malpractice liability under those circumstances was problematic.

At the same meeting, a few doctors expressed their concern for the possible loss of business they would suffer with the opening of the Center's health services program. Although they did not want to care for indigent patients, they were concerned that they would lose some paying patients because the Center will offer more choices in childbirth

(continued)

(continued from previous page)

and a sliding-fee scale. The administrator of General was present at the meeting and said that the hospital would lose obstetric business if the Center and Dr. Stuart gave women the option of delivering their babies at home.

Dr. Samuel Jackson, chief of the OB/GYN department at General, reported that he had reviewed a sample of medical records for patients treated by Dr. Stuart at another hospital, and it was his professional opinion that Dr. Stuart did not provide good-quality care. In addition, he said Dr. Stuart had been sued for medical malpractice two years ago, and her malpractice carrier had settled the case before trial by paying the plaintiff $500,000. After hearing this information at the meeting, the OB/GYN physicians voted to recommend denial of Dr. Stuart's application for medical staff membership and clinical privileges on the grounds that she had failed to demonstrate her professional competence.

The next day, the hospital administrator notified Dr. Stuart in writing of the action taken at the meeting to recommend denial of her application for medical staff membership and clinical privileges. The administrator advised her that she had the right to a hearing on her application before the credentials committee of the medical staff. Dr. Stuart exercised her right to that hearing, at which she testified and was represented by legal counsel.

At the hearing before the credentials committee, the chief of the OB/GYN department, Dr. Jackson, testified that on the basis of his review of medical records, Dr. Stuart did not provide good-quality care. He also told the credentials committee about Dr. Stuart's malpractice settlement. In response, Dr. Stuart testified that her care of patients was appropriate and told her side of the story with regard to the malpractice case. After hearing the evidence, the credentials committee recommended that her application for medical staff membership and clinical privileges be denied, and that recommendation was adopted by the board of trustees of General on December 28, 2012. The next day, the hospital administrator notified Dr. Stuart of the decision and also reported the decision to the Florida State Board of Medical Examiners as required by state law.

One month later, Dr. Jackson and another member of General's OB/GYN staff, Dr. George Alexander, met with a representative of Happy

(continued)

(continued from previous page)

Family Health Plan. The administrator of General was also present at that meeting. The two physicians told the representative of Happy Family that they were concerned about the unsafe practices at the Center's new healthcare program. The two physicians also stated that they hoped Happy Family would not accept the Center and Dr. Stuart as participating providers with eligibility to receive payment from Happy Family. In fact, the doctors said that they were so concerned about the Center's unsafe practices that if Happy Family agreed to pay the Center and Dr. Stuart for services rendered to Happy Family patients, all of the other members of the OB/GYN staff at General would feel ethically bound to stop treating Happy Family patients.

The representative of Happy Family asked the two physicians whether all of the other OB/GYN physicians at General felt the same way. The doctors responded that all of the physicians at the meeting on November 15 had agreed that Dr. Jackson and Dr. Alexander should speak to Happy Family on their behalf. In addition, the administrator of General stated that General might have to reevaluate its contractual arrangement with Happy Family the next time that General's provider contract with Happy Family came up for renewal. One week later, Happy Family wrote to the Center and Dr. Stuart to state that Happy Family would not accept them as participating providers and therefore would not pay the Center or Dr. Stuart for services rendered to Happy Family patients.

Under these facts, what claims could Dr. Stuart assert *against the other physicians*, and what defenses could *the other physicians raise?* Be sure to discuss the elements of each potential claim and defense, as well as your evaluation of the likelihood of success on each claim or defense.

Note: Do not discuss any potential claims against the hospital; however, you may consider the hospital's participation as a possible conspirator.

Relationships Among Healthcare Providers and Third-Party Payers

Competing healthcare providers must act independently in setting their respective prices and negotiating with third-party payers. As a general rule, healthcare providers may not join forces with their competitors in an effort to increase their bargaining power against the insurance companies and other third-party payers who purchase their services.

Many healthcare professionals and managers of healthcare organizations find antitrust laws to be counterintuitive because those laws have the effect of protecting the interests of third-party payers in negotiating with providers of healthcare services. One of the purposes of antitrust law is to ensure the ability of buyers to bargain with sellers and to ensure the ability of buyers to make their own decisions about the trade-off between price and quality, even if some buyers prefer low price over high quality. Antitrust enforcement agencies generally consider the buyers of healthcare services to include third-party payers and not merely individual patients. Therefore, enforcement agencies use antitrust law to protect the ability of third-party payers to negotiate with providers for the lowest possible prices, if that is their preference, regardless of the effect of those low prices on healthcare quality or access to care. As discussed earlier, antitrust laws do not permit a defense that restraining competition was justified by the need to preserve quality or protect the public interest.

Moreover, some physicians and professional organizations have expressed frustration that antitrust laws permit a large insurance company to use its market power to force down the prices for physician services, but nevertheless those laws prohibit physicians from combining forces to level the playing field. The reason for this apparently disparate treatment is that the physicians and medical group practices are independent competitors, whereas a large insurance company is a single entity acting on its own. Of course, a group of third-party payers agreeing among themselves on the prices they would pay for physician services would be unlawful, but a single payer, acting alone, may use its market power to force down the price of physician services.[56]

In the past, some physicians argued that they should be allowed to negotiate jointly in dealing with third-party payers, under the exemption from antitrust laws for collective bargaining by labor unions. However, most physicians in private practice are not bona fide employees of the third-party payers with which they negotiate their prices. Therefore, those independent physicians are not entitled to the protection of the labor union exemption from federal antitrust laws. Some physicians urged Congress to amend the law to begin treating independent, competing physicians in the same manner as employees who are members of labor unions, and bills to that effect were introduced in Congress.[57] However, there is little or no justification for amending the law to treat competing physicians in private practice as if they were members of a bona fide labor union, and no bill to that effect has been enacted by Congress.

In some situations, independent physicians and medical group practices may lawfully work together. In other situations, such collective effort would be unlawful. In situations in which independent physicians are prohibited from negotiating jointly, they would also be prohibited from creating a single organization to negotiate on their behalf because that would have the same practical effect as joint negotiation. For example, some physicians and other providers have established organizations, such as independent practice associations (IPAs), to negotiate on their behalf in selling the services of all of the independent competitors.[58] Some IPAs are lawful and procompetitive, but others are merely vehicles for price fixing by independent competitors. The latter group has been described as "sham IPAs."

Although independent competitors are required to make their own decisions on prices, participants in a single economic entity may legally agree among themselves on the prices that will be charged by that entity. For example, if Physicians A and B decide to form a medical group practice, they may decide together on the prices at which the combined firm will sell the services of each physician. However, if A and B remain independent from each other, they may not agree on prices or use a joint sales agent to sell their services.

Between these two extremes are many business arrangements in which people and organizations work together in some respects but retain their independence for all other purposes. As discussed in Chapter 4, these arrangements may be referred to as joint ventures. For example, physicians and hospitals could establish a joint venture to sell a combined package of physician and hospital services while maintaining their independence for other purposes. As a practical matter, the providers in that joint organization might need to reach an agreement on the prices at which the organization will sell the services of all of its members. From an antitrust perspective, the issue is whether to characterize the providers' agreement on price as (1) an unlawful price-fixing conspiracy among independent competitors or (2) the lawful operation of a single economic entity.

If the new organization is not really an integrated entity, its pricing agreement is merely naked price fixing among independent competitors. It could be characterized as a "sham joint venture," and its conduct would be unlawful per se. However, if the new organization is an integrated joint venture, such as a group of providers who share financial risk for services they provide through the organization, the providers' agreement on price would *not* be viewed as unlawful per se. Rather, the collective pricing of an integrated entity will be evaluated under the more flexible rule of reason. Therefore, the threshold issue is determining whether the entity is sufficiently integrated to qualify for rule of reason treatment.

Qualifying for rule of reason treatment does not necessarily mean the arrangement will be lawful under the antitrust laws, as discussed previously. Even if an organization or joint venture is sufficiently integrated to be analyzed under the rule of reason, it would be lawful only if it has a positive net effect on competition. Therefore, a finding of integration is only the first step, and must be followed by an analysis of the likely competitive effects in the relevant market. This second step is similar to the antitrust analysis of a merger because it requires consideration of the likely effect on competition in the relevant product and geographic markets.

For example, some organizations of physicians and hospitals have tried to include substantially all of the physicians in a particular geographic area. Similarly, an organization might try to include most of the healthcare providers in a particular category, such as most of the primary care physicians in the relevant geographic market. Under those circumstances, the collective pricing by the joint venture would probably prevent third-party payers from forcing physicians and medical group practices to bargain against each other for preferred provider contracts. In addition, other networks might have difficulty finding enough physicians to be able to effectively compete with that joint venture. Therefore, the formation of that joint venture and its collective pricing would probably have an adverse effect on competition and would probably be unlawful even under the more flexible rule of reason. In contrast, a joint venture that included a smaller percentage of providers in each category might aggressively compete with other networks and providers on quality and price, thereby increasing the level of competition in the relevant market. Thus, the first step is to determine whether the entity is significantly integrated. If so, the second step would be to determine whether the entity is too large or too inclusive to have a positive effect on competition.

To develop a joint venture or network that is not too large, excluding some providers that want to participate in the group might be necessary. Although the excluded providers might complain, their exclusion should not create an antitrust problem because excluding a few providers from a network would probably not have an adverse effect on competition. In fact, excluding some providers might promote competition on price and quality and might encourage excluded providers to form a competing network. Therefore, exclusion of providers is usually analyzed under the rule of reason.[59]

Note that forming a lawful joint venture only provides legal protection for those agreements among the participants that are necessary to accomplish the legitimate purposes of the joint venture. It does not allow the participants to make collateral agreements to fix prices or divide markets for unrelated services. For example, two hospitals had made a lawful joint venture, under the supervision of the state, to jointly provide certain high-technology services. However, they later agreed not to compete with each other on other types of healthcare services and fixed the prices for unrelated services by collective negotiation through a joint sales agent. In a challenge by the state attorney general, the federal district court held that the joint negotiations with third-party payers and the market allocation agreement were unlawful per se, regardless of the legality of the original joint venture.[60]

These principles of antitrust law also apply to the formation and operation of ACOs. As discussed in Chapter 8, the 2010 Patient Protection and Affordable Care Act promotes the development of ACOs under the Medicare Shared Savings Program, in which groups of healthcare providers deliver quality care to Medicare patients in a coordinated manner and share the cost savings resulting from those efforts. However, the creation and operation of an ACO require healthcare providers to cooperate and share financial resources in ways that might violate existing laws about antitrust, fraud and abuse, and tax-exempt status. Therefore, federal agencies have issued guidance about the legal issues arising from ACO participation, such as the limited waivers from fraud and abuse laws discussed in Chapter 8.

To address the antitrust issues in ACOs, in 2011 the FTC and DOJ issued their final "Statement of Antitrust Enforcement Policy Regarding Accountable Care Organizations Participating in the Medicare Shared Savings Program."[61] As the FTC and DOJ explained, "the antitrust analysis of ACO applicants . . . seeks to protect both Medicare beneficiaries and commercially insured patients from potential anticompetitive harm while allowing ACOs the opportunity to achieve significant efficiencies."[62] The antitrust enforcement agencies concluded that an organization which meets the ACO eligibility criteria established by the Centers for Medicare and Medicaid Services (CMS) is likely to be a bona fide entity with clinical integration, rather than merely a naked price-fixing scheme by nonintegrated competitors. Therefore, the antitrust enforcement agencies will treat the ACO and its agreements with third-party payers under the rule of reason. The FTC and DOJ also created a safety zone for ACOs that meet specific conditions. If an ACO does not fit within the safety zone, it still might be lawful depending on an analysis of its likely effect on competition.

Conclusion

In applying antitrust laws to the healthcare industry, the underlying question of law and policy is how to address healthcare concerns other than competition, such as quality, access, and care for the indigent. Although we usually rely on the competitive market to improve quality and make services available, most people recognize that, in the healthcare system, competition alone cannot meet all of our policy goals. In fact, as one commentator has pointed out, competition and antitrust law have disrupted the traditional system of financing care for the indigent, under which hospitals had earned supra competitive returns as a result of their market power and then used those returns to cross-subsidize their care for the indigent.[63] Moreover, in the context of mergers between religious hospitals and secular hospitals, serious concerns have been raised about whether antitrust law can adequately protect the availability of women's reproductive services when the merging parties agree to eliminate services to which the religious hospital objects.[64]

Incorporating some of these healthcare policy concerns into the standard antitrust analysis might be possible. For example, antitrust laws encourage healthcare providers to compete on the basis of quality. One way to do that is by limiting participation on a medical staff or network to physicians who provide the highest quality of care. However, the definition of *quality* is broader than medical skill or patient outcomes and includes all types of nonprice competition, such as competition on the basis of amenities, convenience, and individual choice.

Nevertheless, some healthcare policy concerns simply cannot be incorporated into standard antitrust doctrine. Other ways must be found to deal with those policy concerns, such as by means of government regulation. For some situations, explicitly acknowledging the need for legal approaches other than antitrust law would be better. That would be preferable to ignoring healthcare policy concerns or allowing courts to ignore the law to achieve desirable results.

Notes

1. *United States v. Topco Assocs., Inc.*, 405 U.S. 596, 610 (1972).
2. U.S. Federal Trade Commission and U.S. Department of Justice, *Improving Health Care: A Dose of Competition* (July 2004), Chapter 1, page 28. www.ftc.gov/reports/healthcare/040723healthcarerpt.pdf.
3. *Nat'l Soc'y of Prof'l Eng'rs v. United States*, 435 U.S. 679 (1978).
4. *Id.* at 695.
5. *FTC v. Ind. Fed'n of Dentists*, 476 U.S. 447, 462 (1986).
6. *Nat'l Soc'y of Prof'l Eng'rs*, 435 U.S. 695
7. Federal Trade Commission, "Overview of FTC Antitrust Actions in Health Care Services and Products" (March 2013), 121. www.ftc.gov/bc/healthcare/antitrust/hcupdate.pdf.
8. Department of Justice and Federal Trade Commission, "Statements of Antitrust Enforcement Policy in Health Care" (August 1996). www.ftc.gov/bc/healthcare/industryguide/policy/hlth3s.pdf.
9. *Id.* at 5.
10. Department of Justice and Federal Trade Commission, "Statement of Antitrust Enforcement Policy Regarding Accountable Care Organizations Participating in the Medicare Shared Savings Program"

(October 28, 2011), 76 Fed. Reg. 67026. www.ftc.gov/os/fedreg/
2011/10/111020aco.pdf.

11. 15 U.S.C. § 1 (2007).

12. See, e.g., *Oksanen v. Page Memorial Hosp.*, 945 F.2d 696, 703 (4th
Cir. 1991).

13. *Hosp. Bldg. Co. v. Trs. of Rex Hosp.*, 425 U.S. 738, 744 (1976).

14. *Summit Health Ltd. v. Pinhas*, 500 U.S. 322, 333 (1991).

15. See *United States v. N.D. Hosp. Assoc.*, 640 F. Supp. 1028, 1039
(D.N.D. 1986).

16. *Ariz. v. Maricopa County Med. Soc'y*, 457 U.S. 332, 348–51 (1982).

17. See *In re Michigan State Medical Society*, 101 F.T.C. 191, 312–14
(1983).

18. *Nat'l Soc'y of Prof'l Eng'rs*, 435 U.S. at 696.

19. *Ind. Fed'n of Dentists*, 476 U.S. at 458.

20. *Cal. Dental Assoc. v. FTC*, 526 U.S. 756, 779–80 (1999).

21. *Ariz. v. Maricopa County Med. Soc'y*, 457 U.S. at 348–51.

22. See *Goldfarb v. Va. State Bar*, 421 U.S. 773 (1975).

23. *Id.* at 788 n.17.

24. See *Maricopa*, 457 U.S. at 348–49.

25. 526 U.S. 756 (1999).

26. *Id.* at 771–73 and n.10.

27. 15 U.S.C. § 2 (2007).

28. See *United Mine Workers v. Pennington*, 381 U.S. 657 (1965); *Eastern
Railroad Presidents Conference v. Noerr Motor Freight, Inc.*, 365 U.S.
127 (1961).

29. *Prof'l Real Estate Investors, Inc. v. Columbia Pictures Indus., Inc.*, 508
U.S. 49 (1993).

30. 15 U.S.C. § 18 (2007) (emphasis added).

31. B. Kendall (2012). "Regulators Seek to Cool Hospital-Deal Fever,"
Wall Street Journal, March 19, B10.

32. See generally J. C. Appelbaum and J. C. Morrison, "Hospital Mergers
and the Threat to Women's Reproductive Health Services: Applying
the Antitrust Laws." *New York University Review of Law and Social
Change* (2001) 1: 26.

33. T. L. Greaney (2002). "Whither Antitrust? The Uncertain Future of
Competition Law in Health Care." *Health Affairs* (March/April) 21
(2): 185.

34. U.S. Federal Trade Commission and U.S. Department of Justice, *supra*
note 2, Chapter 4, page 1 and note 7.

35. See, e.g., *Tenet Health Care Corp.*, 186 F.3d at 1053–54 ("The FTC's contention that the merged hospitals would have eighty-four percent of the market for inpatient primary and secondary services within a contrived market area that stops just short of including a regional hospital . . . that is closer to many patients than the Poplar Bluff hospitals, strikes us as absurd").

36. See *id.* at 1055 ("Third-party payers have reaped the benefit of a price war . . . at the arguable cost of quality for their subscribers. Antitrust laws simply do not protect that benefit"); *FTC v. Butterworth Health Corp.*, 946 F. Supp. 1285, 1299 (W.D. Mich. 1996), *aff'd per curiam*, 121 F.3d 708 (6th Cir. 1997). See also Greaney, *supra* note 33.

37. U.S. Department of Justice and Federal Trade Commission, "Horizontal Merger Guidelines" (August 19, 2010). www.ftc.gov/os/2010/08/100819hmg.pdf.

38. *Id.* at 7.

39. *FTC v. Indiana Federation of Dentists*, 476 U.S. 447, 460–61 (1986).

40. *Id.*

41. *In re Evanston Northwestern Healthcare Corp. and ENH Med. Group, Inc.*, File No. 011 0234, Docket No. 9315. www.ftc.gov/os/adjpro/d9315/index.htm.

42. Federal Trade Commission, "Overview of FTC Antitrust Actions in Health Care Services and Products" (March 2013), 121. www.ftc.gov/bc/healthcare/antitrust/hcupdate.pdf.

43. *Id.* at 116–17, 120.

44. 15 U.S.C. § 18a (2007).

45. See U.S. Department of Justice and Federal Trade Commission, *Statements of Antitrust Enforcement Policy in Health Care*, statement No. 1. www.justice.gov/atr/public/guidelines/0000.htm#CONTNUM_106.

46. *Parker v. Brown*, 317 U.S. 341, 350–51 (1943).

47. *Cal. Retail Liquor Dealers Ass'n v. Midcal Aluminum, Inc.*, 445 U.S. 97 (1980).

48. See *FTC v. Ticor Title Ins. Co.*, 504 U.S. 621 (1992).

49. See D. M. Harris, "State Action Immunity from Antitrust Law for Public Hospitals: The Hidden Time Bomb for Health Care Reform." *University of Kansas Law Review* (1996), 44: 459–516.

50. *FTC v. Phoebe Putney Health System, Inc.*, 133 S. Ct. 1003 (2013).

51. *Id.* at 1005.

52. 15 U.S.C. §§ 34–36 (2007).

53. *Patrick v. Burget*, 486 U.S. 94 (1988).

54. See 42 U.S.C. §§ 11101–52 (2007).

55. See, e.g., *Austin v. McNamara*, 979 F.2d 728, 733–34 (9th Cir. 1992).

56. See *Kartell v. Blue Shield of Mass., Inc.*, 749 F.2d 922 (1st Cir. 1984).

57. See, e.g., *The Quality Health-Care Coalition Act of 2000*, H.R. 1304, 106th Cong. (2000).

58. See *In re Preferred Physicians, Inc.*, 110 F.T.C. 157 (1988) (consent order).

59. See U.S. Department of Justice and U.S. Federal Trade Commission, *supra* note 45, Statement No. 9.

60. *N.Y. ex rel. Spitzer v. Saint Francis Hosp.*, 94 F. Supp. 2d 399 (S.D.N.Y. 2000).

61. U.S. Department of Justice and Federal Trade Commission, "Statement of Antitrust Enforcement Policy Regarding Accountable Care Organizations Participating in the Medicare Shared Savings Program" (October 28, 2011). 76 Fed. Reg. at 67026, www.ftc.gov/os/fedreg/2011/10/111020aco.pdf.

62. *Id.* at 67026.

63. J. F. Blumstein (1998). "The Application of Antitrust Doctrine to the Healthcare Industry: The Interweaving of Empirical and Normative Issues." *Indiana Law Review* 31: 91, 93–94.

64. See generally Appelbaum and Morrison, *supra* note 32.

PATIENT CARE ISSUES

THE LAW OF TORT LIABILITY

10

O ne of the unfortunate realities of life is that some patients are going to have bad outcomes. Despite the tremendous advances in medical science, some patients are not going to get better but are going to get worse or even die. As a legal matter, how should our society deal with the problem of adverse medical outcomes and medical injuries?

One theoretical alternative would be to prosecute healthcare providers under criminal law in the event of an adverse outcome. When patients die, we could call the police to arrest the physicians and prosecute them for homicide. Certainly, imposing a criminal penalty would create a strong incentive for physicians to exercise their utmost skill and care. However, imposing criminal penalties would be inappropriate because adverse outcomes can occur without any error on the part of the physician. Moreover, criminal prosecution would quickly deplete the nation's supply of practicing physicians because some physicians would be sent to jail and others would drop out of the profession. Although a trend appears to be emerging toward increased use of criminal law in the patient care context, as discussed in Chapter 2, criminal penalties have been imposed on healthcare providers only in extreme cases.

Another theoretical alternative for dealing with a bad result is to allow patients to sue physicians or other providers for breach of contract. However, most healthcare professionals do not guarantee specific results for their patients but merely promise that they will do their best and use the appropriate level of skill and care in treating their patients. Therefore, rather than encouraging patients to sue healthcare professionals for breach of contract, our legal system deals with adverse outcomes under the tort liability system of medical malpractice.

A *tort* is a wrongful act that one person commits against another. In contrast to a breach of contract, a tort is not based on a voluntary contractual obligation. Nor is a tort necessarily a violation of the criminal law, which applies to wrongs against society as a whole. Rather, a tort is a wrongful act performed against another person, such as punching someone in the nose or injuring someone in an automobile accident. In our legal system, the injured person may recover monetary damages from the person who caused the injury to compensate the injured party for medical expenses, lost wages, and intangible losses such as pain and suffering. The law of torts is primarily a matter of state law rather than federal law.

There are different kinds of torts. Some torts, such as battery or defamation, are referred to as **intentional torts** because they require an intentional act, as opposed to mere carelessness. However, unlike intentional torts, the tort of **negligence** does not require proof of intent. Rather, negligence is based on a failure to exercise reasonable care under the circumstances. Thus, if Mr. Jones intentionally ran down Mrs. Smith with his car in an attempt to kill or injure her, that would constitute the intentional tort of battery. However, if Mr. Jones did not intend to hurt Mrs. Smith, but merely ran over her as a result of not exercising proper care, that would constitute the tort of negligence. Because healthcare providers do not intend to injure their patients, medical malpractice is considered to be a type of negligence, rather than an intentional tort.

In the context of medical injuries, the law of tort liability raises important issues of health policy. As discussed later, one of the goals of malpractice law is to improve the quality of care by driving out bad providers and causing other providers to be very careful. However, the deterrent effect of malpractice law is unclear, and the current system of malpractice law in the United States raises other issues of cost, quality, and efficiency. Therefore, in addition to understanding the current law of medical malpractice, it is important to consider the need for change and to evaluate the various proposals for reform.

The Tort of Negligence

Under the law of negligence, a plaintiff must prove four elements of the tort in order to recover damages from a defendant. These four elements are duty, breach of duty, causation, and damages.

1. *Duty.* The element of duty is the legal obligation to exercise reasonable care under the circumstances. We usually allow the jury to determine whether a defendant exercised reasonable care under all of the specific facts of the case. In cases of alleged professional negligence, however, we do not simply allow a jury to decide what it thinks that reasonable care would require. Instead, professionals are required to meet the **standard of care**, which is the routine practice of similar professionals under similar circumstances in the same or similar communities. For example, how do other physicians in the same or similar communities routinely treat patients with a particular medical condition or particular symptoms? Which diagnostic tests do other physicians in the same or

---

Intentional tort
A civil wrong committed deliberately by one person against another for violation of a legal duty other than a contract between the parties.

Negligence
A civil wrong based on a failure to meet the duty imposed by law to exercise reasonable care under the circumstances.

Standard of care
The routine practice of similar professionals under similar circumstances in the same or similar communities.

similar communities routinely use for patients in similar circumstances? Ordinarily, members of a jury would not know what a professional, such as a physician, must do in order to meet the standard of care in particular circumstances. Therefore, the standard of care usually must be established by the testimony of an expert witness, who is familiar with the routine practice of similar professionals in the same or similar communities.

2. *Breach of duty.* The plaintiff must also establish that the healthcare professional breached the duty by failing to meet the applicable standard of care. In most cases, it is necessary to introduce expert testimony on this issue as well. Of course, defendants may respond by introducing the testimony of their own expert witnesses, and the result is often a battle of experts from each side, with the jury evaluating the persuasiveness and credibility of each expert.

3. *Causation.* A plaintiff must prove that the healthcare professional's breach of duty was the *cause* of the plaintiff's injuries. Even if a plaintiff can establish a duty and a breach of duty, the plaintiff may not recover damages if the injuries or death would have occurred anyway, regardless of what the healthcare professional had done.

4. *Damages.* Finally, a plaintiff must prove that she suffered damage. If a plaintiff can prove all four of these elements, monetary damages may be awarded to compensate the plaintiff for tangible losses, such as medical expenses and lost wages, as well as for intangible losses, such as pain and suffering.

Imposing Negligence Liability on the Institution or Organization

If a plaintiff can prove all four elements of negligence with regard to the individual healthcare professional, that professional may be held personally liable for damages. Aside from the liability of the individual healthcare professional, one of the most important and interesting issues in the law of medical malpractice is the extent to which a healthcare organization, such as a hospital or managed care organization (MCO) may be held liable to an injured patient.

As a general rule, our legal system only imposes liability on a person or organization when that person or organization was at fault, not merely because an injury has occurred. However, under a legal doctrine known as **respondeat superior**, organizations may be held *vicariously liable* for the negligent acts of their employees or agents who are acting within the scope of their employment or agency relationship, even if the organization was

Respondeat superior
The legal doctrine that organizations may be held liable for the negligent acts of their employees or agents who are acting within the scope of their employment or agency relationship.

not at fault in any way. In other words, the organization is held liable for the negligent act of its employee or agent, rather than for any negligence or fault of its own. An **agent** is a person who acts on behalf of another person or organization without being an employee of that person or organization.

Agent
A person who acts on behalf of another person or organization without being an employee of that person or organization.

For example, if a truck driver negligently injures another person while driving for a trucking company, the company that employs the driver will be held vicariously liable for its employee's negligence. In fact, the trucking company will be held vicariously liable under those circumstances even if the company had been extremely careful in selecting, training, and supervising its drivers. Although holding the company liable when it did nothing wrong may seem unfair, it would be even more unfair to place all of the loss on the person who was injured in the crash. If the injured person could only sue the truck driver, the injured person might be unable to obtain sufficient compensation because the truck driver might have few assets and little insurance coverage. Therefore, to ensure fair compensation to injured persons, the law will hold the trucking company vicariously liable. Then the company can spread the cost of compensation to society at large by increasing the cost of the goods and services it provides to its customers. In addition, the company can protect itself for the future by purchasing liability insurance. Rather than making the injured person bear the risk of an underinsured truck driver with insufficient assets, society uses the employer as a mechanism to compensate the injured party and spread the costs to society as a whole. In this way, our legal system imposes vicarious liability for reasons of public policy, even though the organization was not at fault.

In the healthcare context, the issue of vicarious liability often arises when patients attempt to impose liability on a hospital or other organization as a result of the negligence of a physician or other healthcare professional. It is relatively easy to impose vicarious liability on a hospital for the negligent acts or omissions of a nurse or technician because those categories of health workers are usually employees of the hospital in which they work. In cases of negligence by an individual physician, however, the legal issue of vicarious liability is more complex because of the relationship between physicians and hospitals or other healthcare organizations. In those cases, it is necessary to consider whether the negligent physician is an employee or agent of the organization. This raises the recurring issue of the legal relationship between physicians and healthcare organizations in the United States, which affects many aspects of healthcare law.

As discussed in Chapter 7, only a minority of those U.S. physicians who perform services in hospitals are employees of those hospitals. Some physicians have contractual relationships with a hospital to provide services in a particular department of the hospital, such as radiology, anesthesiology, pathology, or the emergency department. Generally, those hospital-based physicians are not employees of the hospital but are considered independent contractors. Finally, many physicians in private practice are neither employees of the hospital where they treat patients nor hospital-based physicians but merely members of the hospital's medical staff and have clinical privileges to admit and treat patients at the hospital.

Thus, the first step in determining whether to impose vicarious liability in a particular case is to determine the nature of the relationship between the organization and the allegedly negligent physician. If the physician was acting as an employee or agent of the hospital, the court might hold the hospital vicariously liable for the physician's negligent act. Thus, it is more likely that a court would impose vicarious liability on a hospital for the negligent act of an employed physician than for the negligent act of a physician in private practice who is merely a member of the medical staff. Even if a physician is not an employee or agent of the organization, a court might hold the organization vicariously liable under the doctrine of **ostensible agency**. If a hospital "held out" a physician to the public as its employee or agent by making it appear that he was the hospital's physician, and if the patient reasonably assumed that the physician was an employee or agent of the hospital, the physician will be treated as an employee or agent of the hospital for the purpose of imposing vicarious liability on the hospital. For example, courts might hold that emergency department physicians are ostensible agents of a hospital, even though physicians who work in emergency departments usually are not actual employees or agents of the hospitals in which they work. In those situations, patients go to the hospital for emergency care and the hospital provides a physician who appears to be an employee or agent of the hospital. In holding a hospital vicariously liable on the ground of ostensible agency, the court will not be bound by the terms of the physician's written contract with the hospital, nor by a sign in the emergency department that disclaims any employment or agency relationship between the physician and the hospital.

Ostensible agency
The legal doctrine that organizations may be held liable for the negligent acts of individuals who are not employees or agents if the organizations made it appear to the public that they were employees or agents, and the public reasonably assumed they were.

Under these circumstances, a hospital might be held vicariously liable for the negligence of an individual physician on two separate grounds: on the basis of an actual employment or agency relationship or on the basis of ostensible agency.

Aside from being held vicariously liable for a physician's negligence, hospitals may be held liable for their *own* negligence under the legal theory of corporate negligence. The legal doctrine of corporate negligence is based on a hospital's breach of its own duty to a patient, such as the hospital's duty to exercise reasonable care in permitting physicians to treat patients at that hospital.

In *Bost v. Riley*,[1] an appellate court reviewed the development of the legal doctrine of corporate negligence. The following paragraphs describe the circumstances surrounding the case, and a portion of the judicial decision in that case is also provided.

The name of the patient was Wade Lee Bost. Because Bost died as a result of his injuries, the lawsuit against his healthcare providers was filed by the personal representative of his estate. Therefore, the personal representative is the plaintiff in this case.

Bost died without having made a will, which is referred to as *dying intestate*. Therefore, the court occasionally referred to Bost as "the intestate" or "plaintiff's intestate." These facts are not relevant to the outcome of the case or the legal principles of malpractice liability, but they are helpful in reading and understanding the decision of the court.

At trial, the plaintiff (the personal representative) introduced her evidence in an effort to prove that the healthcare providers were liable for negligence with regard to Bost. Because a plaintiff has the burden of proof, she was required to present her case first.

At the conclusion of the plaintiff's case, defendant Catawba Memorial Hospital asked the trial judge to throw out the plaintiff's case against it, by making a motion for a **directed verdict** in favor of the hospital. The trial judge granted the hospital's motion, which ended the plaintiff's case against the hospital. In other words, the hospital convinced the trial judge that, as a legal matter, it could not be held liable for negligence and should be dismissed as a defendant in that case. Under those circumstances, defendant Catawba Memorial Hospital did not even have to introduce any evidence on its behalf, and the jury was not allowed to consider the case against the hospital.

Directed verdict
A decision by a judge during a trial that the plaintiff has not introduced sufficient evidence to support her claim under applicable law and, therefore, entering a verdict in favor of the defendant without the need for a decision by the jury.

Obviously, the plaintiff was disappointed about that decision and appealed that issue to the state court of appeals. The issue on appeal was whether a hospital could be held liable for negligence, under such circumstances as were presented by the plaintiff in that case. In terms of the technicalities of legal procedure, the plaintiff was appealing the trial judge's decision to grant Catawba Memorial Hospital's motion for a directed verdict at the close of the plaintiff's case.

After the appellate court reviewed the facts and the legal procedure in that case, it reviewed the development of the legal doctrine of corporate negligence, which had not been explicitly adopted by the courts of the state at that time. The court determined that corporate negligence was a recognized basis for liability in that state and described the duty that hospitals owe to their patients. Then the court proceeded to apply the legal rule of corporate negligence to the specific facts of that case. Following is an excerpt from the judicial opinion of the appellate court with regard to that appeal.

Bost v. Riley, 44 N.C. App. 638, 262 S.E. 2d 391 (citations omitted), *cert. denied*, 300 N.C. 194, 269 S.E. 2d 621 (1980)[2] (including the Syllabus by the Reporter of Decisions)

Plaintiff's intestate, Wade Lee Bost (Lee), was involved in a bicycle accident on 23 July 1974 in which he injured the left side of his body. On 25 July 1974 Lee was seen in the emergency room of defendant Catawba Memorial Hospital, Inc. (Catawba) and was admitted to Catawba under the supervision of defendant Dr. William J. Riley. Riley conducted tests and diagnosed Lee's injury as a delayed rupture of the spleen. Riley, a surgeon, performed a splenectomy on Lee and replaced blood lost as a result of the rupture. Following the operation, Lee was placed in the intensive care unit, fed intravenously and given various medications. Defendant Riley went on vacation from 29 July 1974 through 11 August 1974, leaving Lee in the care of his two partners, defendant Drs. Bernard L. Rabold and Louis Hamman.

Lee's progress improved from the time of the operation until the late evening of 29 July 1974, when he began experiencing abdominal pain, increased intraperitoneal fluid, perspiration, decreased blood pressure, rapid breathing and vomiting. Defendants Rabold and Hamman diagnosed Lee's condition as peritonitis, an infection of the peritoneal cavity. The doctors placed Lee on the antibiotic Geopen. Between 3 August 1974 and 4 August 1974 Lee's vital signs improved somewhat and the doctors, sensing an improved condition, removed Lee from the intensive care unit.

On 5 August 1974, Lee's condition took a sudden turn for the worse. His temperature shot up to 104 degrees, his blood pressure dropped substantially, his skin became pale and his abdomen showed a marked increase in distention and tenderness. Defendants Rabold and Hamman operated on Lee on 6 August 1974 and found a volvulus, a twisting of the intestine which blocked the passage of its contents and the blood supply. The doctors resected approximately three feet of gangrenous bowel. Post-operatively, Lee recovered poorly, developing a fecal fistula, malnutrition and septicemia, and was treated with antibiotics, steroids, hyperalimentation and transfusions.

(continued)

(continued from previous page)

On 23 August 1974 Lee was transferred to Baptist Hospital in Winston-Salem, his condition critical, under the care of Dr. Richard T. Myers. Three additional operations were performed on Lee, but his condition continued to deteriorate. On 27 January 1975 Lee died of liver failure induced by sepsis.

Plaintiff administratrix of Lee's estate sued defendants Riley, Rabold, Hamman and Catawba for malpractice. In the complaint it was alleged the defendant surgeons were negligent, inter alia, in failing to take adequate preoperative blood studies prior to the operation of 25 July 1974, damaging organs in the area of this operation, failing to diagnose and adequately treat Lee's intestinal infection, failing to adequately monitor Lee's progress, failing to provide Baptist Hospital with adequate information of Lee's condition, failing to keep plaintiff informed about Lee's true condition, removing an excess quantity of Lee's bowel, and failing to adequately treat Lee's condition both prior and subsequent to the operation performed on 6 August 1974. Plaintiff charged Catawba with negligence in the selection of the defendant surgeons to practice surgery in that hospital and allowing the surgeons to perform such surgery, in failing to adequately supervise and monitor the activities of the defendants, and in failing to adequately monitor the condition of Lee or require the defendant surgeons to keep better progress notes on Lee's condition.

At trial, plaintiff called as adverse witnesses the defendant surgeons and other personnel of Catawba, as well as two radiologists and Dr. Richard T. Myers, the surgeon who treated Lee at Baptist Hospital. Plaintiff also called Dr. Stanley R. Mandel, a surgeon practicing at North Carolina Memorial Hospital at Chapel Hill, who had reviewed Lee's medical records. At the close of plaintiff's evidence, all of the defendants moved for a directed verdict. The trial court granted only the motion of defendant Catawba. . . .

WELLS, Judge.

Plaintiff alleges error by the trial court in the admission and exclusion of evidence, the making of prejudicial remarks before the jury, granting defendant Catawba's motion for a directed verdict, charging the jury, and failing to grant plaintiff's motion for a new trial. . . .

Plaintiff also assigns as error the trial court's granting of defendant Catawba's motion for a directed verdict at the close of plaintiff's

(continued)

(continued from previous page)

evidence. Generally, a directed verdict under G.S. 1A-1, Rule 50(a) may be granted only if the evidence is insufficient to justify a verdict for the nonmovant as a matter of law.

Plaintiff argues that the evidence it presented at trial was sufficient to withstand defendant Catawba's motion under both the theory of respondeat superior and the doctrine of corporate negligence. Catawba could be found vicariously liable under respondeat superior if the negligence of any of its employees, agents, or servants, acting within the scope of their authority, contributed to Lee's death. However, because plaintiff's evidence failed to show that the physicians treating Lee were acting as employees, agents, or servants of Catawba, the principle of respondeat superior is inapplicable to this case.

In contrast to the vicarious nature of respondeat superior, the doctrine of "corporate negligence" involves the violation of a duty owed directly by the hospital to the patient. Prior to modern times, a hospital undertook, "only to furnish room, food, facilities for operation, and attendants, and [was held] not liable for damages resulting from the negligence of a physician in the absence of evidence of agency, or other facts upon which the principle of respondeat superior [could have been] supplied." In contrast, today's hospitals regulate their medical staffs to a much greater degree and play a much more active role in furnishing patients medical treatment. In abolishing the doctrine of charitable immunity, formerly available to charitable hospitals as a defense to negligence actions in North Carolina, Justice (later Chief Justice) Sharp acknowledged the changed structure of the modern hospital, quoting from *Bing v. Thunig*, 2 N.Y. 2d 656, 666, 143 N.E. 2d 3, 8, 163 N.Y.S. 2d 3, 11 (1957):

> *The conception that the hospital does not undertake to treat the patient, does not undertake to act through its doctors and nurses, but undertakes instead simply to procure them to act upon their own responsibility, no longer reflects the fact. Present-day hospitals, as their manner of operation plainly demonstrates, do far more than furnish facilities for treatment. They regularly employ on a salary basis a large staff of physicians, nurses and interns, as well as administrative and manual workers, and they charge patients for medical care and treatment, collecting for such services, if necessary, by legal action. Certainly, the person who avails himself of*

(continued)

(continued from previous page)

"hospital facilities" expects that the hospital will attempt to cure him, not that its nurses or other employees will act on their own responsibility.

There has recently been a great deal of discussion about the liability of a hospital for its corporate negligence.

The proposition that a hospital may be found liable to a patient under the doctrine of corporate negligence appears to have its genesis in the leading case of *Darling v. Hospital*, 33 Ill. 2d 326, 211 N.E. 2d 253 (1965), *cert. denied*, 383 U.S. 946, 16 L.Ed. 2d 209, 86 S.Ct. 1204 (1966). In *Darling*, the plaintiff broke his leg while playing in a college football game and was seen at the defendant hospital's emergency room by the physician on call. With the assistance of hospital personnel the physician put a plaster cast on the plaintiff's leg. The cast was put on in such a manner as to restrict the blood flow in plaintiff's leg. Plaintiff was in great pain and his toes become swollen and dark in color, and later cold. When the doctor removed the cast two days later much of plaintiff's leg tissue had died and the leg had to be amputated below the knee.

The Supreme Court of Illinois affirmed the jury's finding of negligence on the part of the hospital. The Court held that the jury could have found the hospital was negligent, inter alia, in failing to have a sufficient number of trained nurses attending the plaintiff, failing to require a consultation with or examination by members of the hospital staff, and failing to review the treatment rendered to the plaintiff. Since *Darling*, the courts of other states have found that a hospital's corporate negligence extends to permitting a physician known to be incompetent to practice at the hospital.

While the doctrine of corporate negligence has never previously been either expressly adopted or rejected by the courts of our State, it has been implicitly accepted and applied in a number of decisions. The Supreme Court has intimated that a hospital may have the duty to make a reasonable inspection of equipment it uses in the treatment of patients and remedy any defects discoverable by such inspection. The institution must provide equipment reasonably suited for the use intended. The hospital has the duty not to obey instructions of a physician which are obviously negligent or dangerous. We have suggested that a hospital could be found negligent for its failure to promulgate adequate safety rules relating to the handling, storage and

(continued)

(continued from previous page)

administering of medications, or for its failure to adequately investigate the credentials of a physician selected to practice at the facility.

Since all of the above duties which have been required of hospitals in North Carolina are duties which flow directly from the hospital to the patient, we acknowledge that a breach of any such duty may correctly be termed corporate negligence, and that our State recognizes this as a basis for liability apart and distinct from respondeat superior. If, as our Supreme Court has stated, a patient at a modern-day hospital has the reasonable expectation that the hospital will attempt to cure him, it seems axiomatic that the hospital have the duty assigned by the *Darling* Court to make a reasonable effort to monitor and oversee the treatment which is pre-scribed and administered by physicians practicing at the facility.

The plaintiff in the present case has introduced evidence tending to show that the defendant surgeons failed to keep progress notes on Lee's condition for a number of days in succession following the opera-tion of 6 August 1974, in violation of a rule promulgated by Catawba. Catawba took no action against the surgeons for their violation. While this evidence is sufficient to show that Catawba may have violated the duty it owed to Lee to adequately monitor and oversee his treatment, plaintiff has offered no evidence to show that this omission contributed to Lee's death. Where a hospital's breach of duty is not a contributing factor to the patient's injuries, the hospital may not be held liable.

Neither may the previously discussed impeachment testimony of Mr. Bost, which was hearsay, alleging that Dr. Myers called Catawba an "inferior hospital" and that Catawba unreasonably delayed its referral of Lee to Baptist Hospital, be considered substantive evidence of the quality of care administered by Catawba. There was also no evidence at trial that Catawba failed to use reasonable care in selecting the defen-dant surgeons to practice at the hospital. Accordingly, the trial court correctly granted defendant Catawba's motion for a directed verdict. However, as discussed previously, there must be a new trial with respect to the defendant surgeons for the trial court's failure to admit the above testimony as impeachment evidence.

Since plaintiff's other assignments of error are not likely to occur on retrial, we decline to address them here.

As to defendant hospital, affirmed; as to individual defendants, new trial.

Malpractice in the Context of Cost Containment and Managed Care

In an effort to control healthcare costs, health insurance plans and other third-party payers have used various techniques, such as utilization review, selective contracting, and financial incentives, for physicians to provide care in a more cost-effective manner. These techniques may be referred to collectively as managed care, and the health plans that use those techniques may be referred to as managed care organizations (MCOs). Those techniques are discussed in more detail in Chapter 14. At this point, however, recognizing the impact of those techniques on the law of medical malpractice and the liability of healthcare providers is important.

The goal of healthcare cost containment is not a legally recognized defense to a provider's failure to comply with the prevailing standard of care. Thus, a physician could not successfully defend a claim for alleged malpractice by arguing that she decided against using a routine test or treatment because it would not have been an efficient use of society's limited healthcare resources. What if MCOs or other third-party payers, using restrictive policies or utilization review, refuse to pay for services that previously had been covered and had become the standard of medical practice in that community? As discussed, the legal standard of care is established by the routine practice of similar professionals in the same or similar communities, rather than by the payment policies of third-party payers. Eventually, widespread changes in payment guidelines may cause changes in the routine practice of physicians in the community and may result in a "dumbing down" of the standard of care. In the meantime, however, physicians may be held liable for failure to meet the *current* standard of care, even though some of the payers have begun to refuse to pay for that care.

Another aspect of cost containment and managed care that may have an impact on malpractice litigation is the use of financial incentives for physicians to reduce their use of expensive tests and treatments. To reduce the cost of providing healthcare services, some MCOs give financial incentives to physicians, such as capitation arrangements and bonus pools, which shift a portion of the financial risk from the payer to the provider. If the physician is sued for providing inadequate care to the patient, however, the existence of a financial incentive to provide less care will certainly not be a defense for the physician. In fact, the existence of a financial incentive to provide less care might encourage the jury to make a finding of liability and to award a much higher amount of damages.

In some circumstances, an MCO or other health plan might be held vicariously liable for the negligence of a physician who provides services to individuals who are covered by that plan. If the physician is actually an employee of the MCO, it could be held vicariously liable for the negligence of that physician, even if it was careful in selecting and supervising its physicians. Thus, a court is more likely to impose vicarious liability in the context of a staff-model health maintenance organization (HMO) with full-time employed physicians, as opposed to an individual practice association (IPA) model, which is a looser network of independent physicians in private practice. Even if the physician is not an employee or agent of the MCO, courts might hold the MCO vicariously liable on the ground of ostensible agency, especially if the MCO or other health plan requires or encourages individuals who are covered by their plans to use physicians who are on the payer's list of preferred providers. In that type of case, the court may find that the MCO held out the physician to the public and made it appear that he was its physician, and the patient reasonably believed that he was the MCO's physician.[3] As in the case of physicians who work in hospital emergency departments, courts are likely to disregard the MCO's disclaimer of an employment or agency relationship in its contract with the physician or in materials that are provided to enrollees.

Finally, MCOs and other organizations might be held liable under the doctrine of corporate negligence for their own failure to exercise reasonable care in screening and monitoring physicians in their networks. Thus, the legal principles that were developed in the context of hospitals and other healthcare facilities have been extended to apply to new types of healthcare organizations in the system of cost containment and managed care.

Informed Consent

The legal doctrine of **informed consent** is based on the principle that people have a right to make the decisions about their own medical treatment. The classic statement of that principle was set forth in 1914 by Justice Benjamin Cardozo, who served on the New York Court of Appeals and the U.S. Supreme Court. As Justice Cardozo explained, "Every human being of adult years and sound mind has a right to determine what shall be done with his own body; and a surgeon who performs an operation without his patient's consent, commits an assault, for which he is liable in damages."[4] Moreover, for consent to be valid, it must be fully informed. Therefore, the patient must be advised of the risks and benefits of the particular treatment, as well as possible alternatives, before the treatment takes place.

The American Medical Association acknowledges the patient's right to obtain information from the doctor and explains that "[f]rom ancient times, physicians have recognized that the health and well-being of patients depends upon a collaborative effort between physician and patient."[5] However, as one

Informed consent
The legal doctrine that individuals have the right to make their own decisions about medical treatment after receiving the relevant information about risks, benefits, and alternatives.

author has pointed out, in ancient times it was considered ethical to conceal the patient's true condition, and even the American Medical Association's first Code of Ethics, in 1847, urged patients to obey their physicians and ignore their own "crude opinions."[6] Despite those historical attitudes, informed consent is now an accepted part of medical culture and patient expectations.

Of course, practical problems occur in explaining complex medical choices to patients with varying levels of education, especially under the time pressures of cost containment and managed care. In addition, some patients may be worried about their condition and unable to make decisions about treatment, and some patients do not even want to make those decisions for themselves. Even if patients want to make their own decisions, those decisions are susceptible to subtle influence by their physicians. In spite of all these practical problems, informed consent is a worthwhile goal for providers and consumers in the healthcare system, and it is an important expression of the ethical principle of autonomy.

Like medical malpractice, informed consent is primarily a matter of state law. Although state laws differ in some respects, most state courts agree on some general principles. As a general rule, consent may be given expressly, or it may be implied from the circumstances. In an emergency, when a patient cannot communicate and there is no time to contact a surrogate decision maker, consent may be implied and the patient may be deemed to consent to the necessary emergency treatment. However, if a patient who is about to undergo treatment explicitly refuses to consent to a particular type of procedure, then, even if an emergency arises during the treatment, the patient might not be deemed to consent to the performance of that procedure.[7]

Theoretically, one could argue that performing a medical procedure without informed consent constitutes the intentional tort of battery, on the ground that it is a harmful or offensive touching that is committed with intent and without valid consent. However, most courts are extremely reluctant to categorize the lack of informed consent as the intentional tort of battery because of the harsh standards under the law of battery and the possibility that the patient could recover punitive damages from the physician. Therefore, the vast majority of courts consider a lack of informed consent to be a type of negligence, rather than an intentional tort. Even in those jurisdictions that rely on a negligence theory, however, a battery action might be permitted in those rare cases in which the physician obtained no consent whatsoever or performed a different type of operation.[8] In contrast, the usual informed consent case involves an issue as to the adequacy of the information that was provided, and almost all courts evaluate that issue under the law of negligence.

As in any negligence case, a plaintiff must prove the four elements of duty, breach of duty, causation, and damages. Specifically, the plaintiff must prove that the healthcare professional breached the duty to reasonably disclose the risks to the patient and thereby caused the patient to suffer damages. In a claim for lack of informed consent, however, a plaintiff is *not* required to prove that the diagnosis or treatment was performed in a negligent manner, as is required in other negligence cases.

Whenever a medical procedure is performed, a chance exists that something will go wrong, even without any fault on the part of the healthcare provider. If a plaintiff is unable to prove that the treatment was performed in a negligent manner, she may still argue that she would not have undergone the procedure if the risks had been adequately disclosed. In other words, the injured patient may argue that she suffered damages as a result of agreeing to the procedure without adequate disclosure of the risks. A suit for lack of informed consent can be maintained *even if* the medical procedure was performed in a careful and appropriate manner. Under these circumstances, a claim for lack of informed consent is often a second count or a fallback position in a suit, which begins by alleging negligence in diagnosis or treatment and then alleges a lack of informed consent.

As stated previously, the element of duty in this type of case is the duty to reasonably disclose the risks. To determine whether the physician satisfied that duty, the court must determine *which* risks the physician was required to disclose. Obviously, some risks are so significant that they might affect the patient's decision on whether to undergo the procedure, and those risks could be described as "material." However, other risks are so theoretical and statistically insignificant that it would only waste time and create confusion to require their disclosure by the physician.

Courts of different states use different legal standards to evaluate the element of duty in a claim for lack of informed consent. In many states, a physician's duty to disclose the risks of treatment is measured by the standard of practice of similar physicians in similar circumstances. In those states, it would be necessary to introduce expert testimony on the standard of practice for disclosure to patients under circumstances similar to those in the particular case. However, other states measure the duty to disclose by what a reasonable patient would want to know in deciding whether to have the procedure. Under that test, the focus is on a reasonable patient in what the physician knows or ought to know to be the circumstances of the particular patient.

At the present time, most courts view informed consent as requiring only disclosure of the risks, benefits, and alternatives to the treatment recommended by the physician. However, on the cutting edge of the law, a few courts and commentators have indicated that a physician may be required to disclose other types of information to the patient as a prerequisite to obtaining the patient's informed consent. In fact, from the patient's point of view, there may be other types of information that would be material to the decision about whether to undergo the recommended procedure.

For example, some patients may want their physician to disclose his level of experience in performing the particular procedure, as well as his mortality

rate compared with that of other physicians who perform the same procedure.[9] Similarly, patients may want to know if their physician has a disability,
such as alcoholism or drug addiction, that might affect her performance.[10]
In addition, patients may want to know if the surgeon is HIV-positive or has
AIDS. A few courts have considered whether HIV-positive physicians have a
duty to disclose their HIV status to their patients to obtain informed consent
for invasive medical procedures, but that issue is still unresolved.[11]

Similarly, in considering the advice of their physicians, some patients
may want to know if their physicians have financial or other interests that
might affect their independent medical judgment. In one famous case, *Moore
v. Regents of the University of California*,[12] the physician successfully treated
the patient for leukemia by removing his spleen. However, the patient was
not informed that the physician and others were using the patient's discarded
spleen to develop a lucrative cell line, which they patented and sold to bio-
technology and pharmaceutical companies. Under these circumstances, the
patient could not argue that the procedure had been performed in a negligent manner. However, according to the patient, the physician had failed
to obtain his informed consent, because the physician did not disclose the
personal interests that might affect his medical judgment. In that case, the
Supreme Court of California agreed with the patient and held that "a physician who is seeking a patient's consent for a medical procedure must, in order
to satisfy his fiduciary duty and to obtain the patient's informed consent,
disclose personal interests unrelated to the patient's health, whether research
or economic, that may affect his medical judgment."[13]

However, whether the court really appreciated the implications of its
decision for the law of informed consent is unclear. In the modern healthcare
system, physicians have numerous economic interests, such as investments
in healthcare facilities and equipment, that could affect their medical judgment in referring a patient for additional tests and treatments. Moreover, in
the context of cost containment and managed care, some physicians have
financial incentives to reduce the level of care provided to their patients. If
the holding of the California Supreme Court in *Moore* really means what it
says, physicians—at least in California—who fail to disclose their financial
incentives may be held liable for failing to obtain their patients' informed
consent. However, whether the holding in *Moore* will be interpreted literally
or be applied outside its original factual context is unclear, either in California or elsewhere. For example, the Supreme Court of Illinois concluded, "a
physician's failure to disclose HMO incentive plans is significantly unlike the
egregious nature of the alleged behavior at issue in *Moore*."[14]

In fact, despite some cases to the contrary, most courts still interpret
the element of duty as merely requiring disclosure of the risks, benefits, and
alternatives to the treatment that is recommended by the physician. Therefore, most courts would hold that information about the physician does not

need to be disclosed as a prerequisite to obtaining the patient's informed consent. Even if a patient specifically asks the physician about her experience in performing a particular procedure, courts differ as to whether a misrepresentation on that issue by the physician would constitute a lack of informed consent.[15] As stated by the Supreme Court of Pennsylvania, "we hold that information personal to the physician, whether solicited by the patient or not, is irrelevant to the doctrine of informed consent."[16]

Aside from determining what a physician is required to disclose to satisfy the element of duty is a separate issue of how to evaluate the element of causation in a claim for lack of informed consent. In other words, how should the court determine whether the alleged failure to disclose was actually the cause of the patient's injuries? If the patient would have agreed to the procedure, even if the risks had been disclosed, any failure to disclose the risks was not the cause of the patient's injuries.

One alternative is to rely on the testimony of the injured patient, in hindsight, that she would not have undergone the medical procedure if the risks had been fully disclosed. This is referred to as the **subjective test**, because the patient is testifying about what is, or was, in her own mind. Obviously, relying on self-serving testimony by a patient in hindsight on the issue of the patient's subjective belief can lead to a great deal of abuse. Therefore, courts in most states use an **objective test** of whether a reasonable person, in the circumstances of the patient, would have consented to the medical procedure if the risks had been disclosed. In a jury trial, the jury's role is to determine what a reasonable person would have done under the circumstances.

In these ways, the law tries to accommodate the right of the patient to self-determination and the legitimate interest of the provider in avoiding unreasonable claims. In addition, the doctrine of informed consent is more than just a type of claim by an injured patient against a healthcare provider; it is the theoretical basis for a patient's right to refuse treatment, as discussed in Chapter 12. In addition, informed consent is an important part of the federal regulations on experimentation with human subjects.[17]

Subjective test
The legal standard to evaluate the element of causation in a claim for lack of informed consent on the basis of the patient's testimony in hindsight about whether he would have undergone the medical procedure if the risks had been fully disclosed.

Objective test
The legal standard to evaluate the element of causation in a claim for lack of informed consent on the basis of whether a reasonable person, in the circumstances of the patient, would have consented to the medical procedure if the risks had been disclosed.

ACTIVITY 10.1: JOHN PARKER

John Parker, age 35, was a self-employed consultant. When he moved to Littleville in 2012, he purchased health coverage for himself and his family from an MCO known as the Littleville Family Health Plan (the "Plan").

The Plan provides physician services to its enrollees through a network of independent physicians in private practice. Each of those

(continued)

(continued from previous page)

participating physicians has entered into a written agreement with the Plan. The standard agreement explicitly provides that the physicians are not employees or agents of the Plan. The Plan does not provide copies of its participating physician agreements to the patients who are enrolled in the Plan.

However, at the time that he enrolled, the Plan did send Parker an 87-page brochure. On page 54, the brochure from the Plan contained the following language: "We are very happy that you have chosen the Plan to meet all of your health care needs. To obtain services under the Plan, you will need to select a primary care physician (PCP) from the enclosed list of the Plan's participating physicians. Please note that these participating physicians are not employees or agents of the Plan."

Parker did not know any doctors in the area, but he selected Dr. Susan Green as his PCP because she was on the list provided to him by the Plan. Dr. Green is a solo practitioner in private practice, and she leases office space for her practice in a shopping center in the suburbs of Littleville.

On July 15, 2013, Parker began experiencing dizzy spells. He called Dr. Green's office and made an appointment to see her the next day. On July 16, 2013, Dr. Green examined Parker in her office and made a diagnosis of Swinehausen's syndrome. The standard treatment for that medical condition is to prescribe one tablet of pentamite (10 milligrams) once a day for three weeks. In her discussion with Parker, Dr. Green explained the risks and benefits of pentamite as well as the alternative forms of treatment, and Parker consented to take the pentamite as recommended by Dr. Green.

Dr. Green had a large supply of pentamite in her office, because a sales representative for a pharmaceutical company had given her several boxes as free samples. Rather than waste time and money by sending Parker to a pharmacy, Dr. Green simply gave Parker one of the sample boxes of pentamite.

The dosage information from the manufacturer stated that the appropriate dose of pentamite was one tablet (10 milligrams), once a day for three weeks. However, Dr. Green misread the dosage information and instructed Parker, both orally and in writing, to take ten tablets of

(continued)

(continued from previous page)

pentamite (10 milligrams each) once a day for three weeks. Parker did precisely as he was instructed by Dr. Green. At the end of the second week of taking the pentamite as instructed, Parker had a sudden heart attack and died.

As the personal representative of his estate, Parker's wife filed a lawsuit in state court against Dr. Green and the Plan. According to the allegations set forth in the complaint, Dr. Green was negligent in her treatment of Parker by prescribing the wrong dosage of pentamite. In addition, the complaint alleged that Dr. Green had failed to obtain his informed consent to the pentamite treatment. Although Dr. Green had informed Parker about some of the risks of taking pentamite, she failed to inform him of the risk that she might prescribe the incorrect dosage and thereby cause his death. According to the complaint, if Dr. Green had properly advised Parker of the risk of prescribing an incorrect dosage of pentamite, he would not have consented to take that medication, and he would still be alive today.

With regard to the Plan, the plaintiff alleged that it should be held liable for Dr. Green's negligence. In addition, the plaintiff claims that the Plan should be held liable for its own negligence in this case.

Please analyze each of the claims made by the plaintiff against Dr. Green and the Plan. Be sure to discuss all of the elements of each claim as well as your estimate of the likelihood of success on each claim. If you think you need any additional facts, state the facts that you think are needed, and explain how those facts would affect your analysis.

Proposals for Medical Malpractice Reform

The two purposes of the legal liability system for medical injuries are compensation and deterrence. As a society, we want to provide fair compensation to injured persons. In addition, by imposing liability on those healthcare providers that act in a negligent manner, we hope to deter negligent conduct in the future. Many believe that the current liability system does not work and does not accomplish those two policy goals. However, there are wide disagreements as to the reasons for the failure as well as the direction in which the system should be changed. This part of the chapter will evaluate the need for reform in the system of legal liability for medical injuries and then will analyze the advantages and disadvantages of various proposals for reform.

The Need for Reform in the Current System

Many healthcare providers and liability insurance companies complain that patients recover excessive amounts of money, including large awards for pain and suffering, because juries sympathize with injured people and assume that the damages will be covered by liability insurance. In some states and for some specialties, malpractice insurance rates have increased dramatically, and providers periodically encounter what they describe as a "crisis" in the availability of insurance. In a 2002 report, the U.S. Department of Health and Human Services (HHS) wrote that a "litigation crisis" has increased the cost and reduced the availability of malpractice insurance for many physicians, thereby threatening access to care.[18]

In addition to potentially reducing access to care, responding to malpractice litigation can be time consuming and expensive for healthcare providers. Even an unjustified claim can have an adverse effect on a physician's professional reputation.

The current tort liability system also increases healthcare costs by encouraging the practice of defensive medicine, in which physicians order unnecessary tests and treatments to protect themselves against claims of medical malpractice. Once those unnecessary tests and treatments become the routine practice in the community, they are part of the standard of care from which physicians depart at their peril. However, estimates of the cost of defensive medicine vary widely, as do estimates of the extent to which healthcare costs could be reduced by limiting liability for medical malpractice. According to the 2002 HHS report, eliminating defensive medicine would save the federal government and taxpayers between $25.3 billion and $44.3 billion per year.[19] In 2004, however, the U.S. Congressional Budget Office (CBO) concluded that limiting liability for medical malpractice would only lead to small savings in overall healthcare costs.[20] In a more recent analysis, the CBO concluded in 2009 that enacting a package of tort reforms would reduce total healthcare spending in the United States by approximately $11 billion in one year, which is roughly half of 1 percent of total healthcare spending.[21] The 2009 estimate by the CBO includes not only the savings from reduced utilization but also the direct savings from reducing liability insurance premiums. Moreover, the CBO took into account that many states have already adopted some of the malpractice reforms, and, therefore, some of the cost reductions have already been achieved.

Not surprisingly, plaintiffs' lawyers dispute the arguments by proponents of tort reform and insist that malpractice liability is necessary to compensate patients who are severely injured as a result of medical negligence. Moreover, they argue that neither medical licensing boards nor peer-review committees have done a good job of policing the medical profession, and, therefore, private malpractice litigation is the only viable way to drive out the bad physicians and deter negligent conduct in the future. They dispute the claims about the extent of defensive medicine and argue that the malpractice system actually contributes very little to the overall problem of healthcare costs. There are also some indications that the malpractice insurance "crisis" was caused, at least in part, by the failure of insurance companies to charge sufficient premiums in previous years and by the reduction in their investment income from the stock and bond markets.[22]

The empirical evidence on many of these issues is inconclusive, and contradictory studies and reports use different methodologies and assumptions. In 2003, the U.S. General Accounting Office (now known as the Government Accountability Office) concluded that premiums for medical malpractice insurance had increased "dramatically" in some areas and for some specialties and that those increases had resulted from a variety of factors.[23] However, other researchers found that the data contradict the perception of a crisis in malpractice insurance premiums.[24] Similarly, the evidence is inconclusive on the issue of whether the increase in premiums has an adverse effect on access to care.[25]

Whether too many lawsuits for medical malpractice, and, particularly, too many frivolous suits exist is also in dispute. One highly respected study in the *New England Journal of Medicine* concluded that the vast majority of patients who are injured as a result of negligence never even file a medical malpractice claim.[26] In that 1991 study, the researchers looked at more than 30,000 patient records from the state of New York. They determined that 1,133 of those patients had suffered an adverse event, which they defined as an injury resulting from medical management that increased the hospital stay or caused disabilities after discharge, regardless of whether that event was caused by negligence. Of those 1,133 adverse events, the researchers determined that 280 were caused by negligence but only eight of those patients filed a medical malpractice claim.

On the basis of that empirical evidence, the authors of the study concluded that the medical malpractice system was *not* accomplishing its goals of compensating injured persons and deterring negligent conduct in the future. As the authors reasoned, the tort liability system does not really compensate patients who are injured as a result of negligence because approximately 97 percent of those patients never even file a medical malpractice claim. Moreover, because 97 percent of the cases of negligence did not result in a claim, the vast majority of negligent providers were neither identified nor held responsible for their actions.[27]

The failure to hold providers responsible for their negligence raises the question of whether, in the healthcare industry, legal liability can deter negligent performance. Some evidence exists to demonstrate that the threat of legal liability can improve the quality of care. For example, the threat of liability encouraged anesthesiologists in the United States to improve the safety of their medical procedures.[28] However, as other experts have concluded, "the evidence that the system deters medical negligence can be characterized as limited at best."[29] Some of the reasons that malpractice litigation may fail to deter negligent conduct include the availability of liability insurance, the "poor fit" between negligence and the filing of claims, and the ability of hospitals to externalize—or force others to pay—the costs of the hospital's negligence.[30]

Empirical research also contradicts the perception that a large percentage of malpractice claims are frivolous or baseless. In one analysis, about two-thirds of the claims were meritorious in that the patient's injury was caused by an error.[31] The authors of that study also concluded that the litigation process was usually successful in distinguishing valid claims from invalid claims.[32] Based on data in the original study of malpractice claims in New York State, some people have concluded that a high percentage of claims that are filed lack merit, in the sense that the claimant was not injured as a result of negligence. However, a persuasive analysis of the original data demonstrates that the New York study does not support that conclusion, and was not designed to support that type of conclusion.[33] Under these circumstances, underclaiming is a more serious problem than overclaiming, and "portraits of a malpractice system that is stricken with frivolous litigation are overblown."[34]

Another argument in support of malpractice reform is that reducing the extent of legal liability would actually improve the quality of care by facilitating system-based programs of quality improvement. Rather than "shaming and blaming" individual healthcare professionals when something goes wrong, the modern trend in quality improvement is to improve the systems of care. Many people think that the current system of malpractice liability in the United States interferes with system-based efforts to improve the quality of care by discouraging physicians from cooperating with quality improvement efforts and disclosing their medical errors. Under this theory, quality improvement requires disclosure and analysis of medical errors, but physicians are unwilling to disclose their errors because they are afraid of legal liability for malpractice.[35] When they served together as U.S. Senators, Barack Obama and Hillary Rodham Clinton supported that theory in their joint article in the *New England Journal of Medicine*. As Obama and Clinton wrote, "The current tort system does not promote open communication to improve patient safety. On the contrary, it jeopardizes patient safety by creating an intimidating liability environment."[36]

Would reducing the risk of liability really increase the disclosure of medical errors? In theory, disclosure of errors could improve the systems for delivering care. However, available data do not support the claim that reducing liability would increase disclosure of medical errors.[37] For example, doctors in Canada are no more likely to disclose their medical errors, despite having a malpractice system in Canada that is much more favorable to doctors than the system in the United States.[38] The authors of that study concluded that U.S. and Canadian doctors have similar attitudes and experiences about disclosure of errors, and the culture of medicine appears to limit disclosure more than concerns about potential liability.

On the basis of the data, one could argue that the current malpractice liability system should be strengthened to make it *easier* for patients to recover damages and hold providers accountable for their negligence. However, in the debates on comprehensive healthcare reform, most of the proposals for malpractice reform have focused on ways to make it *harder* for patients to recover damages and hold providers liable as a means of reducing overall healthcare costs. Obviously, those proposals raise serious questions of ethics and public policy. First, limiting the ability of patients to recover damages may not actually reduce healthcare costs for society as a whole, as discussed later in regard to limitations on the amount of damages in malpractice cases. Moreover, even if healthcare costs could be reduced by limiting the recovery of damages, solving the cost problem of society at the expense of those patients who were injured as a result of negligence is inappropriate. Instead of reforming the tort liability system as a means of reducing healthcare costs, we should reform the system to better accomplish its original goals of compensation and deterrence. Alternatively, as discussed later, the current system of malpractice liability should be replaced by a new type of system that could accomplish all of these goals in a more efficient and equitable manner.

Advantages and Disadvantages of Various Proposals for Reform

Because medical malpractice is primarily a matter of state law, many of the proposals for reform are at the state government level, as discussed in detail later. Nevertheless, some of the federal proposals for healthcare reform have included changes to the tort liability system for medical injuries, and Congress has considered several specific proposals to limit recovery for medical malpractice. For many years, Republican members of Congress have been attempting to impose federal limitations on claims for medical malpractice, and these efforts have led to an ironic situation. Ordinarily, Republican members of Congress advocate a reduced role for the federal government and expanded authority for the states, but they have been arguing for many years for a federal preemption of many aspects of state liability laws. At the same time, Democratic officials and members of Congress, who often support an active role for the federal government, have argued that medical malpractice should be left under the traditional control of the individual states.

For example, in 1995 the Republican majority in the House of Representatives proposed to limit damages for pain and suffering in malpractice cases and proposed other changes that would have made it more difficult for patients to recover damages for medical malpractice.[39] In 2002, Representative

James Greenwood (R-PA) introduced a bill with 107 cosponsors for federal legislation that would preempt state liability laws unless those state laws were more favorable to healthcare providers.[40] On January 24, 2011, the proposed Help Efficient, Accessible, Low Cost, Timely Healthcare (HEALTH) Act of 2011 (H.R. 5) was introduced in Congress.[41] Among other things, that proposed federal law would set a cap of $250,000 on noneconomic damages; set a three-year statute of limitations on medical malpractice suits; and replace joint-and-several liability with a "fair-share" rule, under which each defendant would only be liable for its share of responsibility. That proposed legislation passed the House of Representatives on March 22, 2012, but did not pass the Senate.

In contrast, President Obama's Patient Protection and Affordable Care Act (ACA), which was enacted by Congress in 2010 and largely upheld by the Supreme Court in 2012, took a different approach to reforming the law of medical malpractice. Rather than imposing an overriding *federal* law of medical liability, the ACA encouraged *states* to develop alternatives to the current system, and provided federal grants for state demonstration programs to resolve disputes and reduce medical errors.[42] Meanwhile, many state legislatures have taken action in recent years to reform their malpractice liability laws, including many provisions that make it more difficult for patients to recover damages or impose limits on the amount of damages.[43] State legislatures have enacted laws that limit the amount of recoverable damages in various ways, as well as laws that limit attorney's fees and impose additional procedural requirements in malpractice cases. In addition to changing the system of liability, several states have taken steps to promote the quality of care, such as requirements to report medical errors. For example, in 2002 the Pennsylvania legislature enacted a statute that requires medical facilities to implement a patient safety plan, including a system for reporting incidents and a legal obligation to notify patients about a "serious event."[44]

One type of reform is to provide by statute that no plaintiff in a medical malpractice case may recover more than a specified amount, which is called a *damage cap*. Depending on the terms of the statute, the limit may apply to all damages or only to noneconomic damages, such as recovery for pain and suffering. For example, California's Medical Injury Compensation Reform Act limits noneconomic damages to $250,000, whereas Indiana's statute imposes a limit on *all* damages in medical malpractice cases. However, as discussed in Chapter 2, some state courts have held that damage caps cannot be enforced because they violate the applicable state constitution.[45]

The argument in favor of damage caps is that they appear to be the most effective way to limit the size of malpractice awards. However, a counterargument is that damage caps are unfair to the most severely injured patients.[46]

Would damage caps be an effective way to reduce healthcare costs for society as a whole? Limiting the amount of damages can be effective in reducing the cost of premiums for physician's malpractice liability insurance. However, those liability insurance premiums are only a small part of overall healthcare costs. The more important issues are whether damage caps would significantly reduce the practice of defensive medicine and how much money that would actually save for the healthcare system. Aside from fear of liability, some physicians might order unnecessary tests for other reasons, such as financial incentives to perform tests or utilize equipment.

As a thought experiment, imagine that you are a physician in a U.S. state that does not have a cap on damages. You know that you can be sued by your patients for all of their economic damages, such as lost wages and medical expenses, as well as for their noneconomic damages, such as pain and suffering. Also, you know that a lawsuit against you will take a lot of your time and will harm your professional reputation. You probably recognize that you might be tempted to practice defensive medicine, in order to protect yourself. Now, imagine that your state government has just adopted a malpractice reform law which limits the amount of damages for which you can be sued. Even after enactment of that law, you can still be sued for medical malpractice, which will harm your reputation and take a lot of your time. However, now the amount of potential damages, or at least the amount of potential noneconomic damages, is limited. In light of this new damage cap, how much less defensive medicine will you practice? Clearly, limiting the amount of damages will not really prevent defensive medicine.

Aside from damage caps, many states have enacted or considered other reforms to reduce the amount of recovery in malpractice cases. For example, under the **collateral source rule**, healthcare providers may be held liable for all of the damages incurred by the patient, including medical expenses and lost wages, even if the patient has already received compensation for those losses through health or disability insurance. The theory behind the collateral source rule is that the negligent provider should not reap the benefit of the insurance premiums that were paid over many years by the patient. However, the rule may allow double recovery by the patient from both the healthcare provider and the collateral source. Therefore, several states have changed the rule to require the court to reduce the damages by the amount of other benefits or to require the court to notify the jury about the patient's other benefits. In addition, several states have enacted limits on legal fees, made legislative changes to legal standards, or imposed strict qualifications for medical expert witnesses.

Each plaintiff in a malpractice case must find an expert witness who is familiar with practice in that community or similar communities, but physicians may be unwilling to testify against their local colleagues. Some people

Collateral source rule
The legal principle that plaintiffs may recover damages from defendants to compensate for losses even if they have already received compensation for those losses from other sources, such as insurance.

refer to this as the "conspiracy of silence." Often, plaintiffs must look elsewhere to find medical experts, but defendants complain about bringing these "hired guns" from another region of the country. Some state governments have responded by raising the standards for medical experts in malpractice litigation. For example, some states now require medical expert witnesses to actively practice in a similar specialty as the defendant, rather than merely being a professional expert witness. Strict requirements for medical expert witnesses are likely to help defendants, by assuring that a plaintiff's expert has sufficient knowledge about the relevant specialty and about medical practice in that type of community. In addition, those requirements can make it more difficult for a plaintiff to find an expert who will be allowed to testify, and can have the effect of reducing lawsuits and payments.

Alternative dispute resolution (ADR) is another widely discussed proposal to reform the procedure for handling medical liability cases. For example, the parties to a case might be required to participate in a mediation process in an effort to reach a negotiated settlement. Moreover, some states have encouraged or required malpractice cases to be screened by a panel before the case may be heard in court, in which instance the panel's decision might be admissible in any subsequent court proceeding. Some people think this type of informal ADR can avoid the time and expense of full-blown civil litigation, but others argue that a requirement for pretrial screening will merely add another step to a lengthy and expensive process.

In addition to mediation and screening panels, binding arbitration by a panel of arbitrators can be an alternative to a trial in court before a judge and jury. Arguably, binding arbitration would be faster and more economical than a trial by jury and would be less likely to be influenced by bias or sympathy. However, because it would deprive the parties of their right to trial by jury, it could only be used when both of the parties agree to do so. Therefore, binding arbitration is purely voluntary.

To encourage fair and efficient resolution of disputes, numerous states have also enacted reforms to promote disclosure and facilitate apologies for medical errors. According to the National Conference of State Legislatures, "In an effort to reduce medical liability/malpractice lawsuits and litigation expenses, state legislators and policymakers are changing the laws to exclude expressions of sympathy, condolences or apologies from being used against medical professionals in court. Proponents of these so-called 'I'm sorry' laws believe that allowing medical professionals to make these statements can reduce medical liability/malpractice litigation."[47]

Finally, some people think we should abandon our current fault-based system of tort liability because it fails to meet its goals and causes serious problems. As discussed previously, the current system fails to meet the goal of fair compensation. It is like a lottery, in which a few people get a lot of

Alternative dispute resolution (ADR) Procedures for handling controversies other than through litigation in court.

money, but most injured people get nothing. The current system also fails to meet the goal of deterrence because no persuasive evidence exists that the fault-based system deters negligent conduct.[48] The current system also fails to promote patient safety or improve quality of care, and it increases health-care costs. Small-scale reforms, such as imposing caps on damages, would not solve the problems of this system. They would not improve fairness in distributing compensation, deter negligence, or significantly reduce costs.

Therefore, some people think we should replace our current system with a no-fault system of guaranteed compensation for medical injuries. In advocating for a no-fault system, people often use the analogy of the current system of workers' compensation for employment-related injuries. In the past, workers who were injured on the job had to sue their employers in a fault-based system, and it was difficult for employees to prevail. Therefore, only a small percentage of injured workers would recover any damages, but those who won their cases might recover a large amount. Because of the obvious inequities of that traditional system, state governments adopted workers' compensation programs, under which employees can receive compensation in limited amounts from an administrative agency of the state without the need to prove that their employer was at fault. However, the employees no longer have the right to sue their employer in court for unlimited damages. Thus, the workers traded the amount of recovery for the certainty of recovery.

By analogy, some people think medical injuries should be compensated through an administrative agency process, without the need for the patient to prove that the healthcare provider was at fault. Like workers' compensation, injured patients would be limited in their amount of recovery but would be assured of some compensation for their injuries. Proponents of a no-fault system argue that it would be faster and fairer than the current tort liability system for medical injuries. In addition, a no-fault system would provide compensation for claims that are too small to pursue through the traditional litigation process. Critics of a no-fault system respond, however, that it would not adequately compensate those patients who suffer severe injuries and require the greatest degree of compensation. In addition, a no-fault system might increase the overall cost of medical claims, although the actual cost is difficult to project. Even without the need to prove fault, going through the process of proving causation would still be necessary because only injuries resulting from medical treatment would be compensated under a no-fault system. Finally, critics argue that a no-fault system would eliminate the deterrent effect of the current system by removing some of the incentive for physicians to exercise care in treating their patients.

Despite these criticisms, a persuasive case can be made for adoption of a no-fault system for compensating medical injuries. It would be fairer because it would compensate more injured patients. It would be more efficient because it would handle disputes in less time and at lower cost. Moreover, a no-fault system would be less antagonistic because patients would not need to prove negligence on the part of their healthcare providers. A no-fault system would not necessarily reduce deterrence because no persuasive evidence exists that the current fault-based system provides deterrence. For all of these reasons, a persuasive case can be made that a no-fault system is the best alternative for handling medical injuries. Creating a partial no-fault system might also be possible by limiting the system to those avoidable adverse events that result from defects in the system or process of care.[49] Clearly, malpractice reform is an important part of the ongoing effort to reduce medical errors, improve patient safety, and increase the overall quality of care. At the same time, developing a system of compensation that would be more efficient and less costly for the parties and the healthcare system as a whole is necessary. The challenge for the future is to make progress toward the goal of a more effective, efficient, and equitable system of compensation and deterrence.

Notes

1. 44 N.C. App. 638, 262 S.E. 2d 391, *cert. denied*, 300 N.C. 194, 269 S.E. 2d 621 (1980).

2. *Id.*

3. See, e.g., *Petrovich v. Share Health Plan of Illinois, Inc.*, 696 N.E.2d 356, 362 (Ill. App. Ct. 1998) (genuine issue of material fact as to whether IPA-model HMO was vicariously liable on a theory of apparent agency), *aff'd*, 719 N.E.2d 756 (Ill. 1999); *Boyd v. Albert Einstein Medical Center*, 547 A.2d 1229, 1235 (Pa. Super. Ct. 1998) (genuine issue of fact as to whether doctors were ostensible agents of the HMO).

4. *Schloendorff v. Society of New York Hospital*, 105 N.E. 92, 93 (N.Y. 1914).

5. American Medical Association, "AMA Code of Medical Ethics: Opinion 10.01—Fundamental Elements of the Patient-Physician Relationship." http://www.ama-assn.org//ama/pub/physician-resources/medical-ethics/code-medical-ethics/opinion1001.page.

6. J. Katz (1994). "Informed Consent—Must It Remain a Fairy Tale?" *Journal of Contemporary Health Law & Policy* 10: 69–91, at 73.

7. *Curtis v. Jaskey*, 759 N.E.2d 962 (Ill. App. Ct. 2001).

8. *Howard v. University of Medicine and Dentistry of New Jersey*, 800 A.2d 73 (N.J. 2002).

9. *Johnson v. Kokemoor*, 545 N.W.2d 495, 506–507 (Wisc. 1996) (trial court properly admitted evidence of defendant physician's lack of experience as comparative mortality and morbidity statistics).

10. Compare *Hidding v. Williams*, 578 So.2d 1192, 1198 (La. Ct. App. 1991) (physician breached the informed consent doctrine by failing to disclose prolonged alcohol abuse), with *Ornelas v. Fry*, 727 P.2d 819, 823–24 (Ariz. Ct. App. 1986) (trial court correctly refused to admit evidence of physician's alcoholism, because of a lack of foundation to establish the relevance of that evidence).

11. See, e.g., *Doe v. Noe*, 707 N.E.2d 588, 589 (Ill. App. Ct. 1998) ("While we acknowledge and follow the holding in *Majca* requiring actual exposure to state a cause of action under these circumstances, we believe that the duty issue now remains unresolved").

12. 793 P.2d 479 (Cal. 1990).

13. *Id.* at 485.

14. *Neade v. Portes*, 739 N.E.2d 496, 505 (Ill. 2000) (holding that a physician's failure to disclose incentives does not give rise to a claim for breach of fiduciary duty, because that would merely duplicate the existing claim for medical malpractice).

15. Compare *Howard v. University of Medicine and Dentistry of New Jersey*, 800 A.2d 73, 83 (N.J. 2002) (allowing plaintiff to attempt to prove that physician's misrepresentations constitute a lack of informed consent, subject to strict criteria), with *Duttry v. Patterson*, 771 A.2d 1255 (Pa. 2001) (evidence of doctor's experience and personal information is not relevant in an informed consent claim, even if patient asks, but patient may have a claim for misrepresentation).

16. *Duttry*, 771 A.2d at 1259 (footnote omitted).

17. See 45 C.F.R. §§ 46.116–46.117 (2006).

18. U.S. Department of Health and Human Services, *Confronting the New Health Care Crisis: Improving Health Care Quality and Lowering Costs by Fixing Our Medical Liability System* (July 24, 2002): 1–29.

19. *Id.* at 7 and n.31.

20. U.S. Congressional Budget Office, *Limiting Tort Liability for Medical Malpractice* (January 8, 2004). www.cbo.gov/sites/default/files/cbofiles/ftpdocs/49xx/doc4968/01-08-medicalmalpractice.pdf.

21. U.S. Congressional Budget Office, *Letter to the Honorable Orrin G. Hatch* (October 9, 2009). www.cbo.gov/sites/default/files/cbofiles/ftpdocs/106xx/doc10641/10-09-tort_reform.pdf.

22. R. A. Zimmerman and C. Oster (2002). "Assigning Liability: Insurers' Missteps Helped Provoke Malpractice 'Crisis,'" *Wall Street Journal*, June 24, A1.

23. U.S. General Accounting Office (2003). *Medical Malpractice Insurance: Multiple Factors Have Contributed to Increased Premium Rates.* GAO-03-702: 3–4. Washington D.C.: GAO.

24. M. A. Rodwin, H. J. Chang, and J. Clausen (2006). "Malpractice Premiums and Physicians' Income: Perceptions of a Crisis Conflict with Empirical Evidence." *Health Affairs* 25 (3): 750–58.

25. See U.S. General Accounting Office, *Medical Malpractice: Implications of Rising Premiums on Access to Health Care,* GAO-03-836 (2003) (confirming some reports of localized service reduction, while finding that some anecdotal reports could not be confirmed); D. Dranove and A. Gron, "Effects of the Malpractice Crisis on Access to and Incidence of High-Risk Procedures: Evidence from Florida," *Health Affairs* (2005), 24 (3): 802–10, 808 ("As might be expected in an area of such debate, our findings provide potential support for both sides of the debate").

26. H. H. Hiatt, B. A. Barnes, and T. A. Brennan (1989). "A Study of Medical Injury and Medical Malpractice: An Overview." *New England Journal of Medicine* 321 (7): 480–84; R. A. Localio, A. G. Lawthers, T. A. Brennan, N. M. Laird, L. E. Hebert, L. M. Peterson, J. P. Newhouse, P. C. Weiler, and H. H. Hiatt (1991). "Relation Between Malpractice Claims and Adverse Events Due to Negligence." *New England Journal of Medicine* 325 (4): 245–51.

27. Localio, et al., *supra* note 26, at 247–50.

28. D. A. Hyman and C. Silver (2005). "Speak Not of Error," *Regulation* 28 (1, Spring): 52–57.

29. D. M. Studdert, M. M. Mello, and T. A. Brennan (2004). "Medical Malpractice." *New England Journal of Medicine* 350 (3): 283–92, at 286.

30. M. M. Mello and T. A. Brennan (2002). "Symposium: What We Know and Do Not Know About the Impact of Civil Justice in the American Economy and Policy. Deterrence of Medical Errors: Theory and Evidence for Malpractice Reform." *Texas Law Review* 80 (7): 1595–637.

31. D. M. Studdert, M. M. Mello, A. A. Gawande, T. K. Gandhi, A. Kachalia, C. Yoon, A. L. Puopolo, and T. A. Brennan (2006). "Claims, Errors, and Compensation Payments in Medical Malpractice Litigation," *New England Journal of Medicine* 354 (19): 2024–33, at 2029.

32. *Id.* at 2029, 2031. See also T. Baker, "Reconsidering the Harvard Medical Practice Study Conclusions About the Validity of Medical Malpractice Claims," *Journal of Law, Medicine & Ethics* (2005), 33 (3): 501–14, 511 ("Negligence matters a great deal to the outcome of

a medical malpractice claim, and the litigation process weeds out most of the weaker claims").

33. T. Baker (2005). "Reconsidering the Harvard Medical Practice Study Conclusions About the Validity of Medical Malpractice Claims." *Journal of Law, Medicine & Ethics* 33 (3): 501–14, at 511.

34. Studdert, et al., *supra* note 31, at 2031.

35. Studdert, et al., *supra* note 29, at 287.

36. H. R. Clinton and B. Obama (2006). "Making Patient Safety the Centerpiece of Medical Liability Reform." *New England Journal of Medicine* 354 (21): 2205–2208.

37. Hyman and Silver, *supra* note 28, at 55; D. A. Hyman and C. Silver, "The Poor State of Health Care Quality in the U.S.: Is Malpractice Liability Part of the Problem or Part of the Solution?" *Cornell Law Review* (2005), 90 (4): 893–993, at 893 ("[T]here is no foundation for the widely held belief that fear of malpractice liability impedes efforts to improve the reliability of health care delivery systems").

38. T. H. Gallagher, A. D. Waterman, J. M. Garbutt, J. M. Kapp, D. K. Chan, W. C. Dunagan, V. J. Fraser, and W. Levinson. (2006). "U.S. and Canadian Physicians' Attitudes and Experiences Regarding Disclosing Errors to Patients." *Archives of Internal Medicine* 166 (15): 1605–11, at 1609.

39. See Medicare Preservation Act of 1995, H.R. 2425, 104th Cong. §§ 15301–15315 (1995).

40. Help Efficient, Accessible, Low-Cost, Timely Health Care (HEALTH) Act, H.R. 4600, 107th Cong. (introduced April 25, 2002).

41. 112th Cong., H.R. 5 (introduced January 24, 2011).

42. Patient Protection and Affordable Care Act, Pub. L. No. 111-148, § 10607 (2010).

43. National Conference of State Legislatures (2011). "Medical Liability/ Medical Malpractice Laws" (updated August 15). www.ncsl.org/issues-research/banking/medical-liability-medical-malpractice-laws.aspx.

44. 40 Pa. Cons. Stat. §§ 1303.307, 1303.308 (2006).

45. See, e.g., *Lucas v. United States*, 757 S.W.2d 687 (Tex. 1988).

46. See, e.g., F. Cornelius, "Crushed by My Own Reform," *New York Times* (1994), October 7, A2. See also D. M. Studdert, Y. T. Yang, and M. M. Mello, "Are Damage Caps Regressive? A Study of Malpractice Jury Verdicts in California," *Health Affairs* (2004), 23 (4): 54–67.

47. National Conference of State Legislatures (2012). "Medical Professionals Apologies 2011 Legislation" (updated August 15). www.ncsl.org/issues-research/banking/medical-professionals-apologies-2011-legislation.aspx.

48. M. M. Mello, A. Chandra, A. A. Gawande, and D. M. Studdert (2010). "National Costs of the Medical Liability System." *Health Affairs* 29 (9): 1569–77, at 1570 ("[r]eliable evidence about the deterrent effect of the tort system does not exist").

49. Mello and Brennan, *supra* note 30, at 1621–28.

LEGAL AND ETHICAL OBLIGATIONS TO PROVIDE CARE

I f you are ever arrested and charged with a crime, you will have the right to a lawyer. In fact, if you cannot afford a lawyer, one will be appointed for you at society's expense.

What if, instead of a lawyer, you need a doctor? Do you have the right to a doctor? If you cannot afford a doctor, will one be appointed for you at society's expense?

These questions raise the broader issue of whether citizens of the United States have a legal right to healthcare. Unlike the right to appointed counsel in criminal cases and unlike the right to a free public education through the twelfth grade, the U.S. system of government generally does not provide a comparable right to healthcare services.

Under the U.S. Constitution, the government cannot take away your life, liberty, or property without due process of law. In other words, the government cannot do bad things *to* you. However, the government generally has no legal obligation to do good things *for* you. According to the U.S. Supreme Court, the government has no constitutional obligation to provide necessary services, even if you would die without those services.[1]

This limited role of government may reflect the eighteenth-century views of the nation's founders, who essentially wanted the king of England and other governmental authorities to leave them alone. In contrast, in the modern social welfare state, government plays a much more active role in protecting and helping individual members of society. Many people believe that government should do things *for* people, rather than merely leaving them alone. However, the U.S. system has not yet developed a legal right to healthcare services, and the Constitution does not require the government to provide or pay for care.

However, Congress, by creating the Medicare and Medicaid programs, chose to pay for specific services for people who are elderly, disabled, or indigent. As discussed in Chapter 8, the government has flexibility under those programs to decide which groups of people will be eligible for benefits, such as persons with end-stage renal disease (ESRD), who are eligible for Medicare regardless of their age. In addition, as discussed in Chapter 8, the government may provide Medicaid coverage for some services, such as labor and delivery, but not for other services, such as elective abortion. In fact,

Congress could terminate the entire Medicare and Medicaid programs by simply repealing the statutes because, again, there is no underlying constitutional obligation to provide or pay for care.

Similarly, the traditional common-law rules provided that doctors and hospitals had no legal obligation to treat people who needed their services, even in an emergency. Although there are now some limited exceptions to those traditional rules, the old rules still apply whenever the situation does not fit within one of the limited exceptions. Therefore, the first step toward analyzing the legal obligation to provide care is to understand the common-law rules, and the second step is to determine the scope of the exceptions to those rules.

Traditional Common-Law Rules for Doctors and Hospitals

The physician–patient relationship is based on a contract, which is a voluntary agreement between the parties. After that voluntary relationship is established, a physician who fails to meet the applicable standard of care may be subject to a negligence claim for breach of duty under the law of torts. However, the physician would not have any duty to that patient until a relationship is voluntarily established in accordance with the law of contracts. In other words, once the relationship is voluntarily formed, a suit for breach of duty is governed by the tort law principles of negligence, but the formation of the relationship is governed by the law of contracts.

The contract between physician and patient may be in writing, but a written agreement is not required. Rather, the contract may be created by the conduct of the parties. If a person requests medical examination or treatment, and if the doctor begins to examine or treat that person, a contract has been created in the eyes of the law. Under some circumstances, physicians might also take on the obligation to provide services to additional patients by voluntarily making a contract with a hospital to be on call or by agreeing to accept patients who have coverage through a particular health plan.

Ordinarily, physicians have no legal obligation to accept a patient, even in an emergency. As a general rule, U.S. law does not impose any legal obligation to help a stranger in distress. If a person sees a drowning swimmer who could be rescued easily and safely, and if the person has no special relationship with that swimmer, such as being a caretaker or lifeguard, the person is not legally required to do anything to save the swimmer and cannot be held legally liable for allowing the swimmer to drown.[2] Similarly, if a person with a gunshot wound crawls to the office of a physician, and if the wounded person has no prior relationship with that physician, the physician has no legal obligation to treat the patient. Although many states have enacted so-called Good Samaritan statutes, those statutes do not require physicians or other healthcare professionals to treat strangers in distress, but merely provide immunity from liability if they voluntarily choose to do so.

Of course, the physician would have an *ethical* obligation to treat the person under those circumstances. According to the Principles of Medical Ethics of the American Medical Association, the physician ordinarily has the right to refuse to treat any particular patient, but that right does not apply in the case of a medical emergency.[3] As a legal matter, however, a physician is ordinarily not obligated to treat a person, even in an emergency, if she does not have a preexisting physician–patient relationship with the person.

Once a physician has made a contractual relationship with a patient, the physician will have certain duties to the patient, as discussed previously. The physician may not simply stop treating the patient, even if the patient is uncooperative or fails to pay the physician's bill. If the physician prematurely stops treating the patient, he could be held liable for abandonment. Therefore, a physician who wishes to terminate the relationship must ordinarily finish treating the patient for the current medical problem, make alternative arrangements for the patient's treatment, or provide the patient with notice and a reasonable opportunity to make other arrangements for medical coverage.

Similarly, hospitals *generally* have no legal obligation to accept and treat any particular patient, even in an emergency.[4] However, there are some exceptions to that general rule. First, as part of the Consolidated Omnibus Budget Reconciliation Act of 1985 (COBRA), Congress enacted the Emergency Medical Treatment and Active Labor Act (EMTALA)[5] and thereby provided a limited obligation to treat patients in the event of a medical emergency. EMTALA is also known as the "COBRA antidumping law" because it prohibits hospitals from improperly transferring or "dumping" emergency patients from one hospital to another as a result of a patient's inability to pay. As described in detail later, EMTALA requires the hospital to provide an appropriate medical screening examination to determine whether a patient has an emergency medical condition. If so, EMTALA requires the hospital to provide further treatment to stabilize the condition or a proper transfer in accordance with the requirements of the statute.

As a second exception to the general rule of no duty to treat, many public and nonprofit hospitals had accepted obligations to provide a certain volume of free care and make their services available to the community, as a condition of grants or loans under the federal Hill-Burton program.[6] However, many of the hospitals that were obligated to provide free care have already fulfilled those obligations, and the remaining obligations under the Hill-Burton program are extremely vague.

Finally, a specific hospital might have legal obligations to provide care as a result of the law or document that established that particular hospital. For example, in enacting a statute to create a public hospital for its residents, a state legislature might have specified that the public hospital will provide services to all persons in need, or at least all residents of the state, regardless of their ability to pay. Similarly, a board of county commissioners might have provided by resolution that its local public hospital shall provide care without regard to a patient's ability to pay. Even if a hospital is owned and operated by a private, nonprofit corporation, the charter or other documents that created the corporation, as well as the deed or lease by which the corporation acquired the hospital property, might stipulate obligations to provide care. However, those obligations, if any, would only apply to that particular hospital. Therefore, the most important exception to the general rule of no duty to treat is the COBRA antidumping law (EMTALA).

The COBRA Antidumping Law (EMTALA)

Historically, people without money or health insurance had serious problems obtaining emergency medical care. In addition to being denied access to some hospitals, indigent patients were often transferred to or "dumped on" public hospitals, despite the risks of delay in receiving emergency treatment. Many indigent women in active labor were transferred or told to go to a different hospital, which caused serious risks to the women and their unborn children. Under state law, those patients often had no legal remedy for harm caused by the denial of care. As already discussed, physicians were not required to enter a relationship with patients, and hospitals were not required to accept and treat patients, even in an emergency. In addition, patient dumping was a financial burden on public hospitals and teaching hospitals that provided a disproportionate share of uncompensated emergency care and maternity care for the indigent. Eventually, enough people came to believe "there ought to be a law," and Congress responded by enacting EMTALA.[7]

Through that law, Congress addressed an important goal of public policy, but it did so by an indirect method that failed to acknowledge the obligation of society as a whole. Rather than compensating local hospitals with federal funds for providing all necessary emergency care, Congress simply declared that hospitals must provide emergency care to all individuals without regard to their ability to pay. Although hospitals may charge patients *after* emergency services are rendered, the practical reality is that many of those bills will be uncollectible, and hospitals will end up providing a large volume of emergency services for free. Of course, that is good for patients who would otherwise go without care, but ultimately the cost of that care will be borne by the healthcare system and all of those who use it. To a large extent, EMTALA is an unfunded mandate or a tax on the hospital industry, which passes on the cost of care for the indigent to other patients and payers through the process of **cost shifting**.

Cost shifting
Charging higher rates to private payers to make up for low payment rates from government programs such as Medicare and Medicaid.

Nevertheless, Congress did accomplish the important policy goal of ensuring that all people will receive necessary emergency treatment, regardless of their ability to pay. To do so, Congress had to find a constitutionally permissible way to require public and private hospitals to give away a portion of their services for free, or at least to provide emergency care regardless of the patient's ability to pay. Even if the government is trying to accomplish an important public purpose, as it was in this case, the government cannot deprive individuals or organizations of their property, including their goods and services, without just compensation. Congress avoided that potential constitutional problem by relying on its power as a large-scale buyer of healthcare services through the federal Medicare program: As a condition of participation in Medicare, the government requires hospitals to provide emergency care without regard to the patient's ability to pay. EMTALA applies, therefore, to every hospital that has an emergency department and chooses to participate in Medicare.

The requirements of EMTALA apply to *all* patients, not merely to senior citizens or persons with disabilities or ESRD who are eligible for Medicare. In fact, EMTALA contains specific provisions for women in active labor, relatively few of whom are eligible for benefits under the Medicare program. EMTALA even applies to patients who have health insurance and those who are covered by managed care plans, as discussed later.

As indicated in Exhibit 11.1, when a person comes to the emergency department and requests examination or treatment, the hospital must provide an appropriate medical screening exam to determine whether an emergency medical condition exists. If the person has no emergency medical condition, the hospital has no further obligation under EMTALA. However, if the patient does have an emergency medical condition, the hospital has two options, as set forth in Exhibit 11.1. The hospital may provide the further medical examination and treatment that is required to stabilize the patient's condition. Alternatively, the hospital could transfer the patient to another medical facility, but that transfer would have to meet all of the strict requirements provided by the federal law.

Under a 1989 amendment to the law, a hospital may not delay the medical screening exam or the additional examination and treatment to inquire about the patient's method of payment or insurance status. For patients covered by managed care plans, the U.S. Department of Health and Human Services (HHS) has repeatedly stated that hospitals must comply with all of their obligations under EMTALA regardless of any requirement of the managed care plan to obtain prior authorization for treatment.[8] In addition, federal law requires each hospital to post a sign in the emergency department that specifies the rights of patients under EMTALA. HHS has developed the model sign in Exhibit 11.2, which it considers sufficient to meet the hospital's notice requirement.

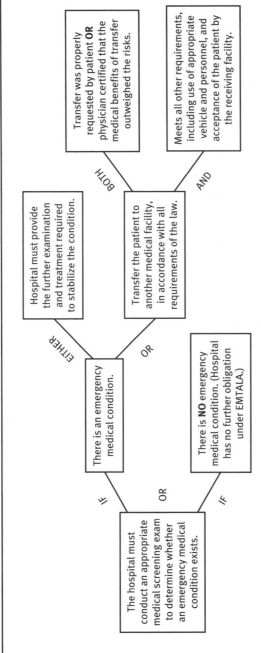

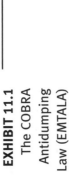

EXHIBIT 11.1
The COBRA
Antidumping
Law (EMTALA)

Note: These requirements apply to all patients and to every hospital that has an emergency department and participates in the Medicare program.

EXHIBIT 11.2
HHS's Model
Sign Entitled
"It's the Law!"

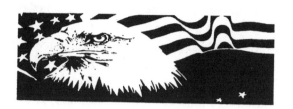

IT'S THE LAW!

IF YOU HAVE A MEDICAL EMERGENCY OR ARE IN LABOR

YOU HAVE THE RIGHT TO RECEIVE, within the capabilities of this hospital's staff and facilities:

- An appropriate medical **SCREENING EXAMINATION**
- Necessary **STABILIZING TREATMENT (including treatment for an unborn child)**

and if necessary

- An appropriate **TRANSFER** to another facility

even if

YOU CANNOT PAY or DO NOT HAVE MEDICAL INSURANCE

or

YOU ARE NOT ENTITLED TO MEDICARE OR MEDICAID

This hospital (does/does not) participate in the Medicaid program

If a hospital fails to meet its obligations under EMTALA, the government may take enforcement action against the hospital, including civil monetary fines and possible termination of the hospital's Medicare provider agreement.[9] In addition, EMTALA may be enforced in a private civil action in federal court by any individual who suffers personal harm as a direct result of a hospital's violation of the law. In a private civil action against a hospital under EMTALA, the plaintiff would need to prove the element of causation by demonstrating that the harm to the patient was a result of the violation.

In enacting the 2010 Affordable Care Act (ACA), Congress emphasized the continuing importance of EMTALA. The new requirements for tax-exempt hospitals under Section 9007 of the ACA provide that a tax-exempt hospital must have a written policy that requires it to provide care required by EMTALA without discrimination and regardless of an individual's eligibility under the hospital's financial assistance policy.

Coming to the Emergency Department

The requirements of EMTALA are triggered when a person "comes to the emergency department."[10] As a policy matter, ensuring that people receive appropriate emergency services is important even if they happen to walk in the wrong door or the wrong building on the hospital campus. Moreover, as seen in the tragic case of Christopher Sercye that was discussed in Chapter 1, no one should lie bleeding outside the door of an emergency department in the driveway or parking lot of a hospital. Clearly, EMTALA obligations should extend beyond the physical walls of the emergency department. However, the federal government has found it difficult to delineate precisely where a hospital's EMTALA obligations apply, especially with regard to separate buildings on the hospital campus or near the hospital, hospital-owned ambulances, and remote outpatient departments that are not equipped to provide any emergency services.

Under the original regulations issued by HHS in 1994, a person was considered to have come to the emergency department if she was "on the hospital property."[11] Later, HHS amended its regulations to explicitly provide that the hospital property includes "the entire main hospital campus . . . including the parking lot, sidewalk, and driveway."[12] In addition, HHS defined the term *campus* to include areas and structures within 250 yards of the main hospital buildings.[13] However, HHS explained that this would not include separate entities, such as restaurants or independent physicians' offices, even if they are located within 250 yards of the main hospital building.[14] Other HHS regulations had applied EMTALA obligations to off-campus facilities of the hospital, such as remote outpatient departments that are classified and paid as hospital based.[15]

Not surprisingly, these regulations resulted in confusion on the part of providers as well as objections to specific requirements. On September 9, 2003, HHS issued final regulations to address some of those concerns and clarify the legal obligations of hospitals under EMTALA.[16] The new regulations limit the types of off-campus facilities that are required to comply with EMTALA.[17]

In the meantime, another important issue in determining the applicability of EMTALA is whether the federal requirements apply to persons who have already been admitted as inpatients of the hospital. If the statute is read literally, it could be interpreted to apply to patients who are admitted as inpatients of the hospital, stabilized, and then have an emergency episode before they are discharged from the hospital. In fact, the statute might even be read to apply to elective, nonemergency patients whose condition deteriorates during the inpatient admission. In 1999, a representative of the HHS Office of Inspector General (OIG) indicated that the OIG considered EMTALA to apply to inpatients,[18] and at least one appellate court had indicated that EMTALA might apply even after several days of hospitalization.[19] However, other appellate courts had rejected attempts to apply EMTALA to inpatients in various situations to reflect their analysis of Congressional intent.[20] As one court had explained,

EMTALA is a limited "anti-dumping" statute, not a federal malpractice statute. Its core purpose is to get patients into the system who might otherwise go untreated and be left without a remedy because traditional medical malpractice law affords no claim for failure to treat. Numerous cases and the Act's legislative history confirm that Congress's sole purpose in enacting EMTALA was to deal with the problem of patients being turned away from emergency rooms for non-medical reasons. Once EMTALA has met that purpose of ensuring that a hospital undertakes stabilizing treatment for a patient who arrives with an emergency condition, the patient's care becomes the legal responsibility of the hospital and the treating physicians. And, the legal adequacy of that care is then governed not by EMTALA but by the state malpractice law that everyone agrees EMTALA was not intended to preempt.[21]

Aside from the availability of a state law remedy, applying EMTALA to inpatients could raise issues of federalism by subjecting an area of traditional state regulation to the rulemaking, investigation, and enforcement authority of federal agencies. As a matter of legislative intent, Congress did not likely intend federal agencies to regulate the practice of medicine and the delivery of hospital care for every inpatient in a code blue situation, such as cardiac arrest.

As part of its final regulations in 2003, HHS considered the applicability of EMTALA to inpatients. The final regulations provide that a hospital's EMTALA obligations end when a patient is admitted as an inpatient in good faith.[22] Moreover, EMTALA obligations do not apply to an inpatient who was admitted to the hospital on a nonemergency basis for elective diagnosis or treatment.[23] The final regulations also clarify that outpatients who are already receiving nonemergency services at the hospital are not covered by EMTALA, even if they have an emergency during the course of the outpatient encounter.[24] Thus, if an outpatient is receiving a nonemergency stress test at the hospital and has a heart attack during the test, the patient would not have the legal protection of EMTALA. However, if the hospital failed to meet the applicable standard of care in treating that patient, the patient would have other legal remedies under the state law of medical malpractice.

After issuing its 2003 final regulations, HHS considered additional comments and recommendations on the issue of applying EMTALA to inpatients, and that process of further consideration lasted for several years. HHS ultimately decided in 2012 that it would continue to follow the policy set forth in its 2003 final regulations.[25] Thus, HHS is continuing to apply the policy that a hospital's EMTALA obligations end when a patient is admitted as an inpatient in good faith. As HHS explained in 2012, "We continue to believe that this policy is a reasonable interpretation of the EMTALA statute and is supported by several Federal courts that have held that an individual's EMTALA protections end upon admission as a hospital inpatient."[26]

The Appropriate Medical Screening Examination

When required by the statute, hospitals must provide an "appropriate medical screening examination." However, the statute does not define that term, nor does it explain what type of screening exam will be considered "appropriate." However, the statute does provide some helpful information. First, it explains that the purpose of the exam is to determine whether the patient has an emergency medical condition. Second, it provides that the exam must be "within the capability of the hospital's emergency department, including ancillary services routinely available to the emergency department."[27] Thus, the hospital may not refuse to provide radiological or laboratory services that are located outside the emergency department if those services are ordinarily available to patients in the emergency department.

In considering whether a medical screening exam was appropriate, the federal courts have also provided some useful standards. To comply with EMTALA, a hospital is required to uniformly apply its standard screening procedure for all patients with the same medical condition. Thus, the EMTALA standard is not the same as the medical malpractice standard of care, which is based on the practice of similar providers in similar communities, as discussed in Chapter 10. In contrast, the EMTALA standard for an appropriate medical screening exam is the particular hospital's own practice. In EMTALA cases, plaintiffs must demonstrate that they received disparate treatment from the hospital's emergency department.[28] In effect, patients must demonstrate that they did not receive the same treatment the hospital ordinarily provides to its paying patients.

A patient or the estate of a patient might be able to assert separate claims in the same lawsuit under the federal law of EMTALA and the state law of medical malpractice. Because the EMTALA standard is different from the malpractice standard of care, a plaintiff might prevail on one claim while losing on the other, depending on the facts of the particular case. A plaintiff might also prevail on both or neither of those claims.

In a claim for alleged violation of EMTALA, is the plaintiff required to prove that the hospital had a bad motive for providing disparate treatment? Federal courts have differing opinions as to whether disparate treatment is sufficient to prove a violation of EMTALA or whether the plaintiff must also show a bad motive for the disparate treatment.[29] In some cases, the hospital might provide disparate treatment because of the patient's race or financial status or because the patient has a particular medical condition, such as AIDS. Each of those reasons would constitute a bad motive for the disparate treatment. However, in other cases, the hospital might provide disparate treatment without intending to do so, and that may simply constitute negligence in the emergency department.

In addressing that issue, some federal courts have concluded that Congress intended EMTALA to provide a legal remedy for *all* cases of disparate treatment. As those courts have reasoned, the language of the statute applies to all patients and is not explicitly limited to patients who are denied access or transferred for an improper reason. In those jurisdictions, the patient is only required to demonstrate that he received disparate treatment and does not have to prove that the disparate treatment was based on an improper motive.

However, other federal courts have reasoned that the intent of Congress in enacting EMTALA was only to protect patients from those denials of access and transfers that were based on their financial status or some other improper motive. According to those courts, Congress never intended to make a federal case out of every instance of negligence in a hospital emergency department, and those cases of ordinary negligence should continue to be governed by the state law of medical malpractice. In those jurisdictions, a patient who received disparate treatment without any improper motive on the part of the hospital could not prevail in a private civil action under EMTALA, but still might be able to prevail in a civil action for medical malpractice under the law of the particular state.

If the hospital provides an appropriate medical screening exam but fails to discover the patient's emergency condition, the hospital will not be held liable under EMTALA. As the Ninth Circuit has explained,

> [t]hus, Plaintiffs argue, in effect, that a hospital should be liable under EMTALA if its staff negligently fails to detect an emergency medical condition. EMTALA, however, was not enacted to establish a federal medical malpractice cause of action nor to establish a national standard of care. Thus, we have held that a hospital has a duty to stabilize only those emergency medical conditions that its staff detects. Every circuit to address this issue is in accord. To restate our ruling in *Jackson*, we hold that a hospital does not violate EMTALA if it fails to detect or if it misdiagnoses an emergency condition. An individual who receives substandard medical care may pursue medical malpractice remedies under state law.[30]

Requirements for a Proper Transfer

For a transfer to meet the requirements of the statute, it would have to be requested by the patient, or a physician would have to certify in writing that the benefits of the transfer outweigh the risks to the patient and any unborn child of the patient. Moreover, the sending facility must provide treatment to minimize the risk, the receiving facility must have space and agree to accept the patient, the records and documents must be sent with the patient, and the transfer must be accomplished with an appropriate vehicle and personnel.

Thus, for a physician to merely state that the patient would be better off at a different facility is not enough.

As demonstrated by *Owens v. Nacogdoches County Hospital District*,[31] the court will not simply defer to the medical judgment of the treating physician with regard to the appropriateness of the transfer. In that case, Rebecca Owens of Nacogdoches County, Texas, was 16 years old, pregnant, and poor. On the afternoon of August 3, 1987, she began to experience labor pains and went to the emergency department of Memorial Hospital. She asked to be admitted to the hospital to deliver her baby.

Owens was examined at the hospital by Dr. Bruce Thompson. After about 30 minutes, Dr. Thompson discharged her and told her to go to a different hospital in Galveston, which was about four hours away. Instead of driving directly to Galveston, Owens went to the office of East Texas Legal Services to get the help of a lawyer. Her lawyer tried to negotiate with Memorial Hospital and then obtained a temporary restraining order from the federal court to require Memorial to admit her. Eventually, she was admitted to Memorial and delivered her baby on August 7, 1987.

Owens sued Memorial Hospital for damages as a result of mental anguish and fear. After hearing the evidence from Ms. Owens and the hospital, the court awarded her $25,000 in damages and another $25,000 in attorneys' fees. In addition, the court granted a permanent injunction requiring Memorial Hospital to admit Ms. Owens for delivery in any future pregnancy as required by law.

At the trial, the hospital argued that the transfer had been medically justified, but the court did not believe the testimony offered by the hospital. Rather, it determined that the only reason for sending her to Galveston was that she could not afford to pay for her care. Moreover, the court noted that Owens and her baby might have died if he had been born on the side of the road.

As a legal matter, the issue in the case was whether Owens had been properly transferred in accordance with the requirements of the statute. Because a proper transfer requires the use of an appropriate vehicle, the court concluded that it was not a proper transfer. As the court explained, "a 1976 Ford Pinto with no medical equipment, whose only other occupant besides the patient is her boyfriend, is not the equivalent of an ambulance for the purposes of the Antidumping Act."[32] Therefore, the transfer was improper, even though the physician claimed that the transfer was medically justified.

Moreover, the court criticized the hospital for its staffing arrangements that, according to the court, would inevitably lead to a pattern of patient dumping. As the court explained, "Memorial Hospital has callously and negligently allowed a situation to develop in which all emergency obstetric and gynecological services to indigent patients—an enormous and ever-increasing load—have been left to on-call private physicians like Dr. Thompson, and the dumping of pregnant women has been the inevitable result."[33] However, the court did not suggest how the hospital ought to arrange for physician staffing to meet the hospital's obligations under EMTALA or who should bear the cost of those arrangements. Should hospitals require physicians in private practice to provide indigent care for free as a condition of medical staff membership? Alternatively, should hospitals compensate physicians for providing indigent care, as an expense to be passed on to all paying patients of the hospital? The *Owens* court did not even suggest any answers to those questions.

ACTIVITY 11.1: JOAN GRANT

Joan Grant was a 45-year-old attorney in private practice. She was enrolled in the GoodHealth health maintenance organization (HMO) through her law firm's self-insured employee benefit plan. Generally, she had been in good health, got plenty of exercise, and ate oat bran for breakfast every morning.

On the evening of April 15, 2013, while she was rushing to finish her tax return, she developed a splitting headache. She decided that she would have to obtain an extension to file her tax return. Because her doctor's office was closed for the night, she asked a friend to drive her to the emergency department of Community General Hospital (Community). She arrived at Community at approximately 9:30 p.m.

Community is an acute-care general hospital licensed by the state; it participates in the Medicare program. It is owned and operated by General Hospital Corporation, which is a for-profit business corporation.

Community has arranged for 24-hour medical coverage of its emergency department by means of a contract with Village Emergency Physicians, P.A. (VEPPA), which employs Dr. Ellen Jones and three other physicians. The contract between Community and VEPPA states that Dr. Jones and the other physician employees of VEPPA are not employees or agents of the hospital and further states that the hospital will not be liable for any negligence by VEPPA or its physician employees. In that regard, the hospital has placed the following sign on the wall in the emergency department:

Community General Hospital wants you to know that the physicians working in the emergency department are employees of VEPPA and are not employees or agents of the hospital. Have a nice day!

(continued)

(continued from previous page)

On her arrival at Community's emergency department, Grant told the nurse on duty that she had a splitting headache, and she was briefly examined by nurse Rebecca Smith. Then she was examined by the doctor on duty, Dr. Jones. Grant had no prior relationship with Dr. Jones.

According to the hospital's written protocols for the emergency department, if an adult patient complains of a splitting headache and if that patient does not appear to be intoxicated, the patient should be given a computed tomography (CT) scan of the head as soon as possible. In addition to being Community's protocol, that method of diagnosis is the ordinary practice at all of the hospitals in the area. However, some of the third-party payers have begun to refuse to pay for CT scans under these circumstances.

Nurse Smith asked Grant about her health insurance. Grant said that she was covered by the GoodHealth HMO and gave Nurse Smith an HMO membership card that contained her policy number and a phone number for the HMO. Nurse Smith called the office of the HMO to verify Grant's coverage and to request authorization for the CT scan. However, the clerk on duty at the HMO informed Nurse Smith that GoodHealth HMO no longer pays for CT scans of the head under these circumstances. Instead, the HMO clerk said that the hospital should instruct Grant to call her primary care physician at the HMO when the office opened at 9:00 a.m. the next day.

Nurse Smith informed Dr. Jones of the HMO's decision, and Dr. Jones discharged Grant at 10:30 p.m. with instructions to call her primary care physician at the HMO the next morning. Dr. Jones did not tell Grant that the usual diagnostic test for her condition was a CT scan, which Grant could have paid for with the credit card that she carried in her wallet.

Grant's friend took her home, where she died of an aneurysm at approximately 11:45 p.m. that night. At the request of the next of kin, an autopsy was performed. According to the autopsy report, Grant died of a rare type of aneurysm that does not show up on a CT scan.

What claims could be asserted against Community by Grant's estate? In discussing each potential claim against Community, be sure to discuss the elements of each claim and the likelihood of success on each claim.

Note: In responding to these questions, do not discuss any potential claims against individual healthcare professionals, VEPPA, the Good-Health HMO, or the law firm's health plan.

Prohibitions Against Discrimination

Ordinarily, healthcare providers may refuse to accept new patients without the need for any reason at all. They may refuse to accept new patients because they already are operating at full capacity, because they want to go on vacation, or because they want to spend more time with their families. However, the law prohibits healthcare professionals and facilities from refusing to accept new patients for a discriminatory reason, such as the prospective patient's race, national origin, or disability.

As recently as the 1960s, some healthcare facilities in the United States practiced overt racial discrimination, including exclusionary admission practices and segregated areas within the facilities. In fact, Congress had allowed recipients of federal Hill-Burton funds to maintain "separate but equal" facilities until that practice was prohibited by the federal courts.[34]

Title VI of the Civil Rights Act of 1964 prohibits discrimination on the basis of race, color, or national origin by any program or activity that receives federal financial assistance (FFA).[35] Most healthcare facilities are subject to the requirements of Title VI because they accept Medicare and Medicaid funds, which are considered FFA.[36] Even if a healthcare facility does not receive FFA, racial discrimination is prohibited by other laws.

The Title VI prohibition against discrimination on the basis of national origin has been interpreted to prohibit discrimination on the basis of a person's inability to speak English.[37] According to a revised policy guidance issued by HHS on August 8, 2003, recipients of FFA, such as healthcare facilities, "are required to take reasonable steps to ensure meaningful access to their programs and activities by LEP [limited English proficient] persons."[38] The extent of a healthcare facility's obligation to provide services such as interpreters depends on facts and circumstances, including the number and percentage of LEP patients and the resources available to the healthcare facility. In some states, laws adopted at the state level might impose additional requirements with regard to access by LEP patients.

Some of the most complex legal issues of prohibiting discrimination involve ensuring access to care for persons with disabilities. In addition to facing architectural barriers, persons with disabilities might need auxiliary aids and services, such as sign-language interpreters or electronic devices. Moreover, some persons with disabilities have been unable to obtain healthcare services because of the unwillingness of providers to treat them.

In § 504 of the Rehabilitation Act of 1973, Congress prohibited discrimination against persons who have a "handicap" in any program that receives FFA.[39] However, the applicability of that 1973 law to individual physicians and other practitioners in private practice was unclear. In addition, other limitations existed and issues remained unresolved with regard to the scope of the 1973 legislation. Under these circumstances, the Rehabilitation Act of 1973 did not solve the problems of access for persons with disabilities.

Eventually, Congress addressed these problems by enacting Title III of the Americans with Disabilities Act (ADA) of 1990.[40] The ADA made a major change in the law of disability discrimination by extending the reach of federal law beyond federally funded programs and into the private offices of physicians, dentists, and other individual practitioners. According to § 12182 of the ADA, "No individual shall be discriminated against on the basis of disability in the full and equal enjoyment of the . . . services . . . of any place of public accommodation."[41] Each word in that statute is carefully defined and loaded with meaning. For example, the term *public accommodation* is defined to include a hospital and the "professional office of a health care provider."[42] In contrast to the Rehabilitation Act of 1973, which only applied to programs that received FFA, the ADA takes a much broader approach by applying to every "place of public accommodation," regardless of the receipt of FFA.

One of the most difficult definitional questions under the ADA is determining whether a particular person has a "disability." According to the federal regulations, *disability* is "a physical or mental impairment that substantially limits one or more of the major life activities of such individual; a record of such an impairment; or being regarded as having such an impairment."[43] Of course, that linguistic formulation raises more questions than it answers. According to the U.S. Department of Justice (DOJ), the phrase *physical or mental impairment* includes "HIV disease (whether symptomatic or asymptomatic)."[44] Moreover, the U.S. Supreme Court held that, on the facts established in the case then before the court, asymptomatic HIV infection caused the plaintiff to have a disability for purposes of the ADA.[45]

Under these circumstances, physicians, dentists, and other individual practitioners cannot refuse to treat HIV-positive patients on the ground of their diagnosis, even in their private professional offices. According to the Centers for Disease Control and Prevention, healthcare professionals can protect themselves from the spread of HIV by using universal precautions. In other words, rather than singling out HIV-positive patients for special treatment, providers should treat all patients as if they might be HIV-positive. In the federal government's view, no scientific justification exists for refusing to perform surgery or other invasive procedures on HIV-positive patients, nor is there any justification for segregating them within healthcare facilities or medical offices. As indicated by the following statement from the DOJ, the government may take action against healthcare providers in cases of alleged refusal to treat HIV-positive patients.

FOR IMMEDIATE RELEASE CR
TUESDAY, MARCH 10, 1998

WASHINGTON, D.C. AREA HOSPITAL AGREES TO NEW POLICY FOR TREATING PATIENTS WITH HIV, UNDER AGREEMENT WITH JUSTICE DEPARTMENT[46]

WASHINGTON, D.C.—After allegedly denying surgical treatment to a patient who is HIV-positive, George Washington University Hospital agreed today to take steps to ensure people with HIV and other infectious diseases are not turned away because of their disabilities, the Justice Department announced.

The agreement stems from a complaint filed with the Justice Department under the Americans with Disabilities Act (ADA) by Ron Flowers, a 32-year-old Washington resident. The complaint alleged that Flowers, who is HIV-positive, was denied surgical treatment at George Washington University Hospital in March 1996.

"People with infectious diseases such as HIV must be able to enter the nation's hospitals and clinics confident that they will receive appropriate medical treatment," said Bill Lann Lee, Acting Assistant Attorney General for Civil Rights. "George Washington University's renewed commitment to serving all members of its community is a model for other hospitals."

Under the terms of the settlement, George Washington University and the Hospital will:

- implement a policy prohibiting its medical staff from making treatment decisions based on a patient's infectious disease status unless medically appropriate;
- provide information regarding this and other non-discrimination policies to patients through pamphlets and other materials posted throughout the hospital;
- provide annual training for its staff regarding this policy and their responsibilities to treat patients with infectious diseases under the Americans with Disabilities Act and the Rehabilitation Act;

(continued)

(continued from previous page)

- sponsor a symposium for cardiothoracic surgeons across the region on cardiothoracic surgery and HIV;
- pay the complainant significant compensatory damages.

The ADA prohibits discrimination against persons with disabilities. Title III of the ADA prohibits discrimination in public accommodations and commercial facilities like hospitals and other medical care facilities.

According to the complaint, Flowers was admitted to George Washington University Hospital after suffering two strokes. Tests revealed that a growth on Flowers' aortic valve was the likely cause. According to the complainant, although the medically appropriate treatment for his condition was open-heart surgery, the cardiothoracic surgeons at the Hospital refused to perform the operation because he is HIV-positive.

Flowers subsequently received the surgery at another local hospital and has fully recovered. As the ADA permits, Flowers filed a private lawsuit, which is being resolved separately.

"Access to medical care should be available to all people, and as advances in medicine extend the lives of people with HIV, compliance with the ADA is even more critical," added Lee.

98–106

With regard to a healthcare facility or practitioner's office, the prohibition against discrimination is broader than merely allowing persons with disabilities in the door. Healthcare providers cannot deny participation, allow participation in an unequal manner, or provide for a different or separate participation on the basis of a person's disability, subject to certain exceptions that are set forth in the statute or regulations.[47] In addition to removing architectural barriers, healthcare facilities may be required to provide auxiliary aids, including special equipment and personnel. For example, in 1998, 32 hospitals in Connecticut agreed with the DOJ and the state government to settle a class action lawsuit under the ADA, by offering to provide auxiliary services such as telecommunication devices and interpreters for hearing-impaired patients.[48]

Preventing Discrimination in Organ Transplantation

In addition to securing adequate treatment for persons with disabilities, issues of access and discrimination may arise in connection with the allocation of scarce human organs for transplantation. At the present time, there simply are not enough donated organs to meet the need, and thousands of people die each year while waiting for an organ.

Some people argue that the best way to make more organs available is to permit individuals to sell their organs in a free, competitive market. For example, proponents of that view think that competent adults should be permitted to sell one of their two kidneys, and they point out that relatives and friends of a patient are permitted to donate one of their kidneys to a particular recipient. In response, many people oppose the concept of an organ market, on the grounds that it would allow organs to go to the highest bidder and would discourage people from donating their organs to the existing transplantation system. To prevent that development of a commercial organ market, Congress has prohibited the purchase or sale of organs for use in human transplantation.[49] Instead, organs are allocated by the United Network for Organ Sharing, which operates the system under contract with HHS.

It is also important to make more organs available for transplantation by encouraging voluntary donation of organs after the death of the donor. If individuals never expressed their desires about donating their organs, the law does not presume their consent to donation. Rather, individuals must affirmatively state their intention to donate their organs, which can be accomplished by signing an organ donor card or other document of gift under their state's version of the Uniform Anatomical Gift Act. Even then, as a practical matter, organ procurement organizations will probably not accept the organs without consent of the donor's family. Therefore, people who want to donate their organs should make their wishes very clear to members of their family.

Hopefully, by encouraging voluntary donation, we will be able to promote access to this form of lifesaving medical treatment. Until there are enough organs to go around, however, we must be careful to avoid discrimination on the grounds of race, national origin, disability, or any other unlawful basis. Patients needing transplants have no legal right to care, except in the limited circumstances discussed in this chapter, but they do have the right to be free from unlawful discrimination.

Notes

1. See *DeShaney v. Winnebago County Department of Social Services*, 489 U.S. 189, 195–96 (1989).
2. See W. L. Prosser, W. P. Keeton, D. B. Dobbs, R. E. Keeton, and D. G. Owen, *Prosser and Keeton on the Law of Torts* (1984), 5th ed., § 56: 375.

3. See American Medical Association, *Code of Medical Ethics, Principles of Medical Ethics*, Preamble, point VI (2001). www.ama-assn.org/ ama/pub/physician-resources/medical-ethics/code-medical-ethics/ principles-medical-ethics.page.

4. See *Brooks v. Maryland General Hospital, Inc.*, 996 F.2d 708, 710 (4th Cir. 1993) (noting that hospitals have no legal duty under state tort law to provide emergency care to everyone).

5. 42 U.S.C. § 1395dd (2006).

6. Hospital Survey and Construction Amendments of 1949, 42 U.S.C. §§ 291 *et seq.* (2006); 42 C.F.R. § 124.4 (2005).

7. See Emergency Medical Treatment and Active Labor Act (EMTALA), 42 U.S.C. § 1395dd (2006).

8. Solicitation of Comments on the OIG/HCFA Special Advisory Bulletin on the Patient Anti-Dumping Statute, 63 Fed. Reg. 67486 (December 7, 1998) (proposed Special Advisory Bulletin); OIG/ HCFA Special Advisory Bulletin on the Patient Anti-Dumping Statute, 64 Fed. Reg. 61353, 61356 (November 10, 1999) (Special Advisory Bulletin); Medicare Program; Changes to the Hospital Inpatient Prospective Payment System and Fiscal Year 2003 Rates, 67 Fed. Reg. 31404, 31471, 31507 (May 9, 2002) (proposed rule).

9. See U.S. General Accounting Office, *Emergency Care: EMTALA Implementation and Enforcement Issues*, GAO-01–747 (June 22, 2001).

10. 42 U.S.C. § 1395dd(a) (2006).

11. Medicare Program; Participation in CHAMPUS and CHAMPVA, Hospital Admissions for Veterans, Discharge Rights Notice, and Hospital Responsibility for Emergency Care, 59 Fed. Reg. 32086, 32121 (June 22, 1994), codified at 42 C.F.R. § 489.24 (2006).

12. Office of Inspector General, Medicare Program; Prospective Payment System for Hospital Outpatient Services, 65 Fed. Reg. 18434, 18548 (April 7, 2000).

13. *Id.* at 18538 (adding a new 42 C.F.R. § 413.65).

14. 67 Fed. Reg. 31506 (May 9, 2002). www.cms.hhs.gov/ QuarterlyProviderUpdates/Downloads/cms1203p2.pdf.

15. See U.S. General Accounting Office, *supra* note 9, at 6, 14.

16. 68 Fed. Reg. 53222–53264 (September 9, 2003).

17. 42 C.F.R. § 413.65(g)(1) (2005).

18. See BNA's Health Care Daily Report, "Emergency Care: HHS Broadly Interprets EMTALA to Include Inpatients of Hospital Grounds," Executive Briefing (June 30, 1999).

19. *Thornton v. Southwest Detroit Hosp.*, 895 F.2d 1131, 1135 (6th Cir. 1990).

20. See, e.g., *Bryant v. Adventist Health System/West*, 289 F.3d 1162, 1167 (9th Cir. 2002) ("the stabilization requirement normally ends when the patient is admitted for inpatient care").

21. *Bryan v. Rectors and Visitors of the University of Virginia*, 95 F.3d 349, 351 (4th Cir. 1996) (citations omitted).

22. 42 C.F.R. § 489.24(d)(2) (2006). See also 68 Fed. Reg. at 53244–53245 (September 9, 2003).

23. 42 C.F.R. § 489.24(d)(2).

24. See 68 Fed. Reg. at 53239.

25. Centers for Medicare & Medicaid Services, Department of Health and Human Services, "Medicare Program; Emergency Medical Treatment and Labor Act (EMTALA): Applicability to Hospital Inpatients and Hospitals with Specialized Capabilities," 77 Fed. Reg. 5213 (February 2, 2012) (request for comments).

26. *Id.* at 5217.

27. 42 U.S.C. § 1395dd(a) (2006).

28. See *Baber v. Hospital Corporation of America*, 977 F.2d 872 (4th Cir. 1992).

29. See *id.* at 880 n.8.

30. *Bryant v. Adventist Health System/West*, 289 F.3d 1162, 1166 (9th Cir. 2002) (citations and footnote omitted).

31. 741 F. Supp. 1269 (E.D. Tex. 1990).

32. *Id.* at 1276.

33. *Id.* at 1280.

34. See *Simkins v. Moses H. Cone Memorial Hospital*, 323 F.2d 959, 967–70 (4th Cir. 1963), *cert. denied*, 376 U.S. 938 (1964).

35. 42 U.S.C. § 2000d (2006).

36. See *United States v. Baylor University Medical Center*, 736 F.2d 1039, 1045–46 (5th Cir. 1984).

37. T. S. Jost (2006). "Racial and Ethnic Disparities in Medicare: What the Department of Health and Human Services and the Centers for Medicare and Medicaid Services Can, and Should Do." *DePaul Journal of Health Care Law* 9: 667–718, 700–702.

38. Department of Health and Human Services, *Guidance to Federal Financial Assistance Recipients Regarding Title VI Prohibition Against National Origin Discrimination Affecting Limited English Proficient Persons*, 68 Fed. Reg. 47311, 47314 (August 8, 2003).

39. Pub. L. No. 93-112, § 504 (1973), codified at 29 U.S.C. § 794 (Supp. 1982).

40. See 42 U.S.C. §§ 12181 *et seq.* (2006).

41. 42 U.S.C. § 12182(a) (2006). See also 28 C.F.R. § 36.201(a) (2006) (Department of Justice regulations).

42. 42 U.S.C. § 12181(7)(F) (2006). See also 28 C.F.R. § 36.104 (2006) (defining "place of public accommodation").

43. 28 C.F.R. § 36.104 (2006).

44. *Id.*

45. *Bragdon v. Abbott*, 524 U.S. 624, 641 (1998).

46. Department of Justice, "Washington, D.C. Area Hospital Agrees to New Policy for Treating Patients with HIV, Under Agreement with Justice Department," No. 98-106 (March 10, 1998). www.justice. gov/opa/pr/1998/March/106.htm.html.

47. See 28 C.F.R. § 36.202 (2006).

48. Consent Decree, Connecticut Association of the Deaf v. Middlesex Memorial Hospital (No. 395-CV-02408, D. Conn., 1998). www. justice.gov/crt/foia/readingroom/frequent_requests/ada_ settlements/cn/ctmiddle.php.

49. See National Organ Transplant Act, 42 U.S.C. § 274e (2006).

12

LEGAL AND ETHICAL ISSUES IN TERMINATION OR REFUSAL OF CARE AND PHYSICIAN-ASSISTED SUICIDE

I n Chapter 11, we considered the extent of the legal right to *obtain* health-care services. Now we are shifting our focus to the right to *refuse* services, including the right to refuse life-sustaining treatment and the right to die. Obviously, decisions to accept or refuse medical treatment are intensely personal and may involve religious and ethical beliefs. Therefore, reasonable people may disagree about the "right" thing to do in a particular case, and beginning the discussion by acknowledging a healthy respect for the diversity of opinion on these sensitive issues is wise.

This area of law provides a fascinating example of the interaction between state and federal authority in the regulation of healthcare services. As a general rule, issues of termination or refusal of care will be governed by the laws of the individual states. However, federal law plays a role in these issues in at least three important ways.

First, the U.S. Supreme Court has recognized, albeit somewhat tentatively, that patients *may* have a right to refuse medical treatment under the federal constitution. As the Supreme Court explained, "We have also assumed, and strongly suggested, that the Due Process Clause protects the traditional right to refuse unwanted lifesaving medical treatment."[1] Such a constitutional right, however, would not necessarily override a state's law that imposes conditions on the refusal of treatment. As discussed in Chapter 2, in *Cruzan* the U.S. Supreme Court held that Missouri's requirement to show clear and convincing evidence of the patient's desires did not violate any right of the patient under the U.S. Constitution.[2]

Second, in addition to the possibility of a federal constitutional right, Congress enacted the Patient Self-Determination Act as part of the Medicare law.[3] That statute requires healthcare facilities participating in Medicare to inform patients of their rights to refuse treatment and make advance directives, even though the rights are provided by the laws of the particular state.[4] Pursuant to that federal statute, facilities must have written policies for advising patients of their rights. Although the original federal legislation from 1990 had already required facilities to document whether the patient had made an advance directive, Congress added a requirement in 1997 that the documentation be placed "in a prominent part of the individual's current medical record."[5]

Third, the U.S. government has attempted to prevent or discourage physician-assisted suicide (PAS), even if a state government decides to permit it. For example, in the Assisted Suicide Funding Restriction Act, Congress has prohibited the use of federal funds in connection with assisted suicide, mercy killing, or euthanasia, even in states where assisted suicide is lawful.[6] Therefore, in a state such as Oregon, which provides a limited right to PAS, the Medicare program will not pay for the lethal drug or the physician's service in writing the prescription. In addition, as discussed in detail later, the federal government grants physicians the authority to write prescriptions for controlled substances and threatened to revoke that authority for any physician who uses federally controlled substances for the purpose of PAS. Aside from these limited assertions of federal authority, however, most issues of termination or refusal of care will be governed by the laws of the particular state.

Living wills and other advance directives have received a great deal of publicity, especially in cases of patients who were terminally ill or in a persistent vegetative state. However, those cases are merely a subset of a broader category of cases that involve the right to refuse any type of unwanted medical care. Therefore, the starting point in analyzing these issues is understanding the legal principles of the right to refuse ordinary medical or surgical care. Those principles can then be applied to the specific problem of withholding or withdrawing artificial means of life support. Finally, we can consider whether those legal principles of the right to refuse treatment can be extended to create a right to have the assistance of a physician in committing suicide.

The Right to Refuse Treatment

Some patients refuse to accept blood transfusions on the grounds of religious beliefs. In other situations, patients refuse to undergo surgery that is recommended by their physicians because they do not want to take the risk of surgery or because they believe they are likely to get better without undergoing the surgical procedure. In light of the practice of defensive medicine, as discussed in Chapter 10, patients may have reason to be skeptical of some tests and treatments recommended by their physicians. Therefore, patients may choose to decline those tests and treatments that pose a significant risk of injury or complications. In each of those cases, the patient is simply exercising her right to say no.

From a legal perspective, the right to refuse treatment is based on the doctrine of informed consent or at least on the same policy goals that led to the development of that doctrine. As discussed in Chapter 10, the focus of informed consent in medical malpractice cases is the patient's right to know the risks, benefits, and alternatives to the course of treatment suggested by the physician. However, the right to know would be meaningless without the other aspect of informed consent, which is the right to say no. In other words, the right of informed consent is more than just the right to be fully informed. Rather, it is the right to consent or, more important, the right to refuse to give one's consent.

In 1914, Benjamin Cardozo, who was then a New York Court of Appeals judge, wrote that "every human being of adult years and sound mind has a right to determine what shall be done with his own body."[7] In the abstract, that proposition is noble and one with which almost everyone would agree. However, many situations are encountered in which our society will *not* allow people to decide what will be done with their own bodies. For example, most states outlaw prostitution. In addition, the government prohibits adults from using controlled substances without a prescription, even in the privacy of their homes. In the healthcare context, the government has the authority to force people to be vaccinated against communicable diseases, even if they are being treated against their will.[8] Also, although most people have two kidneys and need only one, federal law prohibits people from selling one of their kidneys if the sale affects interstate commerce.[9]

Thus, despite the general principle enunciated by Justice Cardozo, individuals of adult years and sound minds will not be allowed to decide what will be done with their own bodies and will not be allowed to refuse medical treatment in some situations. In those cases, the interests of the individual will be outweighed by the interests of society as a whole.

In addition, one must resist the temptation to characterize the refusing person as incompetent or not of sound mind merely because he is rejecting a treatment that almost everyone else would accept. In the past, some courts and some medical professionals have tended to declare that patients refusing lifesaving medical care were mentally incapable of making their own decisions or that they did not understand the facts. Some severely ill or injured patients may lack the mental capacity to understand the situation and make a rational decision. However, judges and medical professionals need to be aware of their bias in favor of medical intervention, particularly if they believe treatment is necessary to save the patient's life. In some cases, the patient may believe she is more likely to be cured by prayer, meditation, diet, herbal remedies, or alternative medicine rather than the drugs or surgery recommended by the physician. In those circumstances, our society should respect the right of the individual to refuse medical treatment for personal, cultural, or religious reasons and should not violate that right by declaring that the person "must be crazy."

Nevertheless, cases will arise in which the patient is mentally incapable of making a rational decision. In those cases, two separate inquiries will be relevant. First, will our society allow an individual to refuse treatment in this situation? Second, if the person is unable to make or communicate a decision, how can medical personnel, family members, or judges determine what the individual would have wanted or find some way to make a decision on behalf of the patient?

The following excerpt is from the classic case of *Application of the President and Directors of Georgetown College*.[10] In reading this case, try to determine which of the two inquiries the court was attempting to answer.

Application of the President and Directors of Georgetown College, Inc., 331 F.2D 1000 (D.C. CIR.) (CITATIONS AND FOOTNOTES OMITTED), *Cert. Denied*, 377 U.S. 978 (1964)

Attorneys for Georgetown Hospital applied for an emergency writ at 4:00 P.M., September 17, 1963, seeking relief from the action of the United States District Court for the District of Columbia denying the hospital's application for permission to administer blood transfusions to an emergency patient. The application recited that "Mrs. Jesse E. Jones is presently a patient at Georgetown University Hospital," "she is in extremis," according to the attending physician "blood transfusions are necessary immediately in order to save her life," and "consent to the administration thereof can be obtained neither from the patient nor her husband." The patient and her husband based their refusal on their religious beliefs as Jehovah's Witnesses. The order sought provided that the attending physicians "may" administer such transfusions to Mrs. Jones as might be "necessary to save her life." After the proceedings detailed in Part IV of this opinion, I signed the order at 5:20 P.M. . . .

The temporary order issued was more limited than the order proposed in the original application, in that the phrase "to save her life" was added, thus limiting the transfusions in both time and number. Such a temporary order to preserve the life of the patient was necessary if the cause were not to be mooted by the death of the patient. . . .

Let us now reconstruct the narrative of events through the medium of the contemporaneous Memorandum of Facts filed in this cause, the

(continued)

(continued from previous page)

substance of which is as follows: Mrs. Jones was brought to the hospital by her husband for emergency care, having lost two thirds of her body's blood supply from a ruptured ulcer. She had no personal physician, and relied solely on the hospital staff. She was a total hospital responsibility. It appeared that the patient, age 25, mother of a seven-month-old child, and her husband were both Jehovah's Witnesses, the teachings of which sect, according to their interpretation, prohibited the injection of blood into the body. When death without blood became imminent, the hospital sought the advice of counsel, who applied to the District Court in the name of the hospital for permission to administer blood. Judge Tamm of the District Court denied the application, and counsel immediately applied to me, as a member of the Court of Appeals, for an appropriate writ.

I called the hospital by telephone and spoke with Dr. Westura, Chief Medical Resident, who confirmed the representations made by counsel. I thereupon proceeded with counsel to the hospital, where I spoke to Mr. Jones, the husband of the patient. He advised me that, on religious grounds, he would not approve a blood transfusion for his wife. He said, however, that if the court ordered the transfusion, the responsibility was not his. I advised Mr. Jones to obtain counsel immediately. He thereupon went to the telephone and returned in 10 or 15 minutes to advise that he had taken the matter up with his church and that he had decided that he did not want counsel.

I asked permission of Mr. Jones to see his wife. This he readily granted. Prior to going into the patient's room, I again conferred with Dr. Westura and several other doctors assigned to the case. All confirmed that the patient would die without blood and that there was a better than 50 per cent chance of saving her life with it. Unanimously they strongly recommended it. I then went inside the patient's room. Her appearance confirmed the urgency which had been represented to me. I tried to communicate with her, advising her again as to what the doctors had said. The only audible reply I could hear was "Against my will." It was obvious that the woman was not in a mental condition to make a decision. I was reluctant to press her because of the seriousness of her condition and because I felt that to suggest repeatedly the imminence of death without blood might place a strain on her religious convictions. I asked her whether she would oppose the blood transfusion if the court

(continued)

(continued from previous page)

allowed it. She indicated, as best I could make out, that it would not then be her responsibility.

I returned to the doctors' room where some 10 to 12 doctors were congregated, along with the husband and counsel for the hospital. The President of Georgetown University, Father Bunn, appeared and pleaded with Mr. Jones to authorize the hospital to save his wife's life with a blood transfusion. Mr. Jones replied that the Scriptures say that we should not drink blood, and consequently his religion prohibited transfusions. The doctors explained to Mr. Jones that a blood transfusion is totally different from drinking blood in that the blood physically goes into a different part and through a different process in the body. Mr. Jones was unmoved. I thereupon signed the order allowing the hospital to administer such transfusions as the doctors should determine were necessary to save her life. . . .

Before proceeding with this inquiry, it may be useful to state what this case does not involve. This case does not involve a person who, for religious or other reasons, has refused to seek medical attention. It does not involve a disputed medical judgment or a dangerous or crippling operation. Nor does it involve the delicate question of saving the newborn in preference to the mother. Mrs. Jones sought medical attention and placed on the hospital the legal responsibility for her proper care. In its dilemma, not of its own making, the hospital sought judicial direction.

It has been firmly established that the courts can order compulsory medical treatment of children for any serious illness or injury, and that adults, sick or well, can be required to submit to compulsory treatment or prophylaxis, at least for contagious diseases. And there are no religious exemptions from these orders. . . .

Of course, there is here no sick child or contagious disease. However, the sick child cases may provide persuasive analogies because Mrs. Jones was in extremis and hardly compos mentis at the time in question; she was as little able competently to decide for herself as any child would be. Under the circumstances, it may well be the duty of a court of general jurisdiction, such as the United States District Court for the District of Columbia, to assume the responsibility of guardianship for her, as for a child, at least to the extent of authorizing treatment to save her life. And if, as shown above, a parent has no power to forbid the

(continued)

(continued from previous page)

saving of his child's life, a fortiori the husband of the patient here had no right to order the doctors to treat his wife in a way so that she would die.

The child cases point up another consideration. The patient, 25 years old, was the mother of a seven-month-old child. The state, as parens patriae, will not allow a parent to abandon a child, and so it should not allow this most ultimate of voluntary abandonments. The patient had a responsibility to the community to care for her infant. Thus the people had an interest in preserving the life of this mother. . . .

The Gordian knot of this suicide question may be cut by the simple fact that Mrs. Jones did not want to die. Her voluntary presence in the hospital as a patient seeking medical help testified to this. Death, to Mrs. Jones, was not a religiously-commanded goal, but an unwanted side effect of a religious scruple. There is no question here of interfering with one whose religious convictions counsel his death, like the Buddhist monks who set themselves afire. Nor are we faced with the question of whether the state should intervene to reweigh the relative values of life and death, after the individual has weighed them for himself and found life wanting. Mrs. Jones wanted to live.

A third set of considerations involved the position of the doctors and the hospital. Mrs. Jones was their responsibility to treat. The hospital doctors had the choice of administering the proper treatment or letting Mrs. Jones die in the hospital bed, thus exposing themselves, and the hospital, to the risk of civil and criminal liability in either case. It is not certain that Mrs. Jones had any authority to put the hospital and its doctors to this impossible choice. The normal principle that an adult patient directs her doctors is based on notions of commercial contract which may have less relevance to life-or-death emergencies. It is not clear just where a patient would derive her authority to command her doctor to treat her under limitations which would produce death. The patient's counsel suggests that this authority is part of constitutionally protected liberty. But neither the principle that life and liberty are inalienable rights, nor the principle of liberty of religion, provides an easy answer to the question of whether the state can prevent martyrdom. Moreover, Mrs. Jones had no wish to be a martyr. And her religion merely prevented her consent to a transfusion. If the law undertook the responsibility of authorizing the transfusion without her consent, no problem would be raised with respect to her religious practice. Thus,

(continued)

> *(continued from previous page)*
>
> the effect of the order was to preserve for Mrs. Jones the life she wanted without sacrifice of her religious beliefs.
>
> The final, and compelling, reason for granting the emergency writ was that a life hung in the balance. There was no time for research and reflection. Death could have mooted the cause in a matter of minutes, if action were not taken to preserve the status quo. To refuse to act, only to find later that the law required action, was a risk I was unwilling to accept. I determined to act on the side of life.

In *Georgetown College*, the court apparently believed that a person in those circumstances should not be allowed to refuse treatment, which relates to the first inquiry discussed earlier. Moreover, even if a person would be allowed to refuse treatment under those circumstances, the court believed this particular patient really wanted to receive the lifesaving blood transfusion. Therefore, the court addressed both inquiries to some extent.[11]

However, the court's analysis may be questioned on several grounds. As a factual matter, was the patient really incapable of making her own decision? Even if she was mentally incompetent, should the court have allowed her husband to make a decision on her behalf because he was her next of kin and certainly knew what she wanted? Finally, did the religious beliefs of the patient and her husband really permit a blood transfusion, as long as it was performed over their objection, or was that merely a convenient rationalization for the decision that the court was determined to make?

Georgetown College is a classic case, and it has long been required reading for students of healthcare law and ethics. Note, however, that attitudes and values in American society have changed somewhat since that case was decided in 1964. Since that time, people have come to expect more freedom to make their own individual decisions, regardless of the interests of society as a whole. In fact, many modern courts would not follow the precedent of *Georgetown College* but rather would allow an individual patient to refuse a blood transfusion on the grounds of religious belief.[12] Nevertheless, modern courts are still likely to order blood transfusions for children over the religious objections of their parents.[13]

Perhaps the most interesting aspect of the *Georgetown College* decision is the court's reliance on society's interest in keeping the patient alive because she had a child who was only seven months old.[14]

However, if we accept the proposition that a parent has a duty to society to accept unwanted medical treatment, it leads to an even more difficult question. Does a female patient who is pregnant with a viable fetus have a duty to society to accept unwanted medical and surgical treatment to preserve the *potential* life of her unborn child? That issue will be addressed in Chapter 13, in connection with the problem of maternal–fetal conflict. First, however, we must apply the legal principles of the right to refuse treatment to cases involving termination of artificial means of life support.

The Right to a Natural Death

As a subset of the right to refuse treatment, the right to a natural death applies the legal principles of informed consent in the context of decisions at the end of life. In many of those cases, however, the patient is unable to expressly give or withhold consent because of her mental or physical condition. For example, if the patient is in a persistent vegetative state and made no living will or other advance directive, determining what she would have wanted with regard to the continuation or termination of artificial life support may be difficult or impossible.

In some circumstances, the law allows consent to be given by someone other than the patient. For example, a parent has the right to consent to surgery on behalf of a minor child. By analogy, it is reasonable that the decision to continue or discontinue life support for an incompetent patient should be made by a surrogate, such as a close relative, legal guardian, or judge. In some jurisdictions, courts make a substituted judgment for the patient by trying to determine what the patient would have wanted. However, other courts take a different approach and try to determine what would be in the best interest of the patient. Regardless of their approach, most courts insist that they will never consider the patient's reduced quality of life in determining whether the patient should be treated or allowed to die. However, those courts probably do consider the patient's quality of life as a practical matter. Finally, some states have statutes that permit the termination of treatment under specified conditions, even without any evidence of the patient's intent.[15]

As a practical matter, terminating artificial means of life support can be difficult if members of the patient's family disagree. That was the situation in the case of Terri Schiavo, who was in a persistent vegetative state. Her husband obtained an order from the Florida court for termination of treatment, but her parents objected and wanted the treatment to be continued. After numerous proceedings in state courts, federal courts, the Florida legislature, and the U.S. Congress, her feeding tube was removed and Schiavo died.

Despite the media attention and political maneuvering, that case was not a significant development in the law on termination of treatment. As one commentator has noted, "The case of Terri Schiavo resulted in no changes in the law, nor were any good arguments made that legal changes were necessary."[16] Although the Florida legislature purported to authorize the governor to take action to prevent withholding of nutrition and hydration,[17] the state statute only applied to that one patient as a practical matter.[18] Moreover, the Florida Supreme Court held that the statute was unconstitutional under the legal doctrine of separation of powers.[19] As the Court explained, "[I]t is without question an invasion of the authority of the judicial branch for the Legislature to pass a law that allows the executive branch to interfere with the final judicial determination in a case."[20] Similarly, the special act that was passed by the U.S. Congress and signed by President George W. Bush had limited significance as precedent for future cases because it was expressly limited to that one patient and did not even affect the outcome of that particular case.[21]

In contrast to the case of Terri Schiavo, courts in other cases have tried to develop legal precedents for handling similar situations in the future. Many courts have tried to articulate a legal standard or formula by which all of these cases could be decided.[22] However, those standards are often illogical and impractical and may be little more than attempts to justify common sense in terms of legal doctrine. For example, the Supreme Judicial Court of Massachusetts applied the **substituted judgment doctrine**, which attempts to determine the preferences of the incompetent person. In that case, the court was considering whether to order or withhold chemotherapy for a profoundly retarded adult with leukemia. As the Massachusetts court explained, "We believe that both the guardian *ad litem* in his recommendation and the judge in his decision should have attempted (as they did) to ascertain the incompetent person's actual interests and preferences. In short, the decision in cases such as this should be that which would be made by the incompetent person, if that person were competent, but taking into account the present and future incompetency of the individual as one of the factors which would necessarily enter into the decision-making process of the competent person."[23]

However, in a similar case, the New York Court of Appeals rejected the Massachusetts substituted judgment approach in considering whether to order blood transfusions for a profoundly retarded adult with bladder cancer. According to the New York court, "John Storar was never competent at any time in his life. He was always totally incapable of understanding or making a reasoned decision about medical treatment. Thus it is unrealistic to attempt to determine whether he would want to continue potentially life prolonging treatment if he were competent. As one of the experts testified at the hearing, that would be similar to asking whether 'if it snowed all summer would it then be winter?' Mentally, John Storar was an infant and that is the only realistic way to assess his rights in this litigation."[24]

In light of these different legal standards, it may be more effective to focus on the specific facts of each case and not merely on the legal formula. In most cases, it appears that the court makes a reasonable decision in light

Substituted judgment doctrine
The legal principle that a court should make a decision on behalf of an incompetent person by trying to determine what she would have decided.

of the facts. Specifically, at least four factual variables have a significant effect on the outcome of a particular case:

1. the patient's mental competence,
2. any formal or informal expression of the patient's desires,
3. the physical condition of the patient, and
4. the type of treatment that might be withheld or withdrawn.

First, as a conceptual matter, distinguishing between those patients who are competent and those who are incompetent is useful.[25] In addition, for those patients who are currently incompetent, a further distinction can be made between those who were formerly competent and those who were never competent.[26] If a patient is competent, she is asked what she wants at the present time, and there is no need to consider whether she had previously executed a living will or other advance directive. However, if the patient is currently incompetent, the relevant questions are whether the patient ever made an advance directive and, if not, whether the patient gave any informal indication of desires with regard to artificial life support. If the patient was never competent, because she is an infant or a person with a developmental disability, evaluating her expressions of intent is useless because she was never legally capable of forming any intent.

Therefore, for those patients who are not currently competent but were formerly competent, the second factual variable is whether the patient made a formal or informal declaration of desires with regard to extraordinary means of life support.[27] Obviously, the best evidence of the patient's desires is a formal advance directive, such as a living will. Under the laws of each state, people may execute these formal documents to specify whether they would wish to continue or discontinue various types of treatment in the event that they are ever in a specified medical condition. In addition, almost all states allow a person to execute a durable power of attorney or a healthcare power of attorney to designate another person as an agent to make those types of treatment decisions for the patient. If the patient did not execute a living will or designate a healthcare agent, it makes sense to consider whether the patient had given any informal indications of intent, such as in conversations with relatives or friends.

The third factual variable is the physical condition of the patient. Although all of the patients in these cases are seriously ill, significant distinctions exist among the individual patients. For example, some of the patients are terminally ill, but others could continue to live for many years in a persistent vegetative state. Although some of the patients are unconscious and oblivious to their surroundings, others are conscious and in continual pain. Finally, some of the patients are capable of breathing on their own, but others depend on mechanical respirators.

The fourth variable is the type of treatment that might be withheld or withdrawn from the patient. In fact, the various types of treatment can be arranged along a spectrum from the most passive to the most active interventions. At the most passive extreme, a decision might be made not to resuscitate the patient in the event that he stops breathing or has a heart attack. This is referred to as a "no code order" or a "do not resuscitate order." Rather than taking active steps to end the life of the patient, this alternative merely lets nature take its course in bringing about the patient's death.

At the other extreme is active euthanasia, including PAS, which is discussed in detail in a later section. Some people have argued that PAS is no different from the withdrawal of life-support equipment, because both actions result in the patient's death. However, the U.S. Supreme Court has recognized a "distinction between letting a patient die and making that patient die."[28]

Between the extremes of passive inaction and active euthanasia are various types of treatment that might be withheld or withdrawn. Decisions could be made to perform or withhold blood transfusions, antibiotics, chemotherapy, surgery, or kidney dialysis for a patient in a particular case. Each of those potential interventions would be intrusive to a greater or lesser degree. In addition, the withholding of each intervention would have a different immediate effect on the patient. For example, removing a patient from a respirator would likely result in death within a short and predictable period of time, whereas withholding chemotherapy may not result in death for several months.

Finally, some people believe there is a distinction between withholding medical treatment and withholding artificial nutrition and hydration. In many cases, the action under consideration is the termination of the patient's food and water through the removal of a nasogastric (NG) tube or other mechanical device. Therefore, it is important to focus on the specific facts about each individual patient in evaluating these cases and in answering Activity 12.1.

ACTIVITY 12.1: CASES ON TERMINATION OF TREATMENT

The facts about several individual patients are set forth here. Each of these patients was the subject of a judicial decision by the court of a particular state. In some cases, the court permitted the withholding or withdrawal of treatment, which presumably resulted in the patient's death. However, in three of these cases, the court held that treatment should be continued, and therefore, the patient was not allowed to die.

(continued)

(continued from previous page)

For each case, the decision of the court is also provided. The goal of this activity is to determine whether the court's decision in each case was reasonable in light of the specific facts of the case.

Read the description of each case and record the details in Exhibit 12.1. With regard to the patients for whom treatment was continued, explain in writing any ways in which those cases were factually distinguishable from the cases in which treatment was terminated.

CASE 1: *Cruzan v. Director, Missouri Department of Health*[29]

After Nancy Beth Cruzan was injured in a car accident, she was in a persistent vegetative state and had virtually no chance of regaining her cognitive function. However, she was not terminally ill and was breathing on her own. Her parents asked hospital employees to terminate the artificial nutrition and hydration, but they refused to do so without a court order. Cruzan had never executed an advance directive, and the only evidence of her desires was a somewhat casual statement to a friend. Specifically, Cruzan had indicated that she would not want to continue living if she were ever in a severely impaired condition.

Cruzan's parents sought an order from a Missouri state court to terminate the artificial nutrition and hydration. The Missouri court refused to order the termination of treatment on the grounds that there was no clear and convincing evidence of the patient's desire to terminate artificial nutrition and hydration. As discussed in Chapter 2, this case became the subject of a famous decision by the U.S. Supreme Court. However, because of the limited role of the federal courts, the U.S. Supreme Court did not consider the broad question of whether Cruzan should be allowed to die. Rather, the U.S. Supreme Court merely determined that the state law of Missouri, which required clear and convincing evidence of the patient's intent, did not violate the U.S. Constitution. Therefore, the Missouri court was entitled to apply its requirement of clear and convincing evidence.

CASE 2: *Bouvia v. Superior Court of Los Angeles County*[30]

Elizabeth Bouvia was a 28-year-old quadriplegic with cerebral palsy. She was almost completely immobile and in continual pain. Her condition was irreversible and although she needed medication for pain, she was mentally competent.

(continued)

(continued from previous page)

Bouvia had to be spoon-fed, and eating sometimes caused nausea and vomiting. If she were fed through an NG tube, she could be kept alive for another 15 to 20 years. However, Bouvia dictated instructions to her lawyers that she did not want an NG tube and signed the document with a pen that she held in her mouth. Nevertheless, the hospital's medical staff inserted an NG tube against her will to prevent her from starving herself to death.

Bouvia asked the California state court to order the hospital and physicians to remove the NG tube. In response, the hospital and physicians argued that the state has legitimate interests in preserving life, preventing suicide, and maintaining the ethical standards of the medical profession. Eventually, the California Court of Appeals held that the hospital and physicians must remove the NG tube, which was inserted against her will. As the court of appeals explained, "It is incongruous, if not monstrous, for medical practitioners to assert their right to preserve a life that someone else must live, or, more accurately, endure, for '15 to 20 years.'"[31] Moreover, the court held that the physicians had a duty to relieve her pain and suffering while she starved herself to death.

CASE 3: *Satz v. Perlmutter*[32]

Abe Perlmutter was a 73-year-old man who was paralyzed by Lou Gehrig's disease. He was terminally ill and needed a respirator to breathe. However, he was competent and could communicate with the judge. He had previously pulled out his respirator, but hospital employees reconnected it. Now he wanted to stop the hospital employees from interfering with the removal of his respirator, which would result in his death within an hour. Perlmutter told the judge, "It can't be worse than what I'm going through now."[33] In that case, the Florida court ordered the hospital not to interfere with removal of the respirator.

CASE 4: *Brophy v. New England Sinai Hospital*[34]

Paul Brophy was permanently comatose as a result of a ruptured aneurysm. Although he was unable to swallow, he could survive for several more years with a tube for nutrition and hydration. Previously, he had made some oral statements that he would not want artificial life support

(continued)

(continued from previous page)

and that under those circumstances he might as well be dead. At the request of the patient's family, the Massachusetts court allowed the withdrawal of the tube.

CASE 5: *In re Eichner*[35]

Brother Joseph Fox was a member of a Catholic religious order. He was in a vegetative state, was on a respirator, and had no reasonable chance of recovery. His superior, Father Eichner, wanted the hospital staff to remove the respirator from Brother Fox.

In formal philosophical and religious discussions, Brother Fox had expressed his desire that he not receive any extraordinary means of life support, and he reiterated that view shortly before his final hospitalization. Therefore, the New York Court allowed the removal of the respirator on the grounds that there was clear and convincing evidence of the patient's desires.

CASE 6: *In re Mary O'Connor*[36]

Mary O'Connor, 77 years old, had suffered several strokes but was not in pain. Although she was incompetent as a result of the strokes, she was not in a coma or persistent vegetative state. Rather, she was conscious and might become more alert in the future.

The hospital wanted to insert an NG tube for nutrition and hydration to avoid a potentially painful death by starvation and thirst. However, the patient's two adult daughters objected to the use of the NG tube. The only evidence of the patient's desires was in conversations with her daughters and coworkers to the effect that she would not want artificial life support. However, she had never discussed the specific issue of nutrition and hydration and had not discussed the possibility of a painful death. In this case, the New York court refused to stop the insertion of the NG tube on the grounds that there was no clear and convincing evidence of the patient's desires.

Some people have compared this case to the decision in *Eichner*, in which the New York court allowed termination of treatment for Brother Joseph Fox. Specifically, critics have charged that the New York court is

(continued)

(continued from previous page)

unfair to ordinary people like Mary O'Connor, who express their desires in conversations with family and friends and do not have the opportunity to participate in formal philosophical discussions as Brother Fox did.

CASE 7: *Superintendent of Belchertown State School v. Saikewicz*[37]

Joseph Saikewicz was profoundly retarded, but he was conscious. Although he was 67 years old, he had a mental age of two years and eight months and had never learned to speak. He had leukemia, and the issue was whether he should be given chemotherapy. Most competent patients with leukemia choose to undergo chemotherapy, which can be successful. However, Saikewicz would not have cooperated with the chemotherapy and would not have understood the reason for the treatment. In this case, the Massachusetts court ruled that chemotherapy should be withheld.

CASE 8: *In re Storar*[38]

John Storar was profoundly retarded and conscious. Although he was 52 years old, he had a mental age of only 18 months. He was terminally ill with bladder cancer and on drugs for the pain. Regardless of any treatment, Storar would die within three to six months. However, he was losing blood in his urine and would die within weeks if he did not receive blood transfusions. The facility wanted to give blood transfusions to Storar, but his mother objected. Although the patient disliked the transfusions, he could be sedated. In this case, the New York court held that the facility should be allowed to give blood transfusions to the patient over the objections of his mother.

Physician-Assisted Suicide

Even if a patient has the right to refuse life-sustaining treatment, that right does not necessarily include the right to have another person, such as a physician, assist in ending his life. Some people think access to PAS should be a right, whereas others strongly disagree. The ethical arguments in favor of PAS are based on the principle of autonomy or self-determination in making important personal decisions as well as the principle of beneficence or mercy in helping to relieve the suffering of terminally ill patients.[39] However, others

Name of Patient	Mental Condition (Competence)	Physical Condition	Type of Treatment at Issue	Patient's Instructions	Court's Decision

EXHIBIT 12.1
Termination
of Treatment
Cases

argue that it is simply immoral to kill an innocent person, even if it is done to relieve suffering; that legalized PAS would be difficult to control; and that killing a patient is an inappropriate role for a physician.[40]

The American Medical Association (AMA) takes the position that for a physician to participate in assisted suicide would be unethical. According to the AMA's Council on Ethical and Judicial Affairs, "Physician-assisted suicide is fundamentally incompatible with the physician's role as healer, would be difficult or impossible to control, and would pose serious societal risks."[41] However, the AMA is merely a private professional organization, and its ethical opinions do not have the force of law. In fact, some physicians believe assisted suicide should be lawful and also believe it would be ethical in appropriate cases. Moreover, evidence has existed for many years that PAS is performed quietly on an underground basis where it cannot be supervised or regulated by law.[42]

At the present time, assisted suicide is a crime in almost every state. Therefore, the state government could send physicians and other healthcare professionals to prison or take away their licenses if they participate in PAS. To challenge those state laws, some physicians, patients, and advocacy groups had argued that the state laws violate their rights under the U.S. Constitution. They asked the federal courts to rule that the state laws are unconstitutional and unenforceable. Although some lower federal courts agreed with the plaintiffs, the U.S. Supreme Court held that the state laws are constitutional and indicated that PAS may be allowed or prohibited at the option of the state.

In *Washington v. Glucksberg*,[43] the Supreme Court explained that the right to refuse unwanted medical treatment, as discussed in *Cruzan*, is not the same as a right to assisted suicide. Therefore, the Supreme Court rejected the notion that patients have a constitutionally protected liberty interest in committing PAS. Moreover, the court concluded that the state has important interests to protect, and the prohibition of assisted suicide is reasonably related to those interests. Therefore, the state law that prohibits assisted suicide does not offend the Fourteenth Amendment to the U.S. Constitution.

On the same day, the U.S. Supreme Court reached a similar conclusion in *Vacco v. Quill*.[44] That case dealt with the New York law that allows patients to refuse lifesaving medical treatment but makes helping someone commit suicide a crime. Therefore, under New York law, patients on life-support equipment can choose to die quickly by having the equipment removed, but patients who need no artificial life support cannot choose to die quickly because they are not allowed to obtain any lethal drugs. According to the federal Court of Appeals for the Second Circuit, the withdrawal of life support is the same as assisted suicide; therefore, the distinction made by the New York law violates the Equal Protection Clause of the Fourteenth Amendment. However, the U.S. Supreme Court disagreed and concluded that there is a "distinction between letting a patient die and making that patient die."[45] Therefore, the Supreme Court held that the New York law prohibiting assisted suicide is consistent with the U.S. Constitution.

In light of these decisions, individuals do not have a constitutional right to PAS, and states may prohibit the practice if they so desire. However, states also have the option of permitting assisted suicide, as a few states, such as Oregon, have done to a limited extent. As former Chief Justice William Rehnquist wrote in *Washington v. Glucksberg*, "Throughout the Nation, Americans are engaged in an earnest and profound debate about the morality, legality, and practicality of physician-assisted suicide. Our holding permits this debate to continue, as it should in a democratic society."[46]

In 1994, the citizens of Oregon voted to approve the state's Death with Dignity Act, which is the first law in the United States to permit a type of PAS.[47] After some legal challenges, the Oregon statute finally became effective on October 27, 1997. In a referendum in November 1997, Oregon citizens reaffirmed their support for the assisted suicide law. In Oregon, physicians may now prescribe lethal drugs under specified conditions. However, physicians may not administer the lethal drugs to the patient.

Between 1997 and 2012, 673 patients in Oregon took lethal drugs for the purpose of PAS.[48] In addition, seriously ill residents of Oregon may take comfort in the availability of the procedure to obtain lethal drugs or the opportunity to request lethal drugs that they might never need to use.

Some federal officials tried to prevent Oregon physicians from participating in PAS in accordance with the Oregon statute. This dispute highlights the effect of policy and politics on the law, as well as the interaction of state and federal law in regulating the U.S. healthcare system. As discussed in Chapter 5, the regulation of medical practice is traditionally a state function. However, the federal government regulates the distribution of controlled substances, such as the lethal drugs that are used in PAS.

At the urging of Senator Orrin Hatch (R-UT) and Congressman Henry Hyde (R-IL), in November 1997 the federal Drug Enforcement Administration (DEA) indicated that Oregon physicians might be sanctioned by federal authorities if they prescribe drugs for assisted suicide in accordance with the Oregon statute. However, the U.S. attorney general in President Bill Clinton's administration, Janet Reno, subsequently overruled the DEA and stated that Oregon physicians will not be penalized by the federal government for actions taken pursuant to the state's assisted suicide law. In the meantime, some members of Congress attempted to enact a statute that would have prohibited physicians from performing assisted suicide with federally controlled drugs.[49]

Later, the U.S. attorney general who replaced Reno in President George W. Bush's administration, John Ashcroft, reversed Reno's position and reinstated the original DEA position. In a memorandum issued on November 9, 2001, Ashcroft wrote that the DEA has the authority to suspend or revoke the registration to dispense controlled substances of any physician who uses those substances for PAS.[50] The state of Oregon sued the U.S. attorney general in federal court for an injunction against enforcing Ashcroft's memorandum. On April 17, 2002, the federal district court ruled in favor of the state of Oregon and issued a permanent injunction to prohibit the attorney general from suspending or revoking the DEA registration of Oregon physicians who participate in PAS in accordance with the terms of the Oregon statute. The U.S. Court of Appeals for the Ninth Circuit essentially agreed with the district court and continued the injunction in effect. Finally, on January 17, 2006, the U.S. Supreme Court affirmed the judgment of the Court of Appeals, and rejected Attorney General Ashcroft's position.[51]

The issue in that case, which is known as *Gonzales v. Oregon*, was not whether patients have a constitutional right to PAS. As discussed previously, the Supreme Court had already resolved that issue by holding that there is no such constitutional right. Instead, *Gonzales v. Oregon* dealt with an issue of statutory interpretation with regard to the authority of federal officials under the federal Controlled Substances Act (CSA).[52] The issues were whether the U.S. attorney general and the DEA have authority under the federal statute to revoke the registration to use controlled substances of a physician who uses those substances to assist in a suicide in accordance with Oregon law, and whether an Oregon physician is subject to federal criminal prosecution under those circumstances. In resolving those issues of statutory interpretation, the Supreme Court concluded that Congress had never intended to give federal officials that type of control over the practice of medicine, which has been regulated traditionally by the government of each state. The following reading is an excerpt from the opinion of the U.S. Supreme Court in that case.

Gonzales v. Oregon, 546 U.S. 243 (2006)[53]
(CITATIONS AND FOOTNOTES OMITTED)

The question before us is whether the Controlled Substances Act allows the United States Attorney General to prohibit doctors from prescribing regulated drugs for use in physician-assisted suicide, notwithstanding a state law permitting the procedure. As the Court has observed, "Americans are engaged in an earnest and profound debate about the

(continued)

(continued from previous page)

morality, legality, and practicality of physician-assisted suicide." The dispute before us is in part a product of this political and moral debate, but its resolution requires an inquiry familiar to the courts: interpreting a federal statute to determine whether Executive action is authorized by, or otherwise consistent with, the enactment.

In 1994, Oregon became the first State to legalize assisted suicide when voters approved a ballot measure enacting the Oregon Death with Dignity Act (ODWDA). ODWDA, which survived a 1997 ballot measure seeking its repeal, exempts from civil or criminal liability state-licensed physicians who, in compliance with the specific safeguards in ODWDA, dispense or prescribe a lethal dose of drugs upon the request of a terminally ill patient.

The drugs Oregon physicians prescribe under ODWDA are regulated under a federal statute, the Controlled Substances Act (CSA or Act). The CSA allows these particular drugs to be available only by a written prescription from a registered physician. In the ordinary course the same drugs are prescribed in smaller doses for pain alleviation.

A November 9, 2001, Interpretive Rule issued by the Attorney General addresses the implementation and enforcement of the CSA with respect to ODWDA. It determines that using controlled substances to assist suicide is not a legitimate medical practice and that dispensing or prescribing them for this purpose is unlawful under the CSA. The Interpretive Rule's validity under the CSA is the issue before us.

We turn first to the text and structure of the CSA. Enacted in 1970 with the main objectives of combating drug abuse and controlling the legitimate and illegitimate traffic in controlled substances, the CSA creates a comprehensive, closed regulatory regime criminalizing the unauthorized manufacture, distribution, dispensing, and possession of substances classified in any of the Act's five schedules. The Act places substances in one of five schedules based on their potential for abuse or dependence, their accepted medical use, and their accepted safety for use under medical supervision. Schedule I contains the most severe restrictions on access and use, and Schedule V the least. Congress classified a host of substances when it enacted the CSA, but the statute permits the Attorney General to add, remove, or reschedule substances. He may do so, however, only after making particular findings, and on scientific and medical matters he is required to accept the findings of

(continued)

(continued from previous page)

the Secretary of Health and Human Services (Secretary). These proceedings must be on the record after an opportunity for comment.

The present dispute involves controlled substances listed in Schedule II, substances generally available only pursuant to a written, nonrefillable prescription by a physician. A 1971 regulation promulgated by the Attorney General requires that every prescription for a controlled substance "be issued for a legitimate medical purpose by an individual practitioner acting in the usual course of his professional practice."

To prevent diversion of controlled substances with medical uses, the CSA regulates the activity of physicians. To issue lawful prescriptions of Schedule II drugs, physicians must "obtain from the Attorney General a registration issued in accordance with the rules and regulations promulgated by him." The Attorney General may deny, suspend, or revoke this registration if, as relevant here, the physician's registration would be "inconsistent with the public interest." When deciding whether a practitioner's registration is in the public interest, the Attorney General "shall" consider:

"(1) The recommendation of the appropriate State licensing board or professional disciplinary authority."

"(2) The applicant's experience in dispensing, or conducting research with respect to controlled substances."

"(3) The applicant's conviction record under Federal or State laws relating to the manufacture, distribution, or dispensing of controlled substances."

"(4) Compliance with applicable State, Federal, or local laws relating to controlled substances."

"(5) Such other conduct which may threaten the public health and safety."

The CSA explicitly contemplates a role for the States in regulating controlled substances, as evidenced by its pre-emption provision.

"No provision of this subchapter shall be construed as indicating an intent on the part of the Congress to occupy the field in which that provision operates . . . to the exclusion of any State law on the same subject matter which would otherwise be within the authority of the

(continued)

(continued from previous page)

State, unless there is a positive conflict between that provision . . . and that State law so that the two cannot consistently stand together."

Oregon voters enacted ODWDA in 1994. For Oregon residents to be eligible to request a prescription under ODWDA, they must receive a diagnosis from their attending physician that they have an incurable and irreversible disease that, within reasonable medical judgment, will cause death within six months. Attending physicians must also determine whether a patient has made a voluntary request, ensure a patient's choice is informed, and refer patients to counseling if they might be suffering from a psychological disorder or depression causing impaired judgment. A second "consulting" physician must examine the patient and the medical record and confirm the attending physician's conclusions. Oregon physicians may dispense or issue a prescription for the requested drug, but may not administer it.

The reviewing physicians must keep detailed medical records of the process leading to the final prescription, records that Oregon's Department of Human Services reviews. Physicians who dispense medication pursuant to ODWDA must also be registered with both the State's Board of Medical Examiners and the federal Drug Enforcement Administration (DEA). In 2004, 37 patients ended their lives by ingesting a lethal dose of medication prescribed under ODWDA.

In 1997, Members of Congress concerned about ODWDA invited the DEA to prosecute or revoke the CSA registration of Oregon physicians who assist suicide. They contended that hastening a patient's death is not legitimate medical practice, so prescribing controlled substances for that purpose violates the CSA. The letter received an initial, favorable response from the director of the DEA, but Attorney General Reno considered the matter and concluded that the DEA could not take the proposed action because the CSA did not authorize it to "displace the states as the primary regulators of the medical profession, or to override a state's determination as to what constitutes legitimate medical practice." Legislation was then introduced to grant the explicit authority Attorney General Reno found lacking; but it failed to pass.

In 2001, John Ashcroft was appointed Attorney General. Perhaps because Mr. Ashcroft had supported efforts to curtail assisted suicide while serving as a Senator, Oregon Attorney General Hardy Myers wrote him to request a meeting with Department of Justice officials should the

(continued)

(continued from previous page)

Department decide to revisit the application of the CSA to assisted suicide. Attorney General Myers received a reply letter from one of Attorney General Ashcroft's advisers writing on his behalf, which stated, "I am aware of no pending legislation in Congress that would prompt a review of the Department's interpretation of the CSA as it relates to physician-assisted suicide. Should such a review be commenced in the future, we would be happy to include your views in that review."

On November 9, 2001, without consulting Oregon or apparently anyone outside his Department, the Attorney General issued an Interpretive Rule announcing his intent to restrict the use of controlled substances for physician-assisted suicide. Incorporating the legal analysis of a memorandum he had solicited from his Office of Legal Counsel, the Attorney General ruled:

> assisting suicide is not a 'legitimate medical purpose' within the meaning of 21 CFR 1306.04 (2001), and that prescribing, dispensing, or administering federally controlled substances to assist suicide violates the Controlled Substances Act. Such conduct by a physician registered to dispense controlled substances may 'render his registration . . . inconsistent with the public interest' and therefore subject to possible suspension or revocation under 21 U.S.C. 824(a)(4). The Attorney General's conclusion applies regardless of whether state law authorizes or permits such conduct by practitioners or others and regardless of the condition of the person whose suicide is assisted.

There is little dispute that the Interpretive Rule would substantially disrupt the ODWDA regime. Respondents contend, and petitioners do not dispute, that every prescription filled under ODWDA has specified drugs classified under Schedule II. A physician cannot prescribe the substances without DEA registration, and revocation or suspension of the registration would be a severe restriction on medical practice. Dispensing controlled substances without a valid prescription, furthermore, is a federal crime.

In response, the State of Oregon, joined by a physician, a pharmacist, and some terminally ill patients, all from Oregon, challenged the Interpretive Rule in federal court. The United States District Court for the

(continued)

(continued from previous page)

District of Oregon entered a permanent injunction against the Interpretive Rule's enforcement.

A divided panel of the Court of Appeals for the Ninth Circuit granted the petitions for review and held the Interpretive Rule invalid. It reasoned that, by making a medical procedure authorized under Oregon law a federal offense, the Interpretive Rule altered the "'usual constitutional balance between the States and the Federal Government'" without the requisite clear statement that the CSA authorized such action. The Court of Appeals held in the alternative that the Interpretive Rule could not be squared with the plain language of the CSA, which targets only conventional drug abuse and excludes the Attorney General from decisions on medical policy.

We granted the Government's petition for certiorari. . . .

Executive actors often must interpret the enactments Congress has charged them with enforcing and implementing. The parties before us are in sharp disagreement both as to the degree of deference we must accord the Interpretive Rule's substantive conclusions and whether the Rule is authorized by the statutory text at all. . . .

The Attorney General has rulemaking power to fulfill his duties under the CSA. The specific respects in which he is authorized to make rules, however, instruct us that he is not authorized to make a rule declaring illegitimate a medical standard for care and treatment of patients that is specifically authorized under state law.

The starting point for this inquiry is, of course, the language of the delegation provision itself. . . . The CSA does not grant the Attorney General this broad authority to promulgate rules. . . .

The Interpretive Rule thus purports to declare that using controlled substances for physician-assisted suicide is a crime, an authority that goes well beyond the Attorney General's statutory power to register or deregister. . . .

The authority desired by the Government is inconsistent with the design of the statute in other fundamental respects. The Attorney General does not have the sole delegated authority under the CSA. He must instead share it with, and in some respects defer to, the Secretary [of HHS], whose functions are likewise delineated and confined by the statute. The CSA allocates decision-making powers among statutory

(continued)

(continued from previous page)

actors so that medical judgments, if they are to be decided at the federal level and for the limited objects of the statute, are placed in the hands of the Secretary. In the scheduling context, for example, the Secretary's recommendations on scientific and medical matters bind the Attorney General. The Attorney General cannot control a substance if the Secretary disagrees.

In a similar vein the 1970 Act's regulation of medical practice with respect to drug rehabilitation gives the Attorney General a limited role; for it is the Secretary who, after consultation with the Attorney General and national medical groups, "determine[s] the appropriate methods of professional practice in the medical treatment of . . . narcotic addiction." . . .

The structure of the CSA, then, conveys unwillingness to cede medical judgments to an Executive official who lacks medical expertise. . . .

The Government contends the Attorney General's decision here is a legal, not a medical, one. This generality, however, does not suffice. The Attorney General's Interpretive Rule, and the Office of Legal Counsel memo it incorporates, place extensive reliance on medical judgments and the views of the medical community in concluding that assisted suicide is not a "legitimate medical purpose." This confirms that the authority claimed by the Attorney General is both beyond his expertise and incongruous with the statutory purposes and design.

The idea that Congress gave the Attorney General such broad and unusual authority through an implicit delegation in the CSA's registration provision is not sustainable. "Congress, we have held, does not alter the fundamental details of a regulatory scheme in vague terms or ancillary provisions—it does not, one might say, hide elephants in mouseholes."

The importance of the issue of physician-assisted suicide, which has been the subject of an "earnest and profound debate" across the country, makes the oblique form of the claimed delegation all the more suspect. Under the Government's theory, moreover, the medical judgments the Attorney General could make are not limited to physician-assisted suicide. Were this argument accepted, he could decide whether any particular drug may be used for any particular purpose, or indeed whether a physician who administers any controversial treatment could be deregistered. This would occur, under the Government's view, despite

(continued)

(continued from previous page)

the statute's express limitation of the Attorney General's authority to registration and control, with attendant restrictions on each of those functions, and despite the statutory purposes to combat drug abuse and prevent illicit drug trafficking.

We need not decide whether . . . deference would be warranted for an interpretation issued by the Attorney General concerning matters closer to his role under the CSA, namely preventing doctors from engaging in illicit drug trafficking. In light of the foregoing, however, the CSA does not give the Attorney General authority to issue the Interpretive Rule as a statement with the force of law.

In any event . . . we follow an agency's rule only to the extent it is persuasive, and for the reasons given and for further reasons set out below, we do not find the Attorney General's opinion persuasive. . . .

In deciding whether the CSA can be read as prohibiting physician-assisted suicide, we look to the statute's text and design. The statute and our case law amply support the conclusion that Congress regulates medical practice insofar as it bars doctors from using their prescription-writing powers as a means to engage in illicit drug dealing and trafficking as conventionally understood. Beyond this, however, the statute manifests no intent to regulate the practice of medicine generally. The silence is understandable given the structure and limitations of federalism, which allow the States "'great latitude under their police powers to legislate as to the protection of the lives, limbs, health, comfort, and quiet of all persons.'"

The structure and operation of the CSA presume and rely upon a functioning medical profession regulated under the States' police powers. The Attorney General can register a physician to dispense controlled substances "if the applicant is authorized to dispense . . . controlled substances under the laws of the State in which he practices." When considering whether to revoke a physician's registration, the Attorney General looks not just to violations of federal drug laws; but he "shall" also consider "[t]he recommendation of the appropriate state licensing board or professional disciplinary authority" and the registrant's compliance with state and local drug laws. The very definition of a "practitioner" eligible to prescribe includes physicians "licensed, registered, or otherwise permitted, by the United States or the jurisdiction in which he practices" to dispense controlled substances. Further

(continued)

(continued from previous page)

cautioning against the conclusion that the CSA effectively displaces the States' general regulation of medical practice is the Act's pre-emption provision, which indicates that, absent a positive conflict, none of the Act's provisions should be "construed as indicating an intent on the part of the Congress to occupy the field in which that provision operates . . . to the exclusion of any State law on the same subject matter which would otherwise be within the authority of the State."

Oregon's regime is an example of the state regulation of medical practice that the CSA presupposes. Rather than simply decriminalizing assisted suicide, ODWDA limits its exercise to the attending physicians of terminally ill patients, physicians who must be licensed by Oregon's Board of Medical Examiners. The statute gives attending physicians a central role, requiring them to provide prognoses and prescriptions, give information about palliative alternatives and counseling, and ensure patients are competent and acting voluntarily. Any eligible patient must also get a second opinion from another registered physician, and the statute's safeguards require physicians to keep and submit to inspection detailed records of their actions.

Even though regulation of health and safety is "primarily, and historically, a matter of local concern," there is no question that the Federal Government can set uniform national standards in these areas. In connection to the CSA, however, we find only one area in which Congress set general, uniform standards of medical practice. Title I of the Comprehensive Drug Abuse Prevention and Control Act of 1970, of which the CSA was Title II, provides that:

> [The Secretary], after consultation with the Attorney General and with national organizations representative of persons with knowledge and experience in the treatment of narcotic addicts, shall determine the appropriate methods of professional practice in the medical treatment of the narcotic addiction of various classes of narcotic addicts, and shall report thereon from time to time to the Congress.

This provision strengthens the understanding of the CSA as a statute combating recreational drug abuse, and also indicates that when Congress wants to regulate medical practice in the given scheme, it

(continued)

(continued from previous page)

does so by explicit language in the statute. In the face of the CSA's silence on the practice of medicine generally and its recognition of state regulation of the medical profession it is difficult to defend the Attorney General's declaration that the statute impliedly criminalizes physician-assisted suicide. This difficulty is compounded by the CSA's consistent delegation of medical judgments to the Secretary and its otherwise careful allocation of powers for enforcing the limited objects of the CSA. The Government's attempt to meet this challenge rests, for the most part, on the CSA's requirement that every Schedule II drug be dispensed pursuant to a "written prescription of a practitioner." A prescription, the Government argues, necessarily implies that the substance is being made available to a patient for a legitimate medical purpose. The statute, in this view, requires an anterior judgment about the term "medical" or "medicine." The Government contends ordinary usage of these words ineluctably refers to a healing or curative art, which by these terms cannot embrace the intentional hastening of a patient's death. It also points to the teachings of Hippocrates, the positions of prominent medical organizations, the Federal Government, and the judgment of the 49 States that have not legalized physician-assisted suicide as further support for the proposition that the practice is not legitimate medicine.

On its own, this understanding of medicine's boundaries is at least reasonable. The primary problem with the Government's argument, however, is its assumption that the CSA impliedly authorizes an Executive officer to bar a use simply because it may be inconsistent with one reasonable understanding of medical practice. Viewed alone, the prescription requirement may support such an understanding, but statutes "should not be read as a series of unrelated and isolated provisions." The CSA's substantive provisions and their arrangement undermine this assertion of an expansive federal authority to regulate medicine. . . .

The Government's interpretation of the prescription requirement also fails under the objection that the Attorney General is an unlikely recipient of such broad authority, given the Secretary's primacy in shaping medical policy under the CSA, and the statute's otherwise careful allocation of decisionmaking powers. Just as the conventions of expression indicate that Congress is unlikely to alter a statute's obvious scope and division of authority through muffled hints, the background

(continued)

(continued from previous page)

principles of our federal system also belie the notion that Congress would use such an obscure grant of authority to regulate areas traditionally supervised by the States' police power. . . . For all these reasons, we conclude the CSA's prescription requirement does not authorize the Attorney General to bar dispensing controlled substances for assisted suicide in the face of a state medical regime permitting such conduct.

The Government, in the end, maintains that the prescription requirement delegates to a single Executive officer the power to effect a radical shift of authority from the States to the Federal Government to define general standards of medical practice in every locality. The text and structure of the CSA show that Congress did not have this far-reaching intent to alter the federal-state balance and the congressional role in maintaining it.

The judgment of the Court of Appeals is affirmed.

In *Gonzales v. Oregon*, the U.S. Supreme Court made a decision that had the practical effect of supporting the proponents of PAS. In contrast, the Supreme Court's previous decisions in *Washington v. Glucksberg* and *Vacco v. Quill* had the practical effect of supporting those who are opposed to PAS. This apparent contradiction can be understood by differences in the types of legal issues that were before the court in those cases. As previously discussed, *Gonzales v. Oregon* addressed with an issue of statutory interpretation of the federal Controlled Substances Act, whereas the previous two cases had addressed the issue of whether a right to PAS exists under the U.S. Constitution.

Another way to reconcile the apparent discrepancy in the effect of these cases is to recognize that, in all three cases, the state government retained the authority to make its own decision about whether to permit PAS in its state. Thus, states that choose to prohibit PAS have the power to do so, because no constitutional right to PAS exists. States that choose to allow PAS may do so without interference by the federal government, because Congress never intended to give federal officials control over the practice of medicine in each state. Under these circumstances, the decision about PAS can be made by the citizens and government of each state.

After the Supreme Court's decision in *Gonzales v. Oregon*, the issue of PAS has been considered in a number of states. The state of Washington adopted its Death with Dignity Act as a result of an initiative that was approved by the voters in 2008.[54] In Montana, on December 31, 2009, the state's Supreme Court held that physicians cannot be prosecuted for providing assistance in dying.[55] As stated by the Montana Supreme Court, "We therefore hold that . . . a terminally ill patient's consent to physician aid in dying constitutes a statutory defense to a charge of homicide against the aiding physician when no other consent exceptions apply."[56] However, the Montana Court did not decide broader constitutional issues because doing so was unnecessary.

In 2012, the citizens of Massachusetts had an opportunity to vote on a proposed Death with Dignity Act, but that proposal was defeated. Although the proposed Massachusetts law had many supporters, it also had many opponents, including the Massachusetts Medical Society, the Catholic Church, and some advocates for the rights of disabled persons. However, the legislature in the nearby state of Vermont enacted a law to permit PAS in 2013.[57]

Notes

1. *Washington v. Glucksberg*, 521 U.S. 702, 719 (1997) (citations omitted).

2. *Cruzan v. Director, Missouri Department of Health*, 497 U.S. 261 (1990).

3. See generally D. M. Harris, "Beyond Beneficiaries: Using the Medicare Program to Accomplish Broader Public Goals," *Washington and Lee Law Review* (2003), 60 (4): 1251–1314, at 1280–84.

4. See Patient Self-Determination Act, Omnibus Budget Reconciliation Act of 1990, § 4206, 42 U.S.C. § 1395cc(f) (2006).

5. Balanced Budget Act of 1997, Pub. L. No. 105-33, § 4641, 111 Stat. 251, 487 (1997) codified as amended at 42 U.S.C. § 1395cc(f)(1)(B).

6. See Assisted Suicide Funding Restriction Act of 1997, Pub. L. No. 105-12, 111 Stat. 23 (1997) (codified as amended at 42 U.S.C. §§ 14401 *et seq.*).

7. *Schloendorff v. Society of New York Hospital*, 211 N.Y. 125, 129–30 (1914).

8. *Jacobson v. Massachusetts*, 197 U.S. 11, 25 (1905) (upholding Massachusetts statute on compulsory vaccination).

9. See 42 U.S.C. § 274e (2006).

10. *Application of the President and Directors of Georgetown College, Inc.*, 331 F.2d 1000 (D.C. Cir.), *cert. denied*, 377 U.S. 978 (1964).

11. *Id.* at 1008–1009.

12. See, e.g., *Public Health Trust of Dade County, Florida v. Wons*, 541 So.2d 96 (Fla. 1989) (a competent adult patient may refuse a blood transfusion, even if the patient is a parent of minor children).

13. See, e.g., *In re Guardianship of L.S. and H.S.*, 87 P.3d 521, 526 (Nevada 2004) ("Other jurisdictions have uniformly held that when medical treatment is available and necessary to save a minor's life, the state may intervene").

14. *Application of the President and Directors of Georgetown College, Inc.*, 331 F.2d at 1008.

15. See, e.g., N.C. Gen. Stat. § 90-322 (2005).

16. G. J. Annas (2005). "'Culture of Life' Politics at the Bedside—The Case of Terri Schiavo." *New England Journal of Medicine* 352 (16): 1710–15, at 1714.

17. See 2003 Fla. Laws, Ch. 418.

18. Annas, *supra* note 16 at 1712. See also *Bush v. Schiavo*, 885 So.2d 321, 336 (Fla. 2004) ("In theory, the Act could have applied during its fifteen-day window to more than one person, but it is undeniable that in fact the criteria fit only Theresa Schiavo").

19. *Bush v. Schiavo*, 885 So.2d at 337.

20. *Id.* at 332.

21. See Annas, *supra* note 16, at 1713–14. See also An Act for the Relief of the Parents of Theresa Marie Schiavo, Pub. L. No. 109-3, 119 Stat. 15 (2005); *Schiavo ex rel. Schindler v. Schiavo*, 403 F.3d 1289 (11th Cir. 2005).

22. See, e.g., *In re Conroy*, 486 A.2d 1209 (N.J. 1985).

23. *Superintendent of Belchertown State School v. Saikewicz*, 370 N.E.2d 417, 431 (Mass. 1977).

24. *In re Storar*, 420 N.E.2d 64, 72–73 (N.Y. 1981).

25. See B. R. Furrow, T. L. Graney, S. H. Johnson, T. S. Jost, and R. L. Schwartz, *Health Law*, 2nd ed., Hornbook Series (St. Paul, MN: West Group, 2000): 838–40.

26. See *id.* at 842, 858.

27. See *id.* at 842–53.

28. *Vacco v. Quill*, 521 U.S. 793, 807 (1997).

29. 497 U.S. 261 (1990).

30. 225 Cal. Rptr. 297 (Cal. Ct. App. 1986).

31. *Id.* at 305.

32. 362 So.2d 160 (Fla. Dist. Ct. App.), *aff'd*, 379 So.2d 359 (Fla. 1980).

33. *Id.* at 161.

34. 497 N.E.2d 626 (Mass. 1986).

35. 420 N.E.2d 64 (N.Y. 1981).

36. 531 N.E.2d 607 (N.Y. 1988).

37. 370 N.E.2d 417 (Mass. 1977).

38. 420 N.E.2d 64 (N.Y. 1981).

39. See J. D. Arras, "Physician-Assisted Suicide: A Tragic View," *Journal of Contemporary Health Law & Policy* (1997), 13: 361–89.

40. *Id.*

41. American Medical Association, Council on Ethical and Judicial Affairs, *Code of Medical Ethics of the American Medical Association: Current Opinions with Annotations* (2006–2007 edition) (Chicago: American Medical Association, 2006): § 2.211.

42. See, e.g., A. D. Lowe, "Facing the Final Exit," *ABA Journal* (September 1997), 83: 48–52.

43. 521 U.S. 702 (1997).

44. 521 U.S. 793 (1997).

45. *Id.* at 807.

46. *Washington*, 521 U.S. at 735.

47. See Or. Rev. Stat. §§ 127.800–127.897 (1997).

48. Oregon Health Authority, Public Health Division, "Annual Report: Year 15-2012" (January 16, 2013) at 2. http://public.health. oregon.gov/ProviderPartnerResources/EvaluationResearch/ DeathwithDignityAct/Documents/year15.pdf.

49. See, e.g., proposed Pain Relief Promotion Act of 1999, H.R. 2260, 106th Cong. (introduced June 17, 1999).

50. Dispensing of Controlled Substances to Assist Suicide, 66 Fed. Reg. 56607, 56607–56608 (November 9, 2001).

51. *Gonzales v. Oregon*, 546 U.S. 243 (2006).

52. 21 U.S.C. §§ 801 *et seq.* (2006).

53. *Gonzales v. Oregon*, 546 U.S. 243 (2006)

54. Rev. Code Wash. (ARCW), Chapter 70.245 (effective March 5, 2009).

55. *Baxter v. Montana*, 224 P. 3d 1211 (2009).

56. *Id.* at 1222.

57. General Assembly of the State of Vermont, No. 39, "An act relating to patient choice and control at end of life" (S.77), codified as 18 V.S.A. chapter 113 (signed by the governor on May 20, 2013).

13

REPRODUCTIVE HEALTH

The U.S. Constitution explicitly protects many important rights, such as freedom of speech and freedom of religion. Although the Constitution explicitly protects the right to bear arms, it is silent on the right to bear children as well as the right *not* to bear children. Although these rights are not explicitly mentioned in the Constitution, the U.S. Supreme Court has stated that the right to bear children is "one of the basic civil rights of man."[1]

This type of implicit individual right is often referred to as the right of privacy. It includes the right to make personal decisions about important issues of individual and family life. As the Supreme Court has explained, "If the right of privacy means anything, it is the right of the *individual*, married or single, to be free from unwarranted governmental intrusion into matters so fundamentally affecting a person as the decision whether to bear or beget a child."[2]

Any attempt by the state to regulate human reproduction raises important constitutional issues. As in cases involving the right to refuse treatment, individuals may allege that their state government is violating their rights under the federal constitution. Under these circumstances, individuals may ask a federal court to declare that the state law violates the U.S. Constitution and may ask the court to issue an injunction against the state's enforcement of its law.

In a number of cases involving the right to refuse treatment, the U.S. Supreme Court has upheld state laws and rejected constitutional challenges. For example, in *Cruzan*, the Supreme Court held that Missouri's state law requirement of clear and convincing evidence for termination of treatment does not violate the U.S. Constitution.[3] Similarly, the Supreme Court held that states may prohibit physician-assisted suicide, as Washington and New York had done.[4]

In the area of reproductive rights, however, the outcome of constitutional litigation has been very different. Rather than leaving reproductive issues to the states, the Supreme Court has struck down state laws and set constitutional limits on the authority of state governments to regulate with regard to reproduction. Within those limits, states have some discretion to enact and enforce their own laws. In the following materials, the issue of what states may and may not regulate is addressed with regard to sterilization, contraception, and abortion. In later sections, the chapter addresses some of the complex issues of emergency contraception and maternal–fetal conflict.

Sterilization

Sterilization generally refers to the surgical procedures of vasectomy for men and tubal ligation for women. Although sterilization prevents reproduction, the procedure may be reversible in some cases.

The legal and ethical issues of sterilization may arise in at least three different contexts. First, sterilization may be the unavoidable result of a procedure that is performed for therapeutic reasons. Under those circumstances, the patient was not seeking to be sterilized as a means of preventing reproduction. Therefore, the primary legal issue is that of informed consent. Before agreeing to the therapeutic procedure, the patient has the right to know the consequences of the procedure, including the effect on future ability to procreate.

In another context, a person may wish to be sterilized as a voluntary decision to avoid having any additional children. In that situation, the state has an interest in ensuring that the person is mentally and legally competent, is fully aware of the consequences of the procedure, and has made a considered decision in requesting to be sterilized. The state has an even stronger interest in protecting a minor from an inappropriate sterilization, especially when the procedure is requested by a parent or guardian of the minor. For all of these reasons, states may choose to regulate voluntary sterilization for adults and may require court approval for sterilization of a minor.

The context that surrounds the most difficult legal and ethical issues is involuntary sterilization of persons who are developmentally disabled, including individuals who were referred to as "mentally retarded." In many of those cases, people have argued that sterilization was in the best interest of the disabled person. The reality, however, is that many persons with disabilities have been sterilized for the convenience of their families or the institutions in which they resided.

Apart from determining whether sterilization is in the best interest of the disabled person, in the past some people argued that society has a legitimate interest in preventing persons with disabilities from having any children. In the 1927 case of *Buck v. Bell*,[5] the U.S. Supreme Court upheld a Virginia statute that authorized the involuntary sterilization of so-called mental defectives, such as Carrie Buck.[6] See the excerpt on page 319.

Today, courts and legislatures have a more enlightened view about sterilization of persons with developmental disabilities, and they would not follow the holding or the analysis of *Buck v. Bell*. In fact, most Americans would strongly object to the suggestion made by Justice Holmes that we should "prevent those who are manifestly unfit from continuing their kind."[7] Modern courts would promote the best interests of the individual by means of detailed procedural requirements and would not sterilize individuals or groups for the supposed "good of society."

Buck v. Bell, 274 U.S. 200 (1927)[8]
(CITATIONS OMITTED)

MR. JUSTICE HOLMES delivered the opinion of the Court.

This is a writ of error to review a judgment of the Supreme Court of Appeals of the State of Virginia, affirming a judgment of the Circuit Court of Amherst County, by which the defendant in error, the superintendent of the State Colony for Epileptics and Feeble Minded, was ordered to perform the operation of salpingectomy upon Carrie Buck, the plaintiff in error, for the purpose of making her sterile. The case comes here upon the contention that the statute authorizing the judgment is void under the Fourteenth Amendment as denying to the plaintiff in error due process of law and the equal protection of the laws.

Carrie Buck is a feeble minded white woman who was committed to the State Colony above mentioned in due form. She is the daughter of a feeble minded mother in the same institution, and the mother of an illegitimate feeble minded child. She was eighteen years old at the time of the trial of her case in the Circuit Court, in the latter part of 1924. An Act of Virginia, approved March 20, 1924, recites that the health of the patient and the welfare of society may be promoted in certain cases by the sterilization of mental defectives, under careful safeguard, etc.; that the sterilization may be effected in males by vasectomy and in females by salpingectomy, without serious pain or substantial danger to life; that the Commonwealth is supporting in various institutions many defective persons who if now discharged would become a menace but if incapable of procreating might be discharged with safety and become self-supporting with benefit to themselves and to society; and that experience has shown that heredity plays an important part in the transmission of insanity, imbecility, etc. The statute then enacts that whenever the superintendent of certain institutions including the above named State Colony shall be of opinion that it is for the best interests of the patients and of society that an inmate under his care should be sexually sterilized, he may have the operation performed upon any patient afflicted with hereditary forms of insanity, imbecility, etc., on complying with the very careful provisions by which the act protects the patients from possible abuse. . . .

(continued)

(continued from previous page)

There can be no doubt that so far as procedure is concerned the rights of the patient are most carefully considered, and as every step in this case was taken in scrupulous compliance with the statute and after months of observation, there is no doubt that in that respect the plaintiff in error has had due process of law.

The attack is not upon the procedure but upon the substantive law. It seems to be contended that in no circumstances could such an order be justified. It certainly is contended that the order cannot be justified upon the existing grounds. The judgment finds the facts that have been recited and that Carrie Buck "is the probable potential parent of socially inadequate offspring, likewise afflicted, that she may be sexually sterilized without detriment to her general health and that her welfare and that of society will be promoted by her sterilization," and thereupon makes the order. In view of the general declarations of the legislature and the specific findings of the Court, obviously we cannot say as matter of law that the grounds do not exist, and if they exist they justify the result. We have seen more than once that the public welfare may call upon the best citizens for their lives. It would be strange if it could not call upon those who already sap the strength of the State for these lesser sacrifices, often not felt to be such by those concerned, in order to prevent our being swamped with incompetence. It is better for all the world, if instead of waiting to execute degenerate offspring for crime, or to let them starve for their imbecility, society can prevent those who are manifestly unfit from continuing their kind. The principle that sustains compulsory vaccination is broad enough to cover cutting the Fallopian tubes. Three generations of imbeciles are enough.

But, it is said, however it might be if this reasoning were applied generally, it fails when it is confined to the small number who are in the institutions named and is not applied to the multitudes outside. It is the usual last resort of constitutional arguments to point out shortcomings of this sort. But the answer is that the law does all that is needed when it does all that it can, indicates a policy, applies it to all within the lines, and seeks to bring within the lines all similarly situated so far and so fast as its means allow. Of course so far as the operations enable those who otherwise must be kept confined to be returned to the world, and thus open the asylum to others, the equality aimed at will be more nearly reached.

Judgment affirmed.

Contraception and Abortion

As recently as the 1960s, using any drug or device for the purpose of preventing conception was a crime in some states. In the state of Connecticut, for example, a physician could be fined or imprisoned for counseling or assisting anyone in using a contraceptive device.

For ten days in 1961, the Planned Parenthood League of Connecticut operated a center in New Haven. Its executive director and medical director were arrested for providing advice on contraception to married persons. After they were found guilty, however, the U.S. Supreme Court reversed their convictions on the grounds that the Connecticut statute violated the U.S. Constitution.[9] Although the justices disagreed about the basis for the constitutional right, Justice William Douglas relied on the right of privacy as applied to the intimate relationship of married couples. As Justice Douglas explained, the Connecticut law "operates directly on an intimate relation of husband and wife and their physician's role in one aspect of that relation."[10]

In 1972, the Supreme Court took the next step by extending that right to unmarried people as a matter of equal protection of the laws.[11] As the Supreme Court explained in that case, unmarried people have the same right of access to contraceptives as married people.[12] The Supreme Court reasoned that all people have the right of privacy "to be free from unwarranted governmental intrusion into matters so fundamentally affecting a person as the decision whether to bear or beget a child."[13] Thus, by 1972, the stage had been set for the most contentious issue of reproductive rights for both married and unmarried persons—the issue of abortion.

One year later, in 1973, the U.S. Supreme Court decided the landmark case of *Roe v. Wade*.[14] In that case, the court considered the constitutionality of a Texas statute that made it a crime to obtain an abortion except when necessary to save the life of the mother. Jane Roe was the fictitious name of a woman who wanted to obtain an abortion in Texas. However, her situation did not fit within the sole exception for an abortion—that which is necessary to save the life of the mother. Therefore, she sued a state official in federal court and asked the federal court to prevent the state from enforcing its law. Ultimately, the U.S. Supreme Court held that the Texas abortion statute violated Ms. Roe's constitutional right of personal privacy and established a framework for analyzing individual rights and state authority in this area of the law.

In addition to focusing on the issue of individual rights, the Supreme Court in *Roe v. Wade* emphasized the physician's right to practice medicine without interference by the state. Until a certain point in the pregnancy, "the attending physician, in consultation with his patient, is free to determine, without regulation by the State, that, in his medical judgment, the patient's pregnancy should be terminated."[15] Moreover, "[t]he decision vindicates the right of the physician to administer medical treatment according to his professional judgment up to the points where important state interests provide compelling justifications for intervention. Up to those points, the abortion decision in all its aspects is inherently, and primarily, a medical decision, and basic responsibility for it must rest with the physician. If an individual practitioner abuses the privilege of exercising proper medical judgment, the usual remedies, judicial and intraprofessional are available."[16]

However, the court also recognized that the state has legitimate interests in protecting maternal health and potential life. According to the court, those state interests become compelling at different points in the pregnancy. The court based its analysis of individual rights and state interests on the concept of trimesters of pregnancy. "For the stage prior to approximately the end of the first trimester, the abortion decision and its effectuation must be left to the medical judgment of the pregnant woman's attending physician."[17] After that point, the state may regulate abortion in ways that protect the health of the mother. Furthermore, after the point of viability, the state may protect potential life by prohibiting abortion except when necessary to preserve the life or health of the mother.

For several years, some people speculated that the Supreme Court might overrule its 1973 decision in *Roe v. Wade*. However, in 1992, the Supreme Court issued its decision in *Planned Parenthood of Southeastern Pennsylvania v. Casey*.[18] In that case, the court reaffirmed the right of a woman to terminate her pregnancy before the point of *viability*, which it described as "the most central principle of *Roe v. Wade*."[19] *Viability* refers to the point in time when the fetus could realistically survive outside of the mother.

However, as explained in the following excerpt from *Casey*, the Supreme Court rejected the trimester framework of *Roe*. Rather, in *Casey* the court emphasized viability as the point at which the state's interest in protecting potential life may override the individual rights of the pregnant woman, subject to important exceptions for abortions that are necessary to protect the life or health of the mother.

Planned Parenthood of Southeastern Pennsylvania v. Casey, 505 U.S. 833 (1992)[20] (CITATIONS OMITTED)

Liberty finds no refuge in a jurisprudence of doubt. Yet 19 years after our holding that the Constitution protects a woman's right to terminate

(continued)

(continued from previous page)

her pregnancy in its early stages, that definition of liberty is still questioned. Joining the respondents as amicus curiae, the United States, as it has done in five other cases in the last decade, again asks us to overrule *Roe*.

At issue in these cases are five provisions of the Pennsylvania Abortion Control Act of 1982, as amended in 1988 and 1989. . . . The Act requires that a woman seeking an abortion give her informed consent prior to the abortion procedure, and specifies that she be provided with certain information at least 24 hours before the abortion is performed. . . . Another provision of the Act requires that, unless certain exceptions apply, a married woman seeking an abortion must sign a statement indicating that she has notified her husband of her intended abortion. The Act exempts compliance with these three requirements in the event of a "medical emergency," which is defined in § 3203 of the Act. . . .

Before any of these provisions took effect, the petitioners, who are five abortion clinics and one physician representing himself as well as a class of physicians who provide abortion services, brought this suit seeking declaratory and injunctive relief. Each provision was challenged as unconstitutional on its face. . . .

It must be stated at the outset and with clarity that *Roe*'s essential holding, the holding we reaffirm, has three parts. First is recognition of the right of the woman to choose to have an abortion before viability and to obtain it without undue interference from the State. Before viability, the State's interests are not strong enough to support a prohibition of abortion or the imposition of a substantial obstacle to the woman's effective right to elect the procedure. Second is a confirmation of the State's power to restrict abortions after fetal viability, if the law contains exceptions for pregnancies which endanger the woman's life or health. And third is the principle that the State has legitimate interests from the outset of the pregnancy in protecting the health of the woman and the life of the fetus that may become a child. These principles do not contradict one another; and we adhere to each.

Constitutional protection of the woman's decision to terminate her pregnancy derives from the Due Process Clause of the Fourteenth Amendment. It declares that no State shall "deprive any person of life, liberty, or property, without due process of law." The controlling word in the cases before us is "liberty." . . .

(continued)

(continued from previous page)

The inescapable fact is that adjudication of substantive due process claims may call upon the Court in interpreting the Constitution to exercise that same capacity which by tradition courts always have exercised: reasoned judgment. Its boundaries are not susceptible of expression as a simple rule. That does not mean we are free to invalidate state policy choices with which we disagree; yet neither does it permit us to shrink from the duties of our office. . . .

Men and women of good conscience can disagree, and we suppose some always shall disagree, about the profound moral and spiritual implications of terminating a pregnancy, even in its earliest stage. Some of us as individuals find abortion offensive to our most basic principles of morality, but that cannot control our decision. Our obligation is to define the liberty of all, not to mandate our own moral code. The underlying constitutional issue is whether the State can resolve these philosophic questions in such a definitive way that a woman lacks all choice in the matter, except perhaps in those rare circumstances in which the pregnancy is itself a danger to her own life or health, or is the result of rape or incest. . . .

The sum of the precedent enquiry to this point shows *Roe*'s underpinnings unweakened in any way affecting its central holding. While it has engendered disapproval, it has not been unworkable. An entire generation has come of age free to assume *Roe*'s concept of liberty in defining the capacity of women to act in society, and to make reproductive decisions; no erosion of principle going to liberty or personal autonomy has left *Roe*'s central holding a doctrinal remnant; *Roe* portends no developments at odds with other precedent for the analysis of personal liberty; and no changes of fact have rendered viability more or less appropriate as the point at which the balance of interests tips. . . .

From what we have said so far it follows that it is a constitutional liberty of the woman to have some freedom to terminate her pregnancy. We conclude that the basic decision in *Roe* was based on a constitutional analysis which we cannot now repudiate. The woman's liberty is not so unlimited, however, that from the outset the State cannot show its concern for the life of the unborn, and at a later point in fetal development the State's interest in life has sufficient force so that the right of the woman to terminate the pregnancy can be restricted. . . .

(continued)

(continued from previous page)

We conclude the line should be drawn at viability, so that before that time the woman has a right to choose to terminate her pregnancy. . . .

We must justify the lines we draw. And there is no line other than viability which is more workable. To be sure, as we have said, there may be some medical developments that affect the precise point of viability, but this is an imprecision within tolerable limits given that the medical community and all those who must apply its discoveries will continue to explore the matter. The viability line also has, as a practical matter, an element of fairness. In some broad sense it might be said that a woman who fails to act before viability has consented to the State's intervention on behalf of the developing child.

The woman's right to terminate her pregnancy before viability is the most central principle of *Roe v. Wade*. It is a rule of law and a component of liberty we cannot renounce.

On the other side of the equation is the interest of the State in the protection of potential life. The *Roe* Court recognized the State's "important and legitimate interest in protecting the potentiality of human life." The weight to be given this state interest, not the strength of the woman's interest, was the difficult question faced in *Roe*. We do not need to say whether each of us, had we been Members of the Court when the valuation of the state interest came before it as an original matter, would have concluded, as the *Roe* Court did, that its weight is insufficient to justify a ban on abortions prior to viability even when it is subject to certain exceptions. The matter is not before us in the first instance, and coming as it does after nearly 20 years of litigation in *Roe*'s wake we are satisfied that the immediate question is not the soundness of *Roe*'s resolution of the issue, but the precedential force that must be accorded to its holding. And we have concluded that the essential holding of *Roe* should be reaffirmed. . . .

Roe established a trimester framework to govern abortion regulations. Under this elaborate but rigid construct, almost no regulation at all is permitted during the first trimester of pregnancy; regulations designed to protect the woman's health, but not to further the State's interest in potential life, are permitted during the second trimester; and during the third trimester, when the fetus is viable, prohibitions are permitted provided the life or health of the mother is not at stake. Most of

(continued)

(continued from previous page)

our cases since *Roe* have involved the application of rules derived from the trimester framework. . . .

We reject the trimester framework, which we do not consider to be part of the essential holding of *Roe*. Measures aimed at ensuring that a woman's choice contemplates the consequences for the fetus do not necessarily interfere with the right recognized in *Roe*, although those measures have been found to be inconsistent with the rigid trimester framework announced in that case. A logical reading of the central holding in *Roe* itself, and a necessary reconciliation of the liberty of the woman and the interest of the State in promoting prenatal life, require, in our view, that we abandon the trimester framework as a rigid prohibition on all previability regulation aimed at the protection of fetal life. The trimester framework suffers from these basic flaws: in its formulation it misconceives the nature of the pregnant woman's interest; and in practice it undervalues the State's interest in potential life, as recognized in *Roe*. . . .

The very notion that the State has a substantial interest in potential life leads to the conclusion that not all regulations must be deemed unwarranted. Not all burdens on the right to decide whether to terminate a pregnancy will be undue. In our view, the undue burden standard is the appropriate means of reconciling the State's interest with the woman's constitutionally protected liberty. . . .

A finding of an undue burden is a shorthand for the conclusion that a state regulation has the purpose or effect of placing a substantial obstacle in the path of a woman seeking an abortion of a nonviable fetus. A statute with this purpose is invalid because the means chosen by the State to further the interest in potential life must be calculated to inform the woman's free choice, not hinder it. And a statute which, while furthering the interest in potential life or some other valid state interest, has the effect of placing a substantial obstacle in the path of a woman's choice cannot be considered a permissible means of serving its legitimate ends. . . .

Some guiding principles should emerge. What is at stake is the woman's right to make the ultimate decision, not a right to be insulated from all others in doing so. Regulations which do no more than create a structural mechanism by which the State, or the parent or guardian of a minor, may express profound respect for the life of the unborn are

(continued)

(continued from previous page)

permitted, if they are not a substantial obstacle to the woman's exercise of the right to choose. Unless it has that effect on her right of choice, a state measure designed to persuade her to choose childbirth over abortion will be upheld if reasonably related to that goal. Regulations designed to foster the health of a woman seeking an abortion are valid if they do not constitute an undue burden.

Even when jurists reason from shared premises, some disagreement is inevitable. That is to be expected in the application of any legal standard which must accommodate life's complexity. We do not expect it to be otherwise with respect to the undue burden standard. We give this summary:

(a) To protect the central right recognized by *Roe v. Wade* while at the same time accommodating the State's profound interest in potential life, we will employ the undue burden analysis as explained in this opinion. An undue burden exists, and therefore a provision of law is invalid, if its purpose or effect is to place a substantial obstacle in the path of a woman seeking an abortion before the fetus attains viability.

(b) We reject the rigid trimester framework of *Roe v. Wade*. To promote the State's profound interest in potential life, throughout pregnancy the State may take measures to ensure that the woman's choice is informed, and measures designed to advance this interest will not be invalidated as long as their purpose is to persuade the woman to choose childbirth over abortion. These measures must not be an undue burden on the right.

(c) As with any medical procedure, the State may enact regulations to further the health or safety of a woman seeking an abortion. Unnecessary health regulations that have the purpose or effect of presenting a substantial obstacle to a woman seeking an abortion impose an undue burden on the right.

(d) Our adoption of the undue burden analysis does not disturb the central holding of *Roe v. Wade*, and we reaffirm that holding. Regardless of whether exceptions are made for particular circumstances, a State may not prohibit any woman from making the ultimate decision to terminate her pregnancy before viability.

(continued)

(continued from previous page)

(e) We also reaffirm *Roe*'s holding that "subsequent to viability, the State in promoting its interest in the potentiality of human life may, if it chooses, regulate, and even proscribe, abortion except where it is necessary, in appropriate medical judgment, for the preservation of the life or health of the mother."

These principles control our assessment of the Pennsylvania statute, and we now turn to the issue of the validity of its challenged provisions. . . .

Our Constitution is a covenant running from the first generation of Americans to us and then to future generations. It is a coherent succession. Each generation must learn anew that the Constitution's written terms embody ideas and aspirations that must survive more ages than one. We accept our responsibility not to retreat from interpreting the full meaning of the covenant in light of all of our precedents. We invoke it once again to define the freedom guaranteed by the Constitution's own promise, the promise of liberty. . . .

It is so ordered.

In *Casey*, the Supreme Court established a framework of rules that can be used to evaluate specific laws that restrict or discourage abortion. This framework includes the recognition that a state has legitimate interests in protecting maternal health and potential life. At any time during the pregnancy, the state may regulate abortion for the purpose of protecting maternal health. In addition, the state may promote its interest in potential life by trying to discourage abortion even before the point of viability. However, before viability, the state may not prohibit abortion and may not place "a substantial obstacle in the path of a woman seeking an abortion of a nonviable fetus."[21]

After the point of viability, the state may prohibit abortion, except when it is necessary to preserve the life or health of the mother. Thus, the state could prohibit abortion after the point of viability even if it is clear that the baby will be born with serious deformities, or even if the pregnancy was the result of rape or incest. However, under *Casey*, a state law that prohibits abortion after viability must contain exceptions that would permit abortion to preserve the *health* of the mother and not merely to save the *life* of the mother.

After establishing its framework of rules, the court in *Casey* applied those rules to specific requirements of Pennsylvania law, and demonstrated how its framework should be applied to laws of that type. The court upheld Pennsylvania's requirement for a 24-hour waiting period to obtain an abortion except in cases of medical emergency. According to the court, the state's requirement of a 24-hour waiting period might cause a woman to choose childbirth over abortion. However, the state's requirement did not impose a substantial obstacle or an undue burden on the legal right to obtain an abortion.

In *Casey*, the court also upheld Pennsylvania's requirement that the doctor or other healthcare professional inform the woman about availability of state-published materials regarding the nature of the fetus and the consequences of abortion to the fetus, as well as information about help that would be available to the woman if she decides not to have an abortion. The court recognized that this type of "informed choice" requirement expresses the preference of the state government for birth rather than abortion and also recognized that this type of requirement might influence the woman to not have an abortion. Nevertheless, this type of requirement is permissible under the court's framework because it is not a substantial obstacle or an undue burden.

What about state requirements to notify the woman's spouse before performing an abortion or to obtain the consent of a parent or guardian before performing an abortion on a minor? In *Casey*, the court held that states may not require married women to notify their husbands before obtaining an abortion. As the court stated, "Women do not lose their constitutionally protected liberty when they marry."[22] However, the court upheld Pennsylvania's requirement to obtain the consent of a parent or guardian before performing an abortion on a woman who is under the age of 18 and not legally emancipated. In addition to providing an exception for medical emergencies, the Pennsylvania law provided an alternative for approval of the abortion by a court. This alternative for approval by a court is referred to as a **judicial bypass procedure**, and it is a necessary condition on any state requirement for parental consent to abortion. Activity 13.1 at the end of this chapter provides an opportunity to apply the rules in *Casey* to a hypothetical state abortion law.

In the years since the Supreme Court decided *Casey* in 1992, the court has neither overruled nor affirmed that decision or its framework of legal rules for abortion. The court had an opportunity in 2007 to reconsider *Casey*, as well as *Roe v. Wade*, in a decision about a federal statute that regulated late-term procedures it called "partial-birth abortions."[23] In that case, the Supreme Court upheld a federal statute prohibiting certain late-term abortions, even though that statute did not contain an exception for abortions necessary to preserve the health of the mother.[24] In that case, the court did not reconsider its holdings in *Roe* and *Casey*, but neither did the majority

Judicial bypass procedure
A process to obtain court approval to perform an abortion on a woman who is under the age of 18 and not legally emancipated, as an alternative to consent of a parent or guardian.

of justices reaffirm the holdings of *Roe* and *Casey*. Instead, the majority merely assumed that the principles of *Roe* and *Casey* were controlling.

The applicability of that 2007 decision on late-term abortion is limited, because other medical procedures were available in that situation. Moreover, the court merely held that the federal statute was constitutional on its face, but the statute might be held in the future to be unconstitutional as actually applied. Under these circumstances, *Casey* is still a valid legal precedent, and laws that restrict abortion are still subject to its framework of rules, including the need to provide an exception for abortions necessary to preserve the health of the mother.

Distinguishing between a woman's constitutional right to terminate her pregnancy and the lack of a constitutional right to government funding to terminate a pregnancy is also important. As discussed in Chapter 8, a longstanding federal law known as the Hyde Amendment prohibits use of federal Medicaid funding for abortion, except in very limited circumstances. The Supreme Court has upheld the Hyde Amendment on the grounds that there is no constitutional right to government funding for abortion.[25]

The prohibition of federal funding for abortion became a controversial issue in debates over the 2010 Affordable Care Act (ACA). That health reform law authorizes the creation of insurance exchanges where many uninsured individuals can purchase health insurance, and it helps those individuals to purchase insurance by providing federal subsidies or tax credits on the basis of their income. However, some people objected that the federal subsidies or tax credits might be used to purchase health insurance policies that provide coverage for abortion and thereby would provide federal funding for abortion. As part of the negotiations for enactment of the ACA in 2010, Congress agreed that the ACA would follow the Hyde Amendment by prohibiting use of federal subsidies or tax credits for abortion, in coverage obtained through a health insurance exchange, subject to the same limited exceptions. In addition, the ACA requires accounting and segregation of funds to ensure that federal funding is not used for abortion, and it allows states to enact laws to prohibit coverage for abortion in policies purchased in an exchange.[26]

Another controversial issue in implementing the ACA involves the mandate for employers to provide insurance coverage for contraceptives, especially as that mandate is applied to religiously affiliated employers. To implement the ACA provisions on insurance coverage for preventive services, HHS issued rules requiring access to certain preventive services with no copayment or deductible and asked the Institute of Medicine (IOM) to recommend necessary preventive services for women. In response, IOM recommended providing coverage for contraceptives, and HHS adopted that recommendation. However, some religious organizations and the owners of some business corporations oppose the use of contraceptives and do not want to provide contraceptive coverage to their employees.

HHS revised its *rules*, allowing officials to exempt *some* religious employers from the guidelines for contraceptive services. Specifically, the federal government provided an exemption for the employees of churches, but not for the employees of church-affiliated organizations, such as universities or hospitals. Also, the rule provides no exemption for private, for-profit businesses that are owned by religious individuals.

The federal government tried to develop a compromise and issued several sets of rules or proposed rules on this topic.[27] The government clarified the exemption and created mechanisms so that religiously affiliated employers would not have to pay directly for contraceptive coverage for their workers. However, the government's attempts at compromise have not satisfied the objections of some opponents of the contraceptive mandate.

This dispute over contraceptive coverage has resulted in strong protests as well as litigation in federal courts. At the time of this writing, litigation is still pending, and federal courts have disagreed among themselves about the legal issues in these cases. Although the cases raise some common arguments, different issues arise in cases filed by religiously affiliated organizations and those filed by for-profit corporations. On November 26, 2013, the U.S. Supreme Court indicated that it would resolve at least some of these issues by agreeing to hear two cases involving for-profit companies.[28]

Emergency Contraception

In recent years, new issues of law and ethics have arisen in regard to emergency contraception (EC), which is a pharmaceutical method of preventing pregnancy after unprotected sex or after failure of another method of contraception. EC is not the same as medical abortion, which is a pharmaceutical method of terminating a pregnancy. In September 2000, the U.S. Food and Drug Administration (FDA) approved the use of mifepristone, commonly known as RU-486, for medical abortion up to 49 days of pregnancy.[29] In contrast to RU-486, which clearly is a method of abortion, EC does not terminate a pregnancy.[30]

At least three important legal and ethical issues exist with regard to EC.[31] First, should EC be available over the counter (OTC) without a prescription to adults and to minors? Second, may pharmacists refuse to fill a prescription for EC or sell EC because of their personal beliefs? Finally, should hospital emergency departments, including those operated by religious organizations, be required to provide EC or advice about the availability of EC to survivors of sexual assault?

The proposal to make EC available without a prescription has been a contentious issue. In May 2004, the FDA refused to switch the status of an EC drug known as Plan B to OTC status, despite the recommendations of FDA's staff and advisory committee.[32] Subsequently, in December 2006, the FDA announced its approval of Plan B on an OTC basis for women over the age of 18 years, but would still require the use of a prescription for women under age 18.[33] Even for women over the age of 18 years, Plan B would only be available in a pharmacy or store that is staffed by a pharmacist, and it would be kept behind the counter under that 2006 policy. As the FDA explained at that time, "This means Plan B will not be sold at gas stations or convenience stores, where other OTC products are routinely available."[34] In 2009, the FDA changed its policy by lowering the age limit to 17 years of age.[35] Subsequently, in 2011, the FDA proposed to make EC available, without a prescription, to all women of child-bearing potential, but the secretary of HHS overruled the FDA.[36]

In 2013, litigation in federal court resulted in a change of federal policy about the availability of Plan B on an OTC basis. As the FDA explained in a press release on June 20, 2013,

> Today, the U.S. Food and Drug Administration announced it has approved the use of Plan B One-Step (levonorgestrel) as a nonprescription product for all women of child-bearing potential. This action complies with the April 5, 2013 order of the United States District Court in New York to make levonorgestrel-containing emergency contraceptives available as an over-the-counter (OTC) product without age or point-of-sale restrictions.
>
> Plan B One-Step is an emergency contraceptive intended to reduce the chance of pregnancy following unprotected sexual intercourse or a known or suspected contraceptive failure (e.g., condom). Plan B One-Step is a single-dose pill (1.5 mg tablet) that is effective in decreasing the chance of pregnancy and should be taken as soon as possible within three days after unprotected sex.
>
> On June 10, 2013, the agency notified a United States District Court judge in New York of its intent to comply with the court's April 5, 2013 order instructing the FDA to make levonorgestrel-containing emergency contraceptives available as an over-the-counter (OTC) product without age or point-of-sale restrictions. To comply, the FDA asked Teva Women's Health, the manufacturer of Plan B One-Step, to submit a supplemental application seeking approval of the one-pill product to be made available without any restrictions. The agency has fulfilled its commitment to the court by promptly completing its review and approval of the supplemental application.[37]

As a practical matter, access to Plan B may depend on the willingness of a pharmacist to dispense the drug to an adult or fill the prescription for a minor. Some pharmacists have refused to fill prescriptions for Plan B on the grounds of their personal or religious beliefs. Many states have enacted so-called conscience clauses that protect the right of healthcare professionals to refuse to participate in procedures to which they object, such as abortion. Depending on their precise wording, some existing and proposed state laws may be broad enough to allow pharmacists to refuse to fill prescriptions for Plan B or sell Plan B without a prescription.[38]

Should hospitals that provide treatment to survivors of sexual assault be required by law to provide access to EC, even if the hospital is owned by a religious organization that is opposed to EC? Over several years, Congress has considered—but has not enacted—various bills that would have prohibited giving any federal funds to a hospital that refuses to provide EC to a victim of sexual assault.[39] However, several states have enacted statutes on this issue. For example, a New Mexico statute requires that "[a] hospital that provides emergency care for sexual assault survivors shall . . . provide emergency contraception at the hospital to each sexual assault survivor who requests it."[40]

Maternal–Fetal Conflict

One of the recurring themes in healthcare law and ethics is determining when the interests of society will outweigh the interests of the individual. The state may force people to be vaccinated against their will and, in some circumstances, force people to accept unwanted blood transfusions. In the *Georgetown College* case discussed in Chapter 12, the court reasoned that the individual had a duty to society to care for her seven-month-old child and that the state had an interest in protecting the life of the mother. Therefore, the mother had a duty to society to accept unwanted medical treatment.

That reasoning raises some serious questions. What is the extent of a parent's duty to society to accept unwanted medical treatment? Moreover, if a parent has a duty to society to care for a child, does a woman who is pregnant with a viable fetus have a similar duty to society to protect the potential life of that viable fetus?

In *Planned Parenthood of Southeastern Pennsylvania v. Casey*, the Supreme Court held that the state has a legitimate interest in protecting the potential life of a viable fetus. Therefore, with few exceptions, the state may prohibit abortion after the point of viability. Should the state also have the power to prohibit a pregnant woman from taking other actions that might injure the viable fetus, such as smoking, skydiving, and abusing drugs and alcohol? Should the state have the power to require a pregnant woman to accept unwanted treatment to protect the potential life of the viable fetus?

Many people believe such assertions of governmental power would violate the individual rights of the pregnant woman and constitute unwarranted interference in private decisions.

Another aspect of this issue is whether a pregnant woman's fetally toxic behavior provides a basis for civil commitment, termination of parental rights, or criminal prosecution for child abuse or delivering drugs to a minor.[41] For example, a state statute in South Dakota provides that a pregnant woman who is intoxicated and abusing drugs or alcohol "may be committed to an approved treatment facility for emergency treatment."[42] Moreover, the Supreme Court of South Carolina held that a pregnant woman's drug abuse constituted criminal child neglect because the defendant's viable fetus was a "person" within a meaning of the applicable statute.[43] Nevertheless, many state courts have held that prenatal conduct does *not* provide a basis for criminal prosecution under the terms of the laws in those states.[44]

In another case that arose in South Carolina, the U.S. Supreme Court considered a state hospital's policy of testing some pregnant women for use of cocaine and providing police with the names of those women who tested positive and failed to cooperate in obtaining treatment.[45] The Supreme Court held that the hospital's system of diagnostic testing and reporting constituted an unreasonable search in violation of the Fourth Amendment because the testing was performed by government employees without a warrant and without probable cause. In addition, the court assumed that the searches were performed without the consent of the patients. Finally, the court held that these searches did not fit within a narrow exception to the warrant requirement for "special needs" searches that are not conducted primarily for the purpose of law enforcement. "In this case, however, the central and indispensable feature of the policy from its inception was the use of law enforcement to coerce the patients into substance abuse treatment."[46]

In that case, the Supreme Court resolved a specific issue with regard to the use of warrantless searches without consent by employees of state government hospitals. However, that narrow ruling left many questions unanswered. The court did not address the issue of searches performed with the consent of the patient or searches by employees of nongovernmental hospitals. Moreover, the court acknowledged that hospital employees and healthcare professionals may have duties to report certain information to authorities about their patients, such as gunshot wounds and child abuse. Finally, the court did not resolve the underlying issues of maternal–fetal conflict, such as the possibility of criminal sanctions for drug abuse or other fetally toxic behavior.

In the meantime, other courts have addressed a different aspect of maternal–fetal conflict by considering whether a pregnant woman should be required to deliver by caesarean section when the attending physician believes the surgery is necessary to protect the life or health of the fetus. For example, the case of *In re A.C.*[47] dealt with whether a forced caesarean should have been performed on a terminally ill cancer patient who was pregnant with a viable fetus. In that case, the mother's wishes were somewhat unclear, but she apparently objected to the procedure. According to the appellate court, the issue should not be resolved by trying to balance the interests of the pregnant woman against the interests of the fetus and the state. Rather, the decision on whether to undergo the surgery should be left up to the pregnant woman, if she is competent. If she is not competent, the court should make a substituted judgment on the basis of what the court believes the patient would have wanted.

In that case, the appellate court relied in part on the legal principle that we do not force one person to undergo an operation for the benefit of another. The court in *A.C.* cited *McFall v. Shimp*,[48] which held that a person could not be forced to donate bone marrow to his relative, even if his relative would probably die without it. As the court in *McFall v. Shimp* explained,

> The common law has consistently held to a rule which provides that one human being is under no legal compulsion to give aid or to take action to save another human being or to rescue. . . . Morally, this decision rests with defendant, and, in the view of the court, the refusal of defendant is morally indefensible. For our law to *compel* defendant to submit to an intrusion of his body would change every concept and principle upon which our society is founded. To do so would defeat the sanctity of the individual, and would impose a rule which would know no limits, and one could not imagine where the line would be drawn. . . .
>
> For a society which respects the rights of *one* individual, to sink its teeth into the jugular vein or neck of one of its members and suck from it sustenance for *another* member, is revolting to our hard-wrought concepts of jurisprudence.[49]

In *A.C.*, the court relied in part on that principle and concluded that courts should not force a pregnant woman to undergo surgery for the benefit of her fetus, even if the fetus is viable and may no longer be aborted. In addition, courts should refrain from ordering forced caesareans for other reasons. Physicians may be incorrect in concluding and testifying that a caesarean is necessary to preserve the life or health of the fetus.[50] Moreover, judicial hearings on this issue may be fundamentally unfair because women in labor are likely to have difficulty obtaining immediate legal representation and an independent medical opinion. Finally, the possibility of being forced to have a caesarean may discourage some women from seeking medical care, especially if they are aware that they have a high risk of complications. For all of these reasons, most courts would not order a caesarean over the objections of the pregnant woman.

ACTIVITY 13.1: STATE ABORTION STATUTE

Please assume the following facts. Recently, the state legislature enacted a statute on the subject of abortion. That statute has been signed by the governor, and it is currently in effect. The new statute provides as follows:

State Protection of Human Life Act

1. After the point of viability, no abortion may be performed in this state unless that abortion is necessary to preserve the life of the mother or the health of the mother.

2. No abortion may be performed in this state if the abortion is sought for the purpose of sex selection.

3. Regardless of the stage of pregnancy, no abortion may be performed in this state until the expiration of a 48-hour waiting period. The 48-hour waiting period will begin at the time of the patient's first visit in person to the facility at which the abortion will be performed. However, the requirement of this section does not apply in cases of medical emergency.

4. No abortion may be performed on a woman who is under 18 years of age unless the physician who will perform the abortion obtains the prior written consent of one parent or guardian of that woman. However, the requirement of this section does not apply in cases of medical emergency. In addition, this requirement does not apply to minors who have been legally emancipated by a court. As an alternative to consent by a parent or guardian, prior written consent to the abortion may be provided by the court.

5. The state Department of Health (DOH) shall conduct a campaign of public education, in an effort to discourage pregnant women from having abortions. The legislature hereby appropriates $10 million from state tax revenues to pay for this campaign of public education for the purpose of discouraging abortion. In addition to using other methods of public education, DOH shall use a portion of those appropriated state funds to put signs on billboards throughout the state which contain a picture of a fetus, together with the words "Don't Kill Your Baby."

(continued)

(continued from previous page)

Please assume further that the Reproductive Rights Association (RRA) has filed a lawsuit in federal court to challenge this state statute. According to RRA, the state statute violates the U.S. Constitution in several ways. RRA did not assert any claims under the state Constitution. Therefore, the federal court will base its decision on the U.S. Constitution as interpreted by the U.S. Supreme Court. You should assume that the rules and analysis set forth by the U.S. Supreme Court in *Planned Parenthood of Southeastern Pennsylvania v. Casey* are still good law.

According to RRA, this state statute violates the U.S. Constitution on five separate grounds, as follows:

1. The state statute does not have an exception to allow abortions after the fetus has become viable in cases of rape or incest.
2. The prohibition of all abortions that are sought for the purpose of sex selection is an unconstitutional prohibition of abortion before the point of viability.
3. The requirement for a 48-hour waiting period places a substantial obstacle and an undue burden on abortion before the point of viability.
4. The requirement for prior written consent by a parent or guardian of a minor, as well as the alternative for prior written consent by the court, places a substantial obstacle and an undue burden on abortion before the point of viability.
5. The use of state tax revenues for the purpose of conducting a campaign to discourage abortion is unconstitutional because it uses state funds to argue in favor of a particular point of view and because it forces all taxpayers to support that campaign with their tax dollars even if they do not agree with that point of view.

Please analyze separately each of the arguments made by RRA. For each of those arguments, be sure to make a prediction about RRA's likelihood of success in federal court, and explain the reasons for your predictions.

Notes

1. *Skinner v. Oklahoma*, 316 U.S. 535, 541 (1942) (Douglas, J.).
2. *Eisenstadt v. Baird*, 405 U.S. 438, 453 (1972) (citations omitted).

3. *Cruzan v. Director, Missouri Department of Health*, 497 U.S. 261, 280–84 (1990).

4. *Washington v. Glucksberg*, 521 U.S. 702, 735 (1997); *Vacco v. Quill*, 521 U.S. 793, 807–808 (1997).

5. 274 U.S. 200 (1927) (Holmes, J.).

6. But see P. A. Lombardo, "Three Generations, No Imbeciles: New Light on *Buck v. Bell*," *New York University Law Review* (1985), 60: 30–62.

7. *Buck v. Bell*, 274 U.S. 200 (1927).

8. *Id.*

9. See *Griswold v. Connecticut*, 381 U.S. 479, 485–86 (1965).

10. *Id.* at 482.

11. See *Eisenstadt*, 405 U.S. at 447.

12. See *id.* at 453 (citations omitted).

13. *Id.*

14. 410 U.S. 113 (1973).

15. *Id.* at 163.

16. *Id.* at 165–66.

17. *Id.* at 164.

18. *Planned Parenthood of Southeastern Pa. v. Casey*, 505 U.S. 833 (1992).

19. *Id.* at 871.

20. *Planned Parenthood of Southeastern Pa. v. Casey*, 505 U.S. 833 (1992).

21. *Id.* at 877.

22. *Id.* at 898.

23. See *Gonzales v. Carhart*, 550 U.S. 124 (2007).

24. *Id.*

25. *Harris v. McRae*, 448 U.S. 297 (1980).

26. Pub. L. No. 111-148, § 1303(a) (2010).

27. *See, e.g.*, 78 Fed. Reg. 39870 (July 2, 2013) (final rules).

28. *Hobby Lobby Stores, Inc. v. Sebelius*, 723 F.3d 1114 (10th Cir. 2013), *cert. granted*, 134 S. Ct. 678 (2013); *Conestoga Wood Specialties Corp. v. Secretary*, 724 F.3d 377 (3rd Cir. 2013), *cert. granted*, 134 S. Ct. 678 (2013).

29. See generally C. E. Borgmann and B. S. Jones, "Legal Issues in the Provision of Medical Abortion," *American Journal of Obstetrics and Gynecology* (2000), 183 (2 suppl.): S84–S94.

30. D. A. Grimes (2002). "Switching Emergency Contraception to Over the Counter Status." *New England Journal of Medicine* 347(11): 846–49.

31. See *id.*

32. U.S. Government Accountability Office, "Decision Process to Deny Initial Application for Over-the-Counter Marketing of the Emergency Contraceptive Drug Plan B Was Unusual," GAO-06-109 (November 2005). www.gao.gov/new.items/d06109.pdf.

33. U.S. Food and Drug Administration, Center for Drug Evaluation and Research, "Plan B: Questions and Answers" (August 24, 2006, updated December 14, 2006). www.fda.gov/Drugs/DrugSafety/PostmarketDrugSafetyInformationforPatientsandProviders/ucm109783.htm.

34. *Id.*

35. U.S. Food and Drug Administration, "Updated FDA Action on Plan B (levonorgestrel) Tablets" (April 22, 2009). www.fda.gov/NewsEvents/Newsroom/PressAnnouncements/2009/ucm149568.htm.

36. U.S. Food and Drug Administration, "Statement from FDA Commissioner Margaret Hamburg, M.D. on Plan B One-Step" (December 7, 2011). www.fda.gov/NewsEvents/Newsroom/ucm282805.htm.

37. U.S. Food and Drug Administration, "FDA approves Plan B One-Step emergency contraceptive for use without a prescription for all women of child-bearing potential" (June 20, 2013). www.fda.gov/NewsEvents/Newsroom/PressAnnouncements/ucm358082.htm.

38. See M. J. Seamon, "Plan B for the FDA: A Need for a Third Class of Drug Regulation in the United States Involving a 'Pharmacist-Only' Class of Drugs," *William and Mary Journal of Women & the Law* (2006), 12: 521–62, at 557–58.

39. See, e.g., Compassionate Assistance for Rape Emergencies Act of 2011, H.R. 1724, 112th Cong. (2011); Compassionate Assistance for Rape Emergencies Act, S. 3945, 109th Cong. (2d Sess. 2006); Compassionate Assistance for Rape Emergencies Act, S. 1564, 108th Cong. (2003).

40. N. M. Stat. Ann. § 24-10D-3 (2006).

41. See generally "Development and Trends in the Law: Synopsis of State Case and Statutory Law," *Yale Journal of Health Policy, Law & Ethics* (2001), 1: 237–96.

42. S.D. Codified Laws § 34-20A-63 (2006). See also *id.* at § 34-20A-70(3) (commitment of pregnant alcoholics or drug abusers who habitually lack self-control).

43. *Whitner v. South Carolina*, 492 S.E.2d 777 (S.C. 1997), *cert. denied*, 523 U.S. 1145 (1998).

44. See *id.* at 782.

45. *Ferguson v. City of Charleston*, 532 U.S. 67 (2001).

46. *Id*. at 80.

47. 573 A.2d 1235 (D.C. 1990).

48. 10 Pa.D. and C.3d 90 (Pa. Commw. Ct. 1978).

49. *Id*. at 91–92 (1978).

50. See, e.g., D. B. Kennedy, "A Public Guardian Represents Fetus: Courts Refuse Request for a C-Section and Boy Is Born Apparently Healthy," *ABA Journal* (1994), 80 (March): at 27.

LEGAL AND ETHICAL ISSUES IN COST CONTAINMENT, HEALTH INSURANCE, AND HEALTH REFORM

LEGAL ISSUES IN HEALTHCARE COST CONTAINMENT

14

Throughout this book, we address the effect of cost containment and managed care on various aspects of the law and ethics of health. For example, Chapter 10 deals with the ways in which cost containment and managed care affect the law of medical malpractice, and Chapter 11 discusses the applicability of the Emergency Medical Treatment and Active Labor Act (EMTALA) to patients covered by managed care plans. In Part IV, the legal principles discussed in previous chapters are applied to the system of health insurance in light of cost containment and managed care.

In an effort to reduce healthcare costs, many third-party payers have adopted various techniques that are collectively referred to as **managed care**. These techniques are not limited to health maintenance organizations (HMOs), but rather they are used by many insurance companies, health plans, and even the government payment programs described in Chapter 8. No uniform model of managed care exists, but a few common techniques are shared by health insurance companies, HMOs, and other managed care organizations (MCOs).

One common technique of cost containment and managed care is referred to as **selective contracting**. Many third-party payers make contracts with preferred providers who are willing to cut their prices to obtain a greater volume of patients. The process of bidding for preferred provider contracts has increased the level of competition in the healthcare industry. However, it raises significant issues for patients as well as for providers who are excluded from a payer's network.

Another common technique is to use financial incentives that encourage physicians to reduce the cost of treatment. As discussed later, these incentives have the effect of aligning the financial interest of the physician with that of the payer rather than the patient. As a matter of law, ethics, and public policy, we may want to prohibit some or all financial incentives to provide less care or at least require disclosure of those incentives to the patient.

Finally, most third-party payers control the cost of care by means of **utilization review** (UR). When payers deny authorization for particular treatments, they insist they are not denying care or telling physicians how to practice medicine. According to the payers, they are merely interpreting the terms of coverage under the contract, and the physicians should provide,

Managed care
A method of cost containment in which third-party payers use various techniques to reduce healthcare costs.

Selective contracting
A technique of cost containment in which third-party payers make contracts with healthcare providers that are willing to reduce their prices and agree to the payer's utilization review procedures.

Utilization review
A technique of cost containment in which a third-party payer determines whether it will pay for treatment under the terms of the applicable plan, including retrospective review for services already rendered and prospective review for authorization of proposed services.

without coverage, whatever treatment they consider to be appropriate. However, as discussed later, that supposed distinction between coverage decisions and treatment decisions is specious, and a denial of payment is likely to result in a denial of treatment. As a practical matter, cost containment and managed care reduce healthcare costs by imposing limits on treatment and thereby raise the complex legal and ethical issues of rationing.

In the past, many healthcare providers and patients objected to the use of these techniques by third-party payers, and a significant backlash against managed care occurred.[1] Many states enacted laws to regulate specific aspects of managed care,[2] and market pressures forced MCOs to be somewhat more flexible in their use of UR and their limitations on provider networks. That flexibility, however, was merely a matter of degree, and the use of those techniques has continued or possibly even increased in recent years. In 2012, the *Wall Street Journal* noted that some health insurance companies were "reaching back to the 1990s and boosting the use of techniques that antagonized patients and doctors alike."[3] Although the 2010 Affordable Care Act (ACA) imposes many new requirements on health insurance companies and group health plans,[4] the ACA generally allows the use of these cost containment techniques, as discussed in more detail later.

Selective Contracting with Providers

Before the development of managed care, insured patients could choose to receive their treatment at almost any doctor's office or hospital. That system was referred to as *free choice of provider*. People became so used to being able to choose their own doctor or hospital that many considered the free choice of provider to be their legal right. As a legal matter, however, freedom of choice in private insurance plans was not a constitutional or statutory requirement but merely a term of a contract that was subject to negotiation and change.

Under the traditional system, patients could choose to go to the most expensive providers in the area, a practice that tended to increase overall healthcare costs. Although insurance companies were required to pay the bills for those expensive providers, they could pass on the costs to policyholders by raising premiums at the next opportunity. In an attempt to control their costs, many insurance companies tried to use charge screens for physicians, a mechanism through which the insurance company refused to pay more than the standard fees in each geographic area. In the long run, however, those mechanisms proved to be largely ineffective in keeping down healthcare costs. Therefore, people and organizations responsible for paying the bills looked for other means to control healthcare expenditures, including selective contracting with particular providers.

In selective contracting, payers make contracts with providers that are willing to grant discounts and agree to the payer's UR procedures. By reducing their prices and becoming the preferred providers for specific third-party payers, those physicians and healthcare facilities can increase their market share, or at least avoid a significant loss of market share. In economic terms, sellers of goods or services may be able to maximize their profits by selling a larger volume at a lower unit price, rather than selling fewer goods or services at a higher price. The financial arrangements between the MCO and the physician may take the form of a monthly capitation or a discounted fee-for-service payment.

Before they would be willing to reduce their prices, however, providers need to have some assurance that the payers can actually deliver additional patients who are covered by their plans. To direct those additional patients to preferred providers, third-party payers use various mechanisms to influence their enrollees' choice of provider.

For example, in some HMOs, patients were essentially required to go to a provider that participated in the plan because the HMO would make no payment whatsoever for services that were rendered by nonplan providers. That restrictive form of managed care met with a great deal of resistance in the competitive marketplace. Therefore, some HMOs now allow their enrollees to be treated by providers outside of the plan if the enrollees pay an additional fee for a "point-of-service" option.

Even without that type of strict limitation, payers can influence their enrollees' choice of provider by manipulating the patients' out-of-pocket costs for copayments and deductibles. For example, a plan could provide that the patient would have to pay a 20 percent copayment for services rendered by a provider who is not participating in the network, but little or no copayment would be required for the services of a participating or preferred provider. In some cases, the patient may be willing to pay the additional money to see a particular physician who is not a part of the network, especially if the patient had an existing relationship with that physician. That practice could become costly, however, in the event of a serious illness or injury. Therefore, in the long run, these types of financial incentives can be effective in causing most patients to switch to participating providers to minimize their own out-of-pocket costs.

The ACA generally allows health insurance companies and health plans to use selective contracting, although the ACA provides some protections for patients in that process. Section 2719A of the ACA states that, if a health insurance plan requires enrollees to choose a primary care provider (PCP) who participates in that plan, "then the plan or issuer shall permit each . . . enrollee to designate any participating primary care provider who is available to accept such individual."[5] This section of the ACA does *not* state that individuals have a right to free choice of provider. Rather, this section indicates that health plans may continue to distinguish between participating and nonparticipating providers, and individuals only have a right to free choice among those PCPs who are both participating and available. Nevertheless, other parts of Section 2719A provide some additional rights for individuals who need emergency services, parents who want to designate a pediatrician in the plan as the PCP for a child, and women who want direct access to obstetrical or gynecological (OB/GYN) care without the need for authorization or referral by a PCP or the plan.[6]

In addition to raising issues for patients, the use of selective contracting raises significant legal and practical issues for healthcare providers. As discussed above, third-party payers have the power to direct a substantial number of patients to those providers that are willing to give them a discount, and providers have a strong interest in being selected as a participating or preferred provider. By definition, all of the providers in the area cannot be preferred providers for a single payer. Therefore, payers have bargaining power to exact substantial discounts from providers as a condition of being selected.

This situation has led to the development of a bargaining process in which payers can force providers to bid against each other for the patients who are covered by each particular payer. If a provider is unwilling to meet or exceed the discount offered by another provider, the first provider will probably not obtain the patients who are covered by that payer. Moreover, if a large number of a provider's existing patients are covered through that payer, the provider may even lose a substantial portion of its existing patient base if it is not selected as one of the payer's preferred providers.

As a general rule, MCOs and other payers do not have a legal obligation to accept every physician who applies for membership in their provider network. Moreover, payers have a strong incentive to carefully review the applications of physicians for membership in the network. An MCO may be held liable in tort on the same legal theories as a hospital, as discussed in Chapter 10 on medical malpractice. For example, an MCO might be held vicariously liable for the negligence of a participating physician on a theory of actual agency or ostensible agency. In addition, an MCO might be held liable under the doctrine of corporate negligence for its own failure to exercise reasonable care in screening and monitoring physicians in its network.

In addition to screening new applicants for network membership, an MCO might decide to terminate its existing relationship with a current member of its network. In some cases, the MCO may want to terminate a physician because of questions about that physician's professional performance. In other cases, however, the termination might be based entirely on business reasons, such as having an excess of physicians in that particular specialty. Regardless of the reason for termination, the practical effects are that the physician will no longer be able to treat the MCO's enrollees and the physician may suffer significant economic loss.

The relationship between a payer and a participating physician is set forth in a contract, which is called a provider agreement. However, the use of contract law principles does not necessarily mean that an MCO will have the right to remove a physician from its network. Even if a written provider agreement exists that permits termination by either party without cause, a court might or might not allow the MCO to strictly enforce the terms of that contract.

A contract is a voluntary agreement between the parties. Ordinarily, the rights and obligations of the parties will be governed by the terms of the contract, including specific provisions on how the contract may be terminated. In some circumstances, however, considerations of public policy may override the written terms of the contract and may provide additional rights or obligations for the parties.

The written contract between an MCO and a physician will often specify that the contract may be terminated by either party, with or without cause. In a termination for cause, one party may terminate the contract as a result of the other party's failure to perform its obligations as set forth in the contract. In contrast, a provision for termination without cause allows either party to terminate the contract, without any reason, by merely giving sufficient notice in advance to the other party. Thus, in a termination without cause, an MCO would have the right to terminate a physician from participation in its network without the need to demonstrate incompetence or unethical behavior on the part of the physician.

In *Harper v. Healthsource New Hampshire, Inc.*,[7] the written contract provided that either party could terminate the agreement without cause by giving six months' notice of intent to terminate. Healthsource terminated its agreement with Dr. Harper without cause, but Dr. Harper sued Healthsource in New Hampshire state court to challenge his termination by the plan. According to Dr. Harper, the provision allowing for termination of the contract without cause was void on the ground that it violated the public policy of the state. In 1996, the Supreme Court of New Hampshire agreed with Dr. Harper.

Under the court's analysis in *Harper*, an MCO may terminate a participating physician for no reason at all, but the physician may not be terminated for an improper reason that violates the public policy of the state. This concept is similar to the public policy exception to the legal doctrine of employment at will, although the physicians in this type of MCO network are not really employees of the MCO. In the employment context, workers may be characterized as employees at will, which means that they may be terminated at any time without cause, and they may leave at any time without penalty. Although employees at will may be terminated for no reason at all, some courts have held that they may not be terminated for an improper reason that would be contrary to public policy. For example, a healthcare facility may have the right to terminate an employee at will without cause, but it may not terminate the employee in retaliation for the employee's refusal to give false testimony in a medical malpractice case.[8] By analogy, a participating physician whose contract was terminated without cause by an MCO should have an opportunity to demonstrate that the contract was terminated for an improper reason that violates the public policy of the state.

Subsequently, in *Potvin v. Metropolitan Life Insurance Company*, the Supreme Court of California cited the *Harper* decision in concluding that a contract provision for termination without cause was unenforceable.[9] It is important, however, to keep that decision by the California Supreme Court in perspective. California law is unique in some respects, and this was a hotly disputed decision, as four justices were in favor of the decision and three justices dissented. Moreover, courts in other states might decide not to follow the analysis in *Potvin* and *Harper*. For example, an intermediate appellate court in Colorado rejected a similar challenge by a physician to the termination of his contract without cause because the Colorado legislature had adopted statutes that explicitly authorized the termination of provider agreements without cause.[10] As the Colorado court explained in that case, "It is not for the courts to enunciate the public policy of the state if, as here, the General Assembly has spoken on the issue."[11]

Financial Incentives to Provide Less Care

In the traditional system of fee-for-service medicine, the financial interest of the physician was aligned with the interest of the patient. In most cases, the patient wanted to receive all potentially beneficial services, and the physician was usually happy to provide those services and receive payment for doing so. The physician decided what services were needed, and the patient's health insurance company would pay all or most of the bill. The patient relied on the physician and was not particularly concerned about the cost.

From the perspective of the insurance company, however, that traditional system suffered from a fundamental conflict of interest. Physicians were paid on a fee-for-service basis; therefore, they received more money by performing more services. The physicians who wanted to be paid for providing more services were also determining that the services should be provided. Under these circumstances, the financial interest of the physician was adverse to the interest of the third-party payer and instead was aligned with the interest of the patient.

Many people believe this traditional alignment of interests was desirable and appropriate. However, the fee-for-service system was inherently inflationary, and it contributed to rapid increases in healthcare costs. When insurance companies had to pay more money for healthcare services, they passed the increased cost to employers, individuals, and groups in the form of higher premiums. Eventually, in an effort to control those costs, third-party payers adopted various techniques of managed care. One of the most common techniques is the use of financial incentives for physicians to provide more cost-effective care.

MCOs and other payers use financial arrangements such as capitation to control the cost of treating the patients enrolled in the plan. In addition, payers use financial incentives such as withholds and bonuses to encourage physicians to make fewer referrals to specialists and fewer admissions to hospitals. As a practical matter, these incentives have the effect of realigning the financial interest of the physician to be consistent with the interest of the payer rather than the interest of the patient.

Although these incentives may reduce healthcare costs for the payer and ultimately for society as a whole, they raise serious legal and ethical concerns for physicians and their patients. As a matter of public policy, we might decide to prohibit financial incentives that encourage physicians to provide less care, or at least prohibit the most extreme types of incentives. Even if we do not want to prohibit the use of incentives, we might want to require those incentives to be disclosed to the patient. If we decide that particular incentives ought to be disclosed, we need to address the further issue of whether disclosure should be made by the physician at the time of treatment or by the MCO at the time of enrollment. It is also important to consider whether disclosure of financial incentives would be practical, whether it would be useful to patients, and whether it would reduce the level of trust in the therapeutic relationship.[12]

Another important issue in cost containment and managed care is the effect of financial incentives on the physician's role as advocate for the patient.[13] Because of the complexity of medical issues, the patient has to rely on the physician to explain to the payer why the proposed treatment is medically necessary. Traditionally, the physician acted as the patient's advocate in negotiating with the payer regarding UR and authorization for care. Now that the physician's financial interest is more aligned with that of the payer, however, whether the physician can continue to be an effective advocate for the patient remains to be seen.[14]

The ethical aspects of these issues were addressed by the Council on Ethical and Judicial Affairs of the American Medical Association (AMA) in its report, "Ethical Issues in Managed Care."[15] According to that report, physicians have an ethical duty to act as advocates on behalf of their patients.

"No other party in the health care system has the kind of responsibility that physicians have to advocate for patients, and no other party is in a position to assume that kind of responsibility."[16] Therefore, if the MCO denies care that would materially benefit the patient, "the physician's duty as patient advocate requires that the physician challenge the denial and argue for the provision of treatment in the specific case."[17] The AMA Council also concluded that, in some cases, physicians even have a duty to initiate appeals for their patients.[18] On the basis of that report, the AMA issued Opinion 8.13 about managed care in 1996 and updated that opinion in 2002.[19]

In light of these issues, examining how financial incentives operate in health insurance and managed care is important. When most people think about the financial incentives of managed care, they think about the system of capitation used by HMOs. Under capitation, the physician would not be paid on a fee-for-service basis for each patient visit. Rather, the HMO would pay the physician a monthly amount for each person under her professional care. The physician would have to provide all of the agreed-on services in exchange for the capitation payment and would bear the risk of excessive utilization. As the U.S. Supreme Court has stated, "[I]n an HMO system, a physician's financial interest lies in providing less care, not more."[20] As explained by Chief Judge Richard Posner of the U.S. Court of Appeals for the Seventh Circuit,

> HMOs, though they have made great strides in recent years because of the widespread concern with skyrocketing medical costs, remain relative upstarts in the market for physician services. Many people don't like them because of the restriction on the patient's choice of doctors or because they fear that HMOs skimp on service since, as we said, the marginal revenue of a medical procedure to an HMO is zero. From a short-term financial standpoint—which we do not suggest is the only standpoint that an HMO is likely to have—the HMO's incentive is to keep you healthy if it can but if you get very sick, and are unlikely to recover to a healthy state involving few medical expenses, to let you die as quickly and cheaply as possible. HMOs compensate for these perceived drawbacks by charging a lower price than fee-for-service plans.[21]

However, one must recognize that financial incentives to provide less care or make fewer referrals are not limited to capitation arrangements or even to HMOs. Those types of incentives can even be incorporated into a fee-for-service arrangement between an MCO and its participating physicians. For example, an MCO could pay its PCPs on a fee-for-service basis but could withhold a specified portion of each payment. Then, the MCO could put the withheld portion into a pool that would be used to pay for specialist and hospital care. If any money was left in the pool at the end of the year, the PCPs would receive at least part of it. In that way, the PCPs would have a financial incentive to avoid hospitalizing their patients or referring them to specialists to avoid depleting the money left in the pool.

In addition, other financial incentives to provide less care are much more subtle but just as effective. Because of decreased payment levels from payers, providers will likely be forced to reduce the time and resources they put into providing each service. Ideally, this might force providers to become more efficient, but it could also contribute to a gradual dumbing down of the standard of care. For example, if physicians have to see more patients every day to maintain their previous levels of income, they probably will not be able to spend as much time as they did in the past with individual patients.

Finally, the system of selective contracting, as discussed previously, contains an inherent incentive for physicians to provide fewer tests and treatments. In developing their networks, MCOs might select physicians whose computer profiles indicate a lower usage of diagnostic tests or a lower rate of hospital admission. After physicians have been selected as preferred providers, the MCO might have the right to terminate their contracts without cause if they fail to practice in a manner the MCO considers to be cost effective. If physicians provide "too many" tests or treatments, if they admit "too many" patients to the hospital, or if they make "too many" referrals to specialists, those physicians could quickly lose a large percentage of their patients and a large percentage of their income. Either consciously or subconsciously, the potential loss of patients and income might influence their treatment decisions, as well as their willingness to advocate on behalf of their patients during UR.

As a matter of public policy, some types of financial incentives to reduce care are more problematic than others.[22] If a physician would gain or lose money as a result of a decision about treating or referring an individual patient, that incentive would be extremely effective and extremely dangerous. At the other extreme, less concern exists about incentives that are based on all of the costs incurred and all of the referrals made by all physicians on the MCO's panel in the aggregate. As stated by the AMA's Council on Ethical and Judicial Affairs, "The strength of a financial incentive to limit care can be judged by various factors, including the percentage of the physician's income placed at risk, the frequency with which incentive payments are calculated, and the size of the group of physicians on which the economic performance is judged."[23] From the AMA's perspective, conflicts of interest could be reduced by limiting the size of financial incentives and by calculating the incentives on the basis of a large group of physicians.[24] In fact, this analysis suggests that some types of incentives to provide less care should be prohibited altogether, and those that are allowed should be limited by specific requirements of law.

In the traditional healthcare system, healthcare providers had financial incentives to provide *more* tests and treatments. Physicians were paid on a fee-for-service basis, had incentives to refer their patients to facilities in which they had some type of ownership interest, and had opportunities to receive kickbacks in exchange for referrals. As a policy matter, those types of incentives were problematic because they tended to increase healthcare costs and posed a risk of interfering with the physician's independent judgment. Therefore, as discussed in Chapter 8 with regard to Medicare and Medicaid, the government responded to those concerns by developing a complex set of statutes and regulations that were designed to prevent fraud and abuse.

At least with regard to government healthcare programs, financial incentives to provide more tests, treatments, admissions, and referrals have been extensively regulated. However, the newer financial incentives that encourage physicians to provide less care or make fewer referrals have been less regulated. These incentives pose a similar risk of interfering with the physician's independent judgment, but they have a tendency to reduce healthcare costs.

Nevertheless, a few attempts have been made to regulate some of those incentives in connection with government payment programs. Under the Medicare prospective payment system, the government pays hospitals a fixed amount for treating patients with a particular diagnosis. The government thereby gives hospitals a financial incentive to provide treatment in the most cost-effective manner and perhaps to discharge patients "quicker and sicker." However, decisions on treating and discharging patients are made by physicians on the medical staff, and hospitals may be tempted to provide incentives for physicians to make those decisions in ways that will benefit the hospital. To protect the interests of Medicare and Medicaid patients, the federal government has prohibited hospitals from giving financial incentives to physicians to encourage them to discharge patients more quickly or order fewer tests and treatments. Specifically, as discussed in Chapter 8, Congress enacted a federal statute that prohibits hospitals from paying physicians to reduce the level of services for Medicare and Medicaid patients.[25]

In 1999, the U.S. Department of Health and Human Services (HHS) Office of Inspector General (OIG) expressed particular concern about so-called gainsharing arrangements, in which hospitals attempt to share their savings from cost reductions with physicians.[26] In a special advisory bulletin, the OIG explained that federal law prohibits gainsharing arrangements that provide incentives to encourage physicians to limit services to Medicare and Medicaid beneficiaries. In 2005, however, the OIG issued a series of advisory opinions in which it approved the use of certain gainsharing arrangements under limited circumstances and subject to specific safeguards.[27] This does not mean all gainsharing arrangements are now allowed by law. Rather, it means some gainsharing arrangements are likely to be permissible, and healthcare providers need to carefully structure their arrangements and consult with their lawyers.[28]

Controlling Utilization of Healthcare Services

MCOs and other third-party payers control the cost of care by limiting consumption of services through the UR process. In the past, UR primarily involved the *retrospective* review of services that already had been rendered. Therefore, UR was generally a vehicle that addressed the issue of money rather than access to care. However, payers now use *prospective* UR to authorize or refuse to authorize proposed treatments, referrals, and hospital admissions. If a patient fails to obtain prior approval or preadmission certification before entering the hospital, the payer might refuse to pay any of the cost or might pay only a reduced percentage of the cost. As a practical matter, if prior approval is denied, the patient might be unable to obtain the proposed course of treatment.

The process of prior approval begins with the patient's PCP, who acts as the gatekeeper for access to other healthcare services and facilities. The gatekeeper system provides some benefits to patients, including continuity and coordination of care, but this system can reduce access to specialized facilities and services. For a patient to see a specialist, the PCP must make a referral in accordance with the procedures of the plan. Moreover, payers might encourage their PCPs to handle patients themselves as long as possible, rather than making immediate referrals to expensive specialists. As discussed above, some PCPs have financial incentives to refrain from referring their patients to specialists.

Even if a PCP thinks a referral, hospital admission, or course of treatment is appropriate, a payer might conduct its own review under the plan's guidelines. The payer's reviewers will determine whether, in their opinion, the proposed treatment is medically necessary. Obviously, many physicians view this process as an interference with their professional judgment. In addition, if a physician is paid on a fee-for-service basis, prospective UR may have the effect of reducing the physician's income.

Payers argue, however, that they need to use prospective UR to prevent unnecessary treatment and reduce the cost of services for all participants in the plan. Payers also insist they are not telling physicians how they should treat their patients but are merely making decisions about payment or coverage under the terms of the contract. In reality, the supposed distinction between coverage decisions and treatment decisions is specious, because most patients cannot afford to pay for their own medical care without third-party coverage. As one court explained, a denial of authorization or payment in prospective UR is tantamount to a denial of treatment.

> The stakes, the risks at issue, are much higher when a prospective cost-containment review process is utilized than when a retrospective review process is used.
>
> A mistake [sic] conclusion about medical necessity following retrospective review will result in the wrongful withholding of payment. An erroneous decision in a prospective review process, on the other hand, in practical consequences, results in the withholding of necessary care, potentially leading to a patient's permanent disability or death.[29]

If a payer's denial of authorization or payment causes the death of a patient, the patient's estate might try to sue the payer and seek damages to compensate the survivors for their loss and deter the payer from similar conduct in the future. However, depending on the circumstances, that type of case might be decided under legal rules that predate the modern systems of cost containment and managed care. Those old legal rules can lead to extremely unfair results when applied in this new context of managed healthcare services. Therefore, we might decide that changing the legal rules about the liability of MCOs and other third-party payers for injuries caused by improper denial of benefits is necessary.

Another important issue in prospective UR is whether the employees or agents of a payer are practicing medicine when they determine that a requested treatment is medically unnecessary. If a payer's medical director may be disciplined for an erroneous decision to deny authorization for care on the grounds that it is a medical decision, MCO medical directors might be more inclined to approve the treatment proposed by the patient's own physician. However, courts and officials in different states have reached different conclusions on this issue.

For example, in Arizona, the state Board of Medical Examiners took disciplinary action against a physician who made UR decisions as medical director of an MCO. In that case, the board's investigation of the medical director was prompted by a complaint from a treating physician whose proposed course of treatment was rejected by the medical director. On appeal, the intermediate appellate court in Arizona held that the board did have jurisdiction to investigate and discipline physicians who make decisions in the process of UR, and the Arizona Supreme Court subsequently refused to hear the case.[30] According to the intermediate appellate court, when a medical director substitutes her judgment for that of the attending physician and determines that a proposed treatment is not medically necessary, the medical director is making a medical decision. Therefore, the court held that a medical director is subject to the disciplinary authority of the state medical licensing board. Courts in some states have agreed with the reasoning of the Arizona court,[31] but the attorneys general of other states have taken contrary positions, at least with regard to the statutes in their respective states.[32]

Legal Liability for Improper Denial of Claims

In the past, insurance companies were tempted to deny and delay the payment of claims because the only penalty for the company was the possibility of being forced to pay all those claims at some time in the future. For example, a life insurance company might have used some excuse to refuse to pay claims for death benefits and force the widows, widowers, or orphans to try to sue the insurance company. Even if the survivors eventually won in court, the insurance company would only be required to pay the death benefits under the policies, which it should have paid in the first place.

To encourage insurance companies to pay claims in a prompt and reasonable manner, the legal system has developed a way to penalize insurers for improper handling and payment of claims. At the state level, courts and legislatures developed a variety of legal remedies against insurance companies, such as state law tort claims for bad-faith denial of benefits. Regardless of how these state law remedies are labeled or characterized, the most significant fact is that they allow a plaintiff to recover damages in an amount that far exceeds the value of benefits under the policy. If an insurance company fails to handle the claim in a prompt and reasonable manner, it could be held liable for much more than the amount of the policy. Therefore, these remedies provide strong incentives to encourage insurers to pay claims in a fair and expeditious manner.

As a general rule, these remedies apply to all types of insurance companies, including life, casualty, and health insurance. However, for participants in benefit plans that are sponsored by employers in the private sector, those state law remedies might be negated by federal legislation. Specifically, the federal Employee Retirement Income Security Act (ERISA) of 1974 severely limits the remedies available to many individuals who are harmed by an improper denial of benefits.[33]

As discussed later, ERISA regulates private employer-sponsored healthcare benefit plans through which many employees and their dependents obtain their coverage. According to that federal law, private employer-sponsored ERISA plans cannot be sued under state laws for wrongful denial of benefits. Instead, the only legal remedy for an employee or dependent is to sue the health plan under the federal ERISA statute, in which case the recovery would be limited essentially to the value of the benefits that should have been paid in the first place. Thus, the practical effect of ERISA is to return some employees and their dependents to the situation existing *before* the development of state law claims for bad-faith denial of benefits.

Congress did not enact ERISA for the purpose of limiting the rights of patients in dealing with third-party payers. However, that has been the inadvertent and ironic result of a federal statute that was intended to protect the interests of employees and their dependents. ERISA was enacted before the growth of managed care, and it can lead to extremely unfair results when applied to such a system.

In fact, Congress enacted ERISA in 1974 to protect the rights of employees with regard to pensions and other employment-related benefits, including employee group health insurance. That federal law also helps employers who have employees in multiple states by facilitating uniformity throughout the country in the structure, administration, and regulation of their employee benefit plans. ERISA provides that, by complying with a single set of federal requirements, an employer in the private sector will be exempt from all state law requirements in structuring and operating its benefit plans.

For example, many states require all health plans that operate in the state to provide coverage for particular procedures and conditions, such as mammograms and prostate cancer screening. These state requirements are called **mandated benefit laws**, and significant differences in benefits are mandated by each particular state. If a large company has employees in all 50 states, it might have to operate 50 different health benefit plans, with a different benefit package for the employees in each state. By enacting ERISA, Congress preempted—or displaced—state laws with regard to employee benefit plans and thereby allowed employers to operate nationwide benefit plans without regard to state mandated benefit laws.

In addition, ERISA provides a uniform federal remedy for employees in the private sector to challenge a denial of their pensions, health insurance, or other benefits. Participants in an ERISA plan have the legal right to sue the plan in federal court to recover the benefits to which they are entitled under the plan. However, the participant's claim under the federal ERISA statute is the exclusive remedy against the ERISA plan. Any other remedy, such as a state law claim for bad-faith denial of benefits, is preempted by federal law. Thus, a participant in an ERISA plan is entitled to recover the full amount of healthcare benefits that are payable under the plan but may *not* recover damages in excess of that amount. A participant in an ERISA plan will *not* be able to recover punitive damages or compensation for pain and suffering as a result of an improper denial of healthcare benefits.

In some circumstances, the limited federal remedy under ERISA might be effective for an employee, retiree, or dependent who failed to receive the benefits that were due under the plan. For example, if pension benefits

Mandated benefit laws
Laws that require all health plans to provide coverage for particular procedures and conditions.

were wrongfully withheld, a retiree could obtain reasonably effective relief by suing under ERISA to recover the amount of pension benefits to which she is entitled under the plan. Similarly, in the traditional healthcare system that relied on retrospective UR, an employee could use the ERISA remedy to recover the money to pay for healthcare services that already had been provided. However, in a healthcare system that relies on prospective UR, the physical injury and emotional harm caused by a patient's inability to obtain necessary medical care cannot be adequately remedied by a subsequent award for the amount of benefits that were wrongfully denied. ERISA might have made sense back in 1974, under the healthcare system in effect at that time, but it is doubtful Congress ever intended to apply that law with regard to healthcare benefits in a system of prospective UR and actively managed care.

As applied to healthcare benefits in a system of managed care, the federal ERISA law creates two serious problems of public policy. First, ERISA plans have little or no financial incentive to authorize or pay for care. Many patients will not challenge their denials, and some of the patients who challenge the plan will ultimately lose. Even if patients or their estates sue the plan and win, the most severe penalty for a wrongful denial would be having to pay the original amount at some time in the future and possibly some attorney's fees. As a result of the federal ERISA law, private employer-sponsored health plans have much to gain and little to lose by finding reasons to deny as many claims and requests as possible. Moreover, those patients and their families will not be adequately compensated for their losses as a result of improper denials of care.

The second problem of public policy is that ERISA has created a disparity in cases of denial of care. In a rational legal system, similar cases should be decided in a similar manner, and the legal rights of individuals should not depend on fortuitous circumstances. However, because of ERISA, similar cases of treatment denial will lead to vastly different results, depending on where the patients obtained their health insurance coverage.

ERISA applies to employer-sponsored health plans in the private sector. It does not apply to health plans for state and local government employees or insurance coverage in the individual market. If a patient is covered under an individual policy or a state or local government plan, the health plan may be liable for huge compensatory and punitive damages under the law of the particular state. For example, in *Fox v. Health Net*,[34] the jury awarded $89 million against an HMO in a non-ERISA plan for improperly denying coverage of a bone marrow transplant for a patient with metastatic breast cancer. However, in a similar case involving a patient who was covered by an ERISA plan, *Spain v. Aetna Life Insurance Company*,[35] the patient's survivors could not recover compensatory or punitive damages for delay in authorizing a bone marrow transplant. An excerpt from that case is shown in the following box. As indicated by these cases, the legal rights of patients and their survivors will depend on the fortuitous circumstance of where the patient happened to obtain health insurance coverage. Moreover, only some types of health plans will be subject to the deterrent effect of potential damage awards.

Spain v. Aetna Life Insurance Company, 11 F.3D 129 (9TH CIR. 1993) (PER CURIAM), CERT. DENIED, 511 U.S. 1052 (1994)[36] (CITATIONS OMITTED).

OVERVIEW

A mother and daughter appeal the district court's dismissal of their wrongful death suit against Aetna Life Insurance Company ("Aetna"), the administrator of their husband's/father's employee benefit plan. They contend the district court erred by deciding that a state common law wrongful death action is preempted by the Employee Retirement Income Security Act ("ERISA") § 514(a), 29 U.S.C. § 1144(a). We do not agree and affirm the judgment.

FACTUAL AND PROCEDURAL BACKGROUND

This suit is brought by Janelle and Margaret Spain (the "Spains"), Steven Spain's wife and daughter, respectively. Steven Spain was a plan participant and beneficiary in a self-funded employee benefit plan within the meaning of ERISA. His plan was administered by Aetna.

Steven Spain was diagnosed as having testicular cancer. His doctors decided that an autologous bone marrow transplant ("ABMT") was necessary to attempt to save his life. Aetna preapproved the first two parts of this three-part procedure. Initially, Aetna also authorized the last part of the procedure. However, Aetna later withdrew its authorization on the grounds that Steven Spain's diagnosed condition did not make him eligible for this procedure. Because Spain could not afford the final part of the procedure on his own, he brought suit against his employee benefit plan and its administrator, Aetna, to compel authorization of treatment. Two days after notification of the suit, the plan and Aetna authorized the last part of the procedure.

Appellants contend that "ABMT procedures can be performed successfully only during a very narrow window of time and by the time

(continued)

(continued from previous page)

Aetna acknowledged its error and approved the procedure, Steven's window had closed." Thus, although the procedure was eventually completed, Appellants argue that Steven Spain's death was negligently caused by Aetna's initial denial in authorizing the procedure. At trial, the district court dismissed the case on the grounds that ERISA preempts Appellants' state law claim for wrongful death. This court has jurisdiction under 28 U.S.C. § 1291.

ANALYSIS

"The interpretation of ERISA, a federal statute, is a question of law subject to de novo review." Specifically, "ERISA preemption is a conclusion of law reviewed de novo."

The sole issue on review is whether ERISA preempts the state common law wrongful death action. ERISA's preemption clause is "deliberately expansive," and "contains one of the broadest preemption clauses ever enacted by Congress." The preemption clause states that the provisions provided by ERISA "shall supersede any and all State laws insofar as they may now or hereafter relate to any employee benefit plan . . ." 29 U.S.C. § 1144(a). Interpreting ERISA's preemption clause, the Supreme Court has instructed that "relates to" is to be "given its broad common-sense meaning." Therefore, a state cause of action relates to an ERISA benefit plan if operation of the law impinges on the functioning of an ERISA plan.

Appellants assert that Aetna's improper withdrawal of authorization for Steven Spain's ABMT procedure caused Steven Spain's death. Although Appellants do not seek benefits under the plan, their state common law cause of action seeks damages for the negligent administration of benefit claims. This circuit, following the lead of the Supreme Court in *Pilot Life Ins. Co. v. Dedeaux*, has held that "state common law causes of action arising from the improper processing of a claim are preempted by federal law." Hence, ERISA preempts Appellants' wrongful death action because the state law in its application directly "relates to" the administration and disbursement of ERISA plan benefits. Both the Fifth Circuit and Tenth Circuit, the only two circuits that have confronted the issue of whether ERISA preempts a state wrongful death action, have reached the same conclusion.

(continued)

(continued from previous page)

Further, a state wrongful death action is not "saved" by the sole exception to ERISA's preemption rule. Although the ERISA preemption clause is broad, Congress created an exception for "any law of any State which regulates insurance, banking, or securities." 29 U.S.C. § 1144(b)(2)(A). Under this exception, a law must not just have an impact on an insurance company, "but must be specifically directed toward that industry." The cause of action for wrongful death at issue in this appeal is a general tort and clearly was not specifically tailored by the state to regulate insurance, banking, or securities.

Congress carefully constructed the civil enforcement provisions allowed under ERISA. As the Court instructed, "the policy choices reflected in the inclusion of certain remedies and the exclusion of others under the federal scheme would be completely undermined if ERISA-plan participants and beneficiaries were free to obtain remedies under state law that Congress rejected in ERISA." As the Fifth Circuit stated, "While we are not unmindful of the fact that our interpretation of the pre-emption clause leaves a gap in remedies within a statute intended to protect participants in employee benefit plans, the lack of an ERISA remedy does not affect a pre-emption analysis."

CONCLUSION

Because ERISA preempts the state common law wrongful death action and is not "saved" under the exception to ERISA's broad preemption, we affirm the judgment.

AFFIRMED.

The Statutory Language of ERISA

Preemption clause
A provision of ERISA specifying that ERISA pre-empts state laws insofar as they relate to employee benefit plans regulated by ERISA.

As enacted by Congress, the language of ERISA is confusing. One federal court described the preemption provision as "a veritable Sargasso Sea of obfuscation."[37] As the Supreme Court put it, the statutory provisions "perhaps are not a model of legislative drafting."[38]

In ERISA, Congress addressed the issue of federal preemption by means of three statutory clauses: the **preemption clause**, the **saving clause**, and the **deemer clause**.[39] Under the preemption clause, ERISA preempts state laws insofar as they relate to employee benefit plans that are regulated by ERISA. Thus, state law claims for wrongful denial of benefits are preempted by ERISA, and participants are limited to the exclusive remedy under the federal ERISA statute.

Under the saving clause, a few types of state laws—including those that regulate insurance—are "saved" from preemption, and, therefore, are not preempted. Therefore, state governments may continue to regulate insurance, which is a traditional state function as described in Chapter 15.

Although states cannot regulate ERISA plans, they can use their power to regulate insurance as an indirect method of controlling those ERISA plans that purchase insurance for their employees and dependents. In effect, state governments can regulate some ERISA plans *indirectly* by regulating the insurance company that provides the group insurance policy for the ERISA plan or by regulating the terms of the group insurance contract. For example, assume that a state legislature has enacted a mandated benefit law that requires all health insurance companies doing business in the state to include coverage for chiropractic services in all health insurance policies issued in the state. Assume further that an employer in the private sector does not want to include coverage for chiropractic services in its employee group health plan under ERISA. When the employer contacts various health insurance companies to inquire about a group policy of health insurance for its employees, it will find that every health insurance company authorized to do business in that state will insist on including coverage for chiropractic services, even though the employer does not want that particular coverage. Although the employer's ERISA plan is not subject to the state insurance law, all insurance companies in the state are subject to that law. In that way, state governments can effectively control the benefits provided by ERISA plans that purchase group policies of insurance.

ERISA plans can avoid the effect of state mandated benefit laws in one way: by using the mechanism of self-insurance. If an ERISA plan is self-insured, the state cannot use that indirect method of regulation because the ERISA plan will not do business with any insurance company and will not obtain any policy of insurance. Under the third clause of the ERISA statute, the deemer clause, self-insured ERISA plans are *not* deemed to be insurance companies or to be in the business of insurance. In self-insured ERISA plans, therefore, no insurance company or insurance contract exists for the state to regulate, and those self-insured ERISA plans are beyond the reach of state authority.

With regard to state mandated benefit laws, an important difference exists between *insured* ERISA plans and *self-insured* ERISA plans. State laws that mandate particular health insurance benefits will apply, albeit indirectly, to ERISA plans that purchase insurance. However, those state laws will not apply at all to ERISA plans that are self-insured.

Saving clause
A provision of ERISA that exempts some types of state laws from preemption.

Deemer clause
A provision of ERISA that self-insured ERISA plans are *not* deemed to be insurance companies or to be in the business of insurance.

For example, legislatures in many states enacted laws to prevent so-called drive-through deliveries by requiring health insurance companies in their states to provide coverage for at least 48 hours of inpatient care after normal delivery and at least 96 hours after caesarean section, subject to certain exceptions.[40] If an ERISA plan purchases a group health insurance policy in a state that has enacted that type of mandated benefit law, the insured ERISA plan would have to offer extended maternity coverage as required by the law in that particular state. However, if the ERISA plan elects to self-insure, it would not be subject to the state mandated benefit law on extended maternity coverage.

Under these circumstances, the only way to require self-insured ERISA plans to provide a particular level of maternity coverage is to enact a federal statute, which would not be preempted by the federal ERISA law. That is precisely what Congress did in 1996 when it enacted a federal law to impose specific requirements for maternity coverage on both insurance companies and self-insured ERISA plans.[41]

The foregoing discussion has focused on the differences between insured and self-insured ERISA plans with regard to the issue of state mandated benefit laws. With regard to other issues, however, all ERISA plans are treated alike, and no practical differences exist between insured ERISA plans and self-insured ERISA plans. For this latter category of issues, the relevant distinction is between ERISA plans and non-ERISA plans. The most important issue in this latter category is the ability of an individual to assert state law claims and remedies against a healthcare benefit plan. According to the U.S. Supreme Court, ERISA preempts state law claims and remedies even for insured ERISA plans.[42] Therefore, they will be preempted for both insured and self-insured ERISA plans.

Federal courts often recognize that ERISA's preemption of state law claims and remedies can result in extreme injustice by depriving patients or their families of any effective remedy for serious injury or death.[43] However, courts also recognize that their role in this type of case is limited to interpreting and enforcing the ERISA statute in accordance with the intent of Congress. Even if they considered ERISA to be unfair and unwise as a matter of public policy, many courts have reluctantly concluded that their hands were tied and have strongly urged Congress to amend the statute.

For example, in concluding that a plaintiff's state law claims were preempted by ERISA (in *Andrews-Clarke v. Travelers Ins. Co.*), one federal court wrote that "[t]he tragic events set forth in Diane Andrews-Clarke's Complaint cry out for relief."[44] The court continued, "Nevertheless, this Court had no choice but to pluck Diane Andrews-Clarke's case out of the state court in which she sought redress (and where relief to other litigants is available) and then, at the behest of Travelers and Greenspring, to slam the courthouse doors in her face and leave her without any remedy."[45]

In some cases, however, courts attempted to provide relief to patients or their survivors by characterizing the claim as a type of medical malpractice. Although ERISA preempts state law claims for improper denial of benefits, it does not preempt claims for medical malpractice. Patients who are covered by ERISA plans have the same right as any other patients to sue their healthcare providers for medical malpractice, and they may recover compensatory and punitive damages to the extent allowed by state law.

Some courts tried to extend that reasoning to the next logical step by allowing patients in ERISA plans to assert medical malpractice claims against their MCOs. Under that theory, a plaintiff would argue that the claim is not based on the MCO's denial of benefits, but rather on the MCO's failure to provide appropriate medical care. In other words, those plaintiffs insisted that they were complaining about the *quality* rather than the *quantity* of care. In addition, some state legislatures enacted statutes that provided a cause of action for people to sue an MCO for damages that were caused by an MCO's negligence in making certain types of treatment decisions.[46]

However, in its 2004 decision in *Aetna Health Inc. v. Davila*, the U.S. Supreme Court severely restricted those attempts to circumvent ERISA, by holding that claims under those state statutes were preempted and that plaintiffs' sole remedy was to sue under ERISA for the amount of benefits that had been denied.[47] Thus, a participant in an ERISA plan cannot get around the effect of ERISA preemption by suing under a state managed care law or by trying to recharacterize a claim for denial of benefits as a type of medical malpractice. As the Supreme Court explained, "[I]f an individual, at some point in time, could have brought his claim under ERISA . . . , and where there is no other independent legal duty that is implicated by a defendant's actions, then the individual's cause of action is completely preempted by ERISA."[48]

The Supreme Court left a small opening to bring state law claims against those MCOs that employ physicians or are owned and operated by physicians.[49] However, the practical implication of the Supreme Court's opinion in *Davila* is that neither state legislatures nor lower federal courts will be able to solve the problems caused by ERISA preemption; any solution will have to come from Congress.[50] To achieve a comprehensive solution, therefore, Congress would have to amend the federal ERISA statute.

In amending ERISA, one alternative would be to eliminate the federal preemption of state law claims and remedies for improper denial of benefits. Another alternative would be to retain the federal remedy under ERISA as the exclusive remedy for denial of benefits, but expand it to permit the recovery of damages in excess of the benefits owed under the plan. In addition, compromise might be possible by making incremental changes to ERISA. For example, ERISA could be amended to permit the recovery of *some* additional types of damages, such as lost wages and other economic losses, but still retain certain limitations, such as placing a cap on damages for pain and suffering or limiting the recovery of punitive damages.[51]

Part of the difficulty in reaching an agreement on amending ERISA has been determining the cost to health plans and society of allowing recovery of additional damages. Those opposed to amending ERISA argued that the change would lead to a significant escalation of healthcare costs. The issue of cost is not merely a question of projecting the total amount of jury verdicts and settlements that ERISA plans would be required to pay under an amended law. Rather, the issue is the extent to which healthcare costs would increase throughout the country if the law were changed to put ERISA plans at risk of substantial damages for improper denial of benefits.

In 1998, the Congressional Budget Office (CBO) issued a cost estimate on a proposal for managed care reform, including a proposed amendment of ERISA to permit state law claims for damages.[52] With regard to the proposed amendment of ERISA, the CBO stated, "The cost of this provision depends on assumptions for which the supporting data are extremely limited or nonexistent."[53] Nevertheless, the CBO estimated that amending ERISA would cause the premiums for employer-sponsored health plans to increase by only 1.2 percent.[54] At about the same time that the CBO issued its report, the U.S. General Accounting Office (GAO) issued its own report to Congress with regard to the likely consequences of amending ERISA.[55] The GAO's most significant finding was that not enough data exist to determine the effect of amending ERISA on the quality and cost of care.

The Alternative Approach of External Review

In its report, the GAO recognized the potential advantages of using an upstream approach in attempting to resolve disputes over healthcare benefits without the need for litigation. The upstream approach would include a realistic opportunity for a patient to appeal a health plan's denial of benefits and receive a prompt and fair reconsideration of the claim.

For health plans that are sponsored by private employers under ERISA, the U.S. Department of Labor (DOL) adopted rules that require specific procedures for filing claims, providing notice of decisions, and appealing "adverse benefit determinations."[56] Those federal rules apply to *all* ERISA plans, regardless of whether they are insured or self-insured. However, those federal rules only apply to *internal* review-of-benefit decisions within the plan and do not impose any requirement for independent, *external* review.[57] Some state governments enacted laws to require external review of benefit denials, but a problem existed in attempting to apply those state laws to self-insured ERISA plans.

Under these circumstances, a comprehensive requirement for independent, external review required some action by Congress, and that was achieved as part of the ACA. Under Section 2719(b) of the ACA,[58] both insurance companies and group health plans must provide an external review procedure that meets specific requirements. The specific requirements will depend on whether a particular health plan is subject to a state law that mandates an adequate process of binding external review. The federal requirements under the ACA are explained in the following excerpt from a statement by the Centers for Medicare & Medicaid Services' Center for Consumer Information and Insurance Oversight. After that excerpt, Activity 14.1 presents a specific situation and provides an opportunity to analyze the legal issues under ERISA.

THE CENTER FOR CONSUMER INFORMATION & INSURANCE OVERSIGHT

HHS-Administered Federal External Review Process for Health Insurance Coverage[59]

BACKGROUND

The Affordable Care Act (ACA) ensures that consumers have the right to appeal health insurance plan decisions. This means they are able to ask that the plan reconsider its decision to deny payment for a service or treatment. New rules spell out how plans must handle an appeal (usually called an "internal appeal"). These rules apply to health insurance policies that were first sold or significantly modified after March 23, 2010. These plans are calls non-grandfathered plans. If the plan still denies payment after considering the internal appeal, the law permits a consumer another step. Consumers may choose to have an independent review organization (an outside independent decision-maker) decide whether to uphold or overturn the plan's decision. This additional check is often referred to as an "external review." Rules issued by the U.S. Departments of Health and Human Services (HHS), Treasury, and Labor (DOL) provide for three different ways to process external reviews. In some states, consumers will use their state's external review process. This method is for states determined by the federal

(continued)

(continued from previous page)

government to have a process that meets the federal standards for consumer protections. . . .

If the state's process does not meet the federal consumer protection standards, issuers must use a federally-administered external review process and may choose one of the following external review processes to offer to consumers:

- The accredited Independent Review Organization (IRO) contracting process or
- The HHS-Administered Federal External Review Processes.

The federally-administered external review processes apply to denials (called "adverse benefit determinations") that involve medical judgment (including, but not limited to, those based on the plan's or issuer's requirements for medical necessity, appropriateness, health care setting, level of care, or effectiveness of a covered benefit; or its determination that a treatment is experimental or investigational) and rescissions of coverage (whether or not the rescission has any effect on any particular benefit at that time).

The HHS-Administered Federal External Review Process is available at no cost to the health insurance plan, the consumer, or a consumer's authorized representative. Issuers that elect to use the HHS-Administered Federal External Review Process and consumers whose plan is participating in the HHS-Administered Federal External Review Process, will work with the designated federal contractor which performs all functions of the external review. . . .

A GENERAL OVERVIEW OF THE HHS-ADMINISTERED FEDERAL EXTERNAL REVIEW PROCESS

If a health insurance plan denies a benefit or refuses to pay for a service that has already been received, this is called an adverse benefit determination. If a health insurance plan upholds its earlier decision to deny a benefit or payment for a service, this is called a final internal adverse benefit determination.

Consumers may ask for an external review of a final internal adverse benefit determination. In some instances, consumers may ask for an

(continued)

(continued from previous page)

external review when the initial denial (adverse benefit determination) is made.

A consumer or their authorized representative (called the "claimant") may file a written request for an external review. . . .

For urgent care situations, claimants may file an expedited external review for either an adverse benefit determination or a final internal adverse benefit determination if:

1. An adverse benefit determination involves a medical condition of the claimant for which the timeframe for completion of an expedited internal appeal would seriously jeopardize the life or health of the claimant, or would jeopardize the claimant's ability to regain maximum function and the claimant has filed a request for an expedited internal appeal; or

2. A final internal adverse benefit determination involves a medical condition where the timeframe for completion of a standard external review would seriously jeopardize the life or health of the claimant or would jeopardize the claimant's ability to regain maximum function, or if the final internal adverse benefit determination concerns an admission, availability of care, continued stay or health care service for which the claimant received emergency services, but has not been discharged from a facility.

ACTIVITY 14.1: ALBERT CRENSHAW

Albert Crenshaw, aged 45 years, was employed as a computer specialist. Through his employer in the private sector, he obtained health coverage with the Happy Family Health Plan, which is an MCO. Happy Family has a network of participating physicians who have agreed to provide services to Happy Family enrollees.

Each enrollee is required to choose a PCP from Happy Family's list of participating physicians. Because Crenshaw had recently moved to the

(continued)

(continued from previous page)

area, he did not know any doctors. Therefore, he chose Dr. Julia Smith as his PCP because she was on the list for Happy Family's network.

Dr. Smith is a physician in private practice. Happy Family entered into a participating physician contract with her because she was willing to provide services at a discount. In paying Dr. Smith, Happy Family withholds 20 percent of her fee for each visit and puts that 20 percent into a risk pool. At the end of the year, Dr. Smith will share in any money left in the pool.

Happy Family's participating physician agreement is a standard form contract. It specifies that participating physicians are independent contractors, rather than employees or agents of Happy Family. In addition, the contract between Happy Family and Dr. Smith provides that it may be terminated by either party, with or without cause, on 30 days' notice to the other party.

In the community in which Dr. Smith practices, it has been routine medical practice for many years to give an electrocardiogram (EKG) to any patient older than 40 years who complains of chest pains. However, on October 5, 2013, Happy Family sent a bulletin to Dr. Smith and the other participating physicians with regard to Happy Family's new policy on EKGs. Under that new policy, EKGs will only be covered by the plan if the patient is older than 50 years.

Approximately three weeks later, on October 25, 2013, Crenshaw began experiencing chest pains after working out at his gym during his lunch hour. He immediately went to Dr. Smith's office. She knew Crenshaw was covered by the Happy Family Health Plan, and she remembered the recent bulletin she had received from the plan. Dr. Smith examined Crenshaw but did not perform an EKG, even though performing an EKG under those circumstances was the routine practice in the community at that time.

Dr. Smith advised Crenshaw that it was safe for him to go back to work. Mr. Crenshaw did go back to work, where he died of a heart attack two hours later.

As soon as Dr. Smith heard about Crenshaw's death, she called the president of Happy Family Health Plan. Dr. Smith told him that from now on she was going to order an EKG for every patient who needs it, regardless of age. The next day, Happy Family responded by giving Dr. Smith

(continued)

(continued from previous page)

30 days' notice of termination from the plan, which would effectively prevent her from treating any Happy Family patients.

Subsequently, Crenshaw's widow sued Dr. Smith for medical malpractice in state court. The plaintiff (Victoria Crenshaw) had an expert witness who testified that Albert Crenshaw would not have died if he had been given an EKG instead of being sent back to work. Mrs. Crenshaw also claimed that Happy Family gave financial incentives to Dr. Smith to encourage her to provide less care to patients covered by the plan. According to Mrs. Crenshaw and her lawyer, those financial incentives should be illegal and, at the very least, should have been fully disclosed to Albert Crenshaw.

In response, Dr. Smith denied that she was liable for the death of Crenshaw. According to Dr. Smith, she satisfied the new standard of care as established by the Happy Family Health Plan. In addition, Dr. Smith's lawyer argued that the financial arrangements between Dr. Smith and Happy Family were entirely lawful and that Dr. Smith had no legal obligation to disclose her financial arrangements to Crenshaw. Finally, Dr. Smith's lawyer contended that the medical malpractice case should be thrown out of court because of the federal law known as ERISA, which regulates employer-sponsored health plans such as Crenshaw's plan.

In addition, Mrs. Crenshaw sued the Happy Family Health Plan in state court for damages caused by Happy Family's improper denial of benefits. According to Mrs. Crenshaw, Happy Family's refusal to pay for a necessary diagnostic test was a substantial cause of her husband's death. Therefore, Mrs. Crenshaw claimed that she is entitled to $1 million from Happy Family to compensate her and her children for 20 years of her husband's lost wages. In addition, she asked the court to make Happy Family pay $10 million in punitive damages to teach them a lesson and encourage them to change their policy for the future. However, Happy Family's defense lawyer responded that the case against Happy Family may only be heard in federal court because of the federal ERISA law on employee health plans. Moreover, according to Happy Family's lawyer, even if Mrs. Crenshaw wins her case, she cannot recover $1 million in lost wages or $10 million in punitive damages from Happy Family. Rather, the most that she can possibly recover against Happy Family is the cost of the EKG exam, which should have been covered by the plan.

Who is likely to prevail on each claim, and why?

Notes

1. See, e.g., R. J. Blendon, et al., "Understanding the Managed Care Backlash," *Health Affairs* (1998), 17 (4): 80–94.

2. F. A. Sloan and M. A. Hall (2002). "Market Failures and the Evolution of State Regulation of Managed Care." *Law and Contemporary Problems* 65 (4): 169–206.

3. A. Mathews (2012). "Medical Care Time Warp." *Wall Street Journal*, August 2, B1.

4. Patient Protection and Affordable Care Act, Pub. L. No. 111-148 (2010); Health Care and Education Reconciliation Act of 2010, Pub. L. No. 111-152 (2010).

5. Pub. L. No. 111-148 (2010), § 2719A(a).

6. *Id.* at § 2719A(b)–(d).

7. *Harper v. Healthsource New Hampshire, Inc.*, 674 A.2d 962 (N.H. 1996).

8. See, e.g., *Sides v. Duke University*, 328 S.E.2d 818, 826 (N.C. Ct. App. 1985).

9. *Potvin v. Metropolitan Life Insurance Company*, 997 P.2d 1153 (Cal. 2000).

10. *Grossman v. Columbine Medical Group, Inc.*, 12 P.3d 269 (Colo. Ct. App. 2000).

11. *Id.* at 271.

12. See generally T. E. Miller and C. R. Horowitz, "Disclosing Doctors' Incentives: Will Consumers Understand and Value the Information?" *Health Affairs* (2000), 19 (4): 149–55.

13. See generally E. H. Morreim, "Economic Disclosure and Economic Advocacy: New Duties in the Medical Standard of Care," *Journal of Legal Medicine* (1991), 12: 275.

14. But see W. M. Sage, "Physicians as Advocates," *Houston Law Review* (1999), 35 (5): 1529–630, at 1534–35 ("Physician advocacy should neither be taken for granted nor saddled with expectations which potentially are inconsistent with one another or with normative goals for the health care system").

15. See Council on Ethical and Judicial Affairs of the American Medical Association, "Ethical Issues in Managed Care," *Journal of the American Medical Association* (1995), 273: 330–35 [hereinafter Council on Ethical and Judicial Affairs].

16. *Id.* at 331.

17. *Id.* at 334.

18. See *id.* at 333.

19. American Medical Association, "AMA Code of Medical Ethics, Opinion 8.13—Managed Care" (updated 2002). www.ama-assn.org/ama/pub/physician-resources/medical-ethics/code-medical-ethics/opinion813.page?#.

20. *Pegram v. Herdrich*, 530 U.S. 211, 219 (2000).

21. *Blue Cross and Blue Shield United of Wisconsin v. Marshfield Clinic*, 65 F.3d 1406, 1410 (7th Cir. 1995) (as amended on denial of rehearing).

22. E. B. Hirshfeld (1990). "Should Third Party Payors of Health Care Services Disclose Cost Control Mechanisms to Potential Beneficiaries?" *Seton Hall Legislative Journal*, 14: 127.

23. Council on Ethical and Judicial Affairs, *supra* note 15.

24. See *id.* at 333, 335.

25. 42 U.S.C. § 1320a–7a(b) (2000).

26. Publication of the OIG, "Special Advisory Bulletin on Gainsharing Arrangements and CMPs for Hospital Payments to Physicians to Reduce or Limit Services to Beneficiaries," 64 Fed. Reg. 37985 (July 14, 1999).

27. See U.S. Department of Health and Human Services, Office of Inspector General, Advisory Opinions Nos. 05-01 (2005). oig.hhs.gov/fraud/docs/advisoryopinions/2005/ao0501.pdf.

28. See C. Logarta, "Introduction: Fifth Annual Health Law & Policy Colloquium: Provider Response to Cost Containment: Fraud & Abuse Issues," *Annals of Health Law* (2006), 15: 373–78, at 376 ("[T]he legal climate surrounding gainsharing remains unclear").

29. *Wickline v. State of California*, 239 Cal. Rptr. 810, 811–812 (Cal. Ct. App. 1986).

30. See *Murphy v. Board of Medical Examiners of the State of Arizona*, 949 P.2d 530, 532 (Ariz. Ct. App. 1997), *cert. denied*, December 15, 1997.

31. See, e.g., *State Board of Registration for the Healing Arts v. Fallon*, 41 S.W.3d 474 (Mo. 2001).

32. See 1999 Ohio Op. Atty. Gen. 265 (1999) (citing attorney general opinions from a number of states).

33. 29 U.S.C. §§ 1001 *et seq.* (2006).

34. 29 Trials Digest 54, 1993 WL 794305 (Cal. Super. Ct. 1993).

35. 11 F.3d 129 (9th Cir. 1993) (per curiam), *cert. denied*, 511 U.S. 1052 (1994).

36. *Spain v. Aetna Life Ins. Co.*, 11 F.3d 129 (9th Cir. 1993) (per curiam), *cert. denied*, 511 U.S. 1052 (1994).

37. *Travelers Ins. Co. v. Cuomo*, 14 F.3d 708, 717 (2d Cir. 1993), *rev'd. sub nom New York State Conf. of Blue Cross & Blue Shield Plans v. Travelers Ins. Co.*, 514 U.S. 645 (1995).

38. *Metropolitan Life Ins. Co. v. Massachusetts*, 471 U.S. 724, 739 (1985).

39. See 29 U.S.C. § 1144(a)–(b) (2006).

40. See generally W. H. Dow, D. M. Harris, and Z. Liu, "Differential Effectiveness in Patient Protection Laws: What Are the Causes? An Example from the Drive-Through Delivery Laws," *Journal of Health Politics, Policy and Law* 31(6): 1107–27 (2006); D.A. Hyman, "Drive-Through Deliveries: Is 'Consumer Protection' Just What the Doctor Ordered?" *North Carolina Law Review* 78 (1999): 5–99.

41. See Newborns' and Mothers' Health Protection Act of 1996, Pub. L. No. 104-204, tit. VI § 711, 110 Stat. 2874, 2935 (1996) (codified at 29 U.S.C. § 1185).

42. *Pilot Life Ins. Co. v. Dedeaux*, 481 U.S. 41 (1987) (state law claim was preempted even with regard to the insurance company that had issued the group policy).

43. See, e.g., *Corcoran v. United Healthcare, Inc.*, 965 F.2d 1321, 1338–39 (5th Cir. 1992), *cert. denied*, 506 U.S. 1033 (1992).

44. *Andrews-Clarke v. Travelers Ins. Co.*, 984 F. Supp. 49, 52 (D. Mass. 1997).

45. *Id.* at 53 (footnote omitted).

46. See, e.g., Texas Health Care Liability Act, Tex. Civ. Prac. & Rem. Code Ann., §§ 88.001–88.003 (West 1998).

47. *Aetna Health Inc. v. Davila*, 542 U.S. 200 (2004).

48. *Id.* at 210.

49. T. S. Jost (2004). "The Supreme Court Limits Lawsuits Against Managed Care Organizations." *Health Affairs* (Web Exclusive), August 11: W4-417, at W4-423 to W4-424.

50. *Id.* at W4-425 ("This leads to the final ramification of *Davila*. If anyone is going to permit tort actions to be brought against managed care organizations, it will have to be Congress").

51. See, e.g., H.R. 2563, 107th Cong, § 402 (2001); S. 374, 106th Cong., tit. III, § 302 (1999).

52. U.S. Congressional Budget Office, *Cost Estimate: H.R.3605/S.1890: Patient Bill of Rights Act of 1998* (July 16, 1998). www.cbo.gov/sites/default/files/cbofiles/ftpdocs/6xx/doc668/s1890.pdf.

53. *Id.* at 16.

54. *Id.* at 3–4 (Table 2).

55. U.S. General Accounting Office, *Employer-Based Managed Care Plans: ERISA's Effect on Remedies for Benefit Denials and Medical Malpractice*, GAO/HEHS-98-154 (July 13, 1998). www.gao.gov/assets/230/226032.pdf.

56. 29 C.F.R. § 2560.503–1(b) (2006).

57. See *id.* at § 2560.503–1(k)(2)(ii) (recognizing that procedures for external review are not encompassed within § 503 of ERISA, 29 U.S.C. § 1133, pursuant to which the Secretary of Labor adopted the claims procedure rules).

58. Pub. L. No. 111-148, § 2719(b) (2010).

59. Centers for Medicare & Medicaid Services (CMS), Center for Consumer Information & Insurance Oversight, "HHS-Administered Federal External Review Process for Health Insurance Coverage" (2013). www.cms.gov/CCIIO/Programs-and-Initiatives/Consumer-Support-and-Information/csg-ext-appeals-facts.html.

LEGAL ISSUES IN HEALTH INSURANCE AND HEALTH REFORM

Throughout this book, we have approached healthcare law as a tool to achieve our health policy goals. Chapter 1 analyzed the alternative ways of using the law to accomplish our goals and evaluated the advantages and disadvantages of each alternative. For example, can a particular problem be handled more effectively by means of a single federal law or a series of separate state laws? As discussed in that chapter, each level of government has its own legal powers and its own practical advantages. Chapter 5 applied the different legal powers and advantages of federal and state governments to solving problems such as prevention of disease, improving the quality of care, reducing healthcare costs, and increasing access to care. Chapter 6 analyzed the use of federal and state laws as tools to protect the privacy of health information. This chapter analyzes the use of law as a tool to achieve universal coverage and reform the healthcare system.

The solution is not as simple as merely passing a law to require all insurance companies to provide coverage to all applicants at the same rate. If we were to enact a law that requires all insurers to charge everyone the same rate, which is called **community rating**, people who are young and healthy would have to pay higher premiums to subsidize people who are old and sick. Many of the young and healthy may be unwilling or unable to pay the higher community-rated premium and would simply forgo purchasing any health insurance. Removing many of the young and healthy people from the risk pool would cause premiums to rise even more for those who remain in the system. Therefore, passing a law to require community rating would not be sufficient.

Similarly, adding a legal requirement to cover all applicants, regardless of their health status, would not be sufficient. If we were to enact a law to require insurance companies to cover everyone who applies and prohibit exclusion on the basis of health status, which is called **guaranteed issue**, the rates would increase as older and sicker people are brought into the risk pool. Again, many of the young and healthy would drop out of the system and simply go without insurance coverage. If the uninsured young people ever become seriously ill or injured, they could purchase health insurance at that point and could not be denied on the basis of their medical condition. Because healthy people would have no incentive to buy health insurance, the rates for everyone else would increase. That would cause even more people

Community rating
A method of pricing health insurance in which premiums do not vary on the basis of individual health status.

Guaranteed issue
A legal requirement that health insurance companies provide coverage to all applicants regardless of their health status.

375

to drop out, and eventually the entire health insurance system would self-destruct in a so-called death spiral. For these reasons, reforming the health insurance market to extend coverage to the uninsured is not as simple as merely enacting laws to require community rating or prohibit exclusion on the basis of health status.

As a practical matter, accomplishing the policy goal of universal access to affordable coverage requires a system in which the young and healthy cannot simply choose to drop out. One way to achieve this goal is the Canadian-style single-payer system, which is funded by tax revenues. However, universal coverage can be achieved in other ways. For example, President Bill Clinton proposed a system of employer mandates, which would have required all employers to provide health insurance. In response, some Congressional opponents of the Clinton administration's plan proposed a system of individual mandates, in which each person would be legally obligated to purchase health insurance.[1] Of course, employer mandates would have to be accompanied by subsidies for the unemployed, and individual mandates would have to be accompanied by subsidies for those unable to afford coverage. These legal and practical issues led eventually to the enactment of the Patient Protection and Affordable Care Act (ACA), which is discussed in detail later. First, we must understand the important role of state governments in regulation and reform of health insurance, as well as the federal health reforms that were enacted prior to 2010.

State Regulation and Reforms

In addition to regulating providers of healthcare services, as discussed in Chapter 5, state governments have traditionally regulated health insurance companies for the protection of the public. After individuals and groups pay for health insurance coverage, ensuring that the benefits will be available when people become sick or injured is important. In addition, states can protect consumers by regulating the rates, contract terms, marketing, disclosures, and claims practices of insurance companies.

In light of these important policy concerns, it is not surprising that insurance has been one of the most intensively regulated industries in the United States. Because insurance companies operate in interstate commerce, they clearly fall within the regulatory power of the federal government. However, in the McCarran-Ferguson Act of 1945,[2] Congress chose to leave the regulation of the insurance business primarily to the states. For many years, insurance companies have been regulated by state insurance commissioners in each state. In addition, state officials regulate health maintenance organizations (HMOs) as well as Blue Cross and Blue Shield plans in their states. Nevertheless, federal laws may be applied to the insurance industry if those laws specifically relate to the business of insurance or if those laws are consistent with state policies and regulation.[3]

One of the most important goals of state insurance regulation is to ensure that an insurance company is solvent and financially responsible. Under a contract of insurance, individuals or groups pay premiums to a company in advance, and they rely on that company to remain in business and have sufficient assets to pay the claims that arise in the future. Therefore, state insurance laws require companies to demonstrate that they have sufficient assets before they can obtain a license to do business in a particular state. In addition, state insurance commissioners will audit the companies on a periodic basis and will require companies to maintain adequate reserves. If an insurance company is at risk of becoming insolvent, the state insurance commissioner might appoint a rehabilitator or receiver to manage the affairs of the company for the protection of the policyholders. As a last resort, claims for benefits might be paid by a state insurance guaranty association, which is funded by all of the other insurance companies that have obtained authority to do business in that state.

In addition to ensuring the solvency of health insurance companies, state officials might regulate the level of premiums and the terms of the insurance contract. For example, many states have enacted statutes that require all health insurance contracts to provide coverage for specific services, such as mammograms, Pap smears, and prostate cancer screening. However, as discussed in Chapter 14, these state "mandated benefit laws" do *not* apply to self-insured employee benefit plans that are covered by the federal Employee Retirement Income Security Act (ERISA).[4]

Some state governments have also enacted laws to expand health insurance coverage in their respective states. In fact, a few state and local governments enacted laws that attempted to create universal or near-universal coverage. Prior to 2010, Congress had not succeeded in enacting comprehensive health reform at the federal level, and, to some extent, the focus of reform had shifted to the individual states. In January 2007, the *Washington Post* described "a wave of experiments at the state level."[5] State experiments can be very useful by trying alternatives for which a consensus cannot be reached at the national level. In addition, successful experiments at the state level can provide models for subsequent adoption on a national basis. Both Congress and the Supreme Court have recognized that the states can serve as laboratories for experimentation in healthcare reform.[6]

For example, in 2006 the Maryland legislature took the approach of requiring large nongovernmental employers in that state to pay at least 8 percent of their employee wages on health insurance, or, alternatively, to pay the shortfall in health insurance costs to the state.[7] The Maryland legislature understood that the only company that would be affected by the new law was Wal-Mart Stores, Inc.[8] However, a retail trade association, which included Wal-Mart as a member, sued a Maryland state official for declaratory and injunctive relief. The federal district court held that the Maryland law is unenforceable because it is preempted by the federal ERISA law. As discussed in Chapter 14, ERISA preempts state laws insofar as they relate to the benefit plans of employers in the private sector. To allow multistate employers to operate a uniform set of benefits for all of their employees in various states, Congress provided that those employers only need to comply with the federal law, and they are exempt from state requirements in developing and operating their employee benefit plans. Although states retain the power to regulate insurance companies, many ERISA plans are self-insured and beyond the reach of state authority. On January 17, 2007, the U.S. Court of Appeals for the Fourth Circuit agreed with the district court, and held that the federal ERISA law preempts the Maryland law.[9]

However, that decision of the Fourth Circuit in the Maryland case is not binding on federal courts in other circuits, and the laws of other state or local governments might be distinguishable on the facts. After that decision by the Fourth Circuit in the Maryland case, the U.S. Court of Appeals for the Ninth Circuit upheld a local health reform law in the City of San Francisco and concluded that the city's law was not preempted by ERISA.[10] These different outcomes might be attributable to different judicial philosophies in those circuit courts as well as to factual differences between the Maryland and San Francisco laws.

In 2006, Massachusetts adopted a comprehensive law on health reform.[11] That law imposed requirements on employers, and it required individuals to obtain health insurance coverage if they can afford do so. The law created a system of subsidies for those whose income is too high to qualify for Medicaid but too low as a practical matter to be able to purchase health insurance. Rather than continuing to use large amounts of public funds to pay hospitals for providing care for the indigent, the new system shifted some of those funds to providing subsidies for uninsured individuals to purchase health insurance coverage.[12] It was unclear whether the Massachusetts law would be preempted by the federal ERISA law. What was clear, however, is that the Massachusetts law provided a model for Congress in enacting the 2010 federal health reform legislation.

Federal Regulation and Reforms Before 2010

Health reform at the federal level includes the important steps of creating the Medicare, Medicaid, and SCHIP programs, which are discussed in detail in

Chapter 8. Subsequent federal initiatives include efforts to prevent the loss of coverage as a result of a change in employment or family status.

In 1996, President Bill Clinton signed the Health Insurance Portability and Accountability Act (HIPAA).[13] This federal statute has also been called Kassebaum-Kennedy, because it was sponsored by Senators Nancy Kassebaum (R-KS) and Edward Kennedy (D-MA). In addition to its well-known privacy provisions, HIPAA imposed significant requirements on self-insured employee health plans as well as on insurance companies that provided coverage to large groups, small groups, and individuals.

In the group insurance market, health plans could only exclude coverage of preexisting conditions for a maximum of 12 months in most cases. Moreover, that 12-month period of exclusion had to be reduced by the individual's prior periods of creditable coverage, so long as no break in coverage lasted more than 63 days. For example, a new employee at Company X may have been subject to a 12-month preexisting condition exclusion under Company X's employee health plan. However, that employee was generally entitled to credit against that 12-month exclusion period for any time that he was covered under a previous employer's plan, provided there was no break in coverage of more than 63 days.

This provision for credit against the new employer's period of exclusion is referred to as group-to-group portability. This type of "portability," however, did not mean employees would take their old insurance coverage with them to their new jobs. Rather, group-to-group portability under HIPAA referred to getting credit against the period of exclusion for preexisting conditions when the employee obtained coverage under the *new* employer's plan. HIPAA portability, therefore, was different from continuation coverage under the federal Consolidated Omnibus Budget Reconciliation Act (COBRA), in which former employees may elect to continue their *old* coverage for a limited period of time at their own expense.[14]

In the individual insurance market, HIPAA specified that all health insurers that sell individual policies in the state were required to provide individual coverage, upon request, to all persons who qualify as eligible individuals. This concept was called group-to-individual portability because it applied to people who lost their group coverage and wish to buy coverage in the individual market. However, the definition of *eligible individual* in HIPAA was restrictive and generally included only those people who were covered for a substantial period of time before losing their coverage. Moreover, federal law did not limit the premiums that insurers may charge eligible individuals, but those rates may be regulated by state law.[15]

Originally, the proposed legislation had contained a provision for parity of mental health benefits, which would have required a health plan to provide the same level of benefits for mental illness as it provided for physical illness. Congress deleted that provision from the final HIPAA legislation. A few weeks later, however, Congress enacted a limited provision for mental health parity, as well as a requirement for maternity coverage of at least 48 hours in the hospital after normal delivery and at least 96 hours after caesarean section.[16] The federal requirements for 48-hour and 96-hour maternity coverage are discussed in Chapter 14.

In 2008, Congress took an additional step toward equality of mental health benefits by enacting the Mental Health Parity and Addiction Equity Act (MHPAEA).[17] As explained by the U.S. Department of Labor, this 2008 law "requires group health plans and health insurance issuers to ensure that financial requirements (such as co-pays, deductibles) and treatment limitations (such as visit limits) applicable to mental health or substance use disorder (MH/SUD) benefits are no more restrictive than the predominant requirements or limitations applied to substantially all medical/surgical benefits."[18]

Prior to 2010, Congress was attempting to reform the health insurance system on an incremental basis, such as by promoting parity of benefits under existing coverage and by protecting people who already had coverage from losing their coverage when they change jobs or lose their jobs. In some ways, incremental reform is more difficult than developing a comprehensive system of universal coverage because of the danger that incremental reforms will cause young and healthy people to simply forgo coverage. The practical problem of incremental reform, therefore, is to develop ways to improve access to coverage and portability of coverage for as many people as possible without raising premiums so much that healthy people would drop out of the system.

Ultimately, the goal of universal coverage requires a system in which young and healthy people cannot simply choose to drop out. At the very least, this goal requires some significant incentives for young and healthy people to participate in the system. These are the practical and legal issues which confronted Congress as it considered and enacted the 2010 health reform legislation.

The 2010 Federal Affordable Care Act

Enactment of the 2010 Federal Law
In Congress, serious disagreements arose about several issues. Some members of Congress wanted to create a public health insurance plan similar to Medicare as an option for the general public, but others were strongly opposed to that idea. In addition, members of Congress disagreed about the cost of health reform and how we should pay for it. Conflicts also occurred about using government funds to help people buy health insurance that

would cover abortion. In many ways, the legislation that was finally enacted represented a compromise among conflicting views.

The legislation was enacted in two parts. First, Congress enacted HR 3590 as the Patient Protection and Affordable Care Act (PPACA),[19] which was signed by President Obama on March 23, 2010. A few days later, Congress resolved some outstanding issues by enacting HR 4872 as the Health Care and Education Reconciliation Act of 2010,[20] which the president signed on March 30, 2010. For convenience, the two parts of that legislation are often referred to collectively as the Affordable Care Act or the ACA.

Some critics have argued that the ACA is an example of excessive government intervention in the healthcare system. However, it is important to recognize what the ACA does *not* do. The ACA does not establish a Canadian-style single-payer system or a United Kingdom-style national health system. The ACA continues the system in which millions of people obtain coverage through their place of employment. It continues to allow the sale of private health insurance policies in a competitive market, and it does not establish a public option for all residents of the country.

Before enactment of the ACA, the U.S. system of healthcare financing was fragmented, with different sources of coverage for different groups of people, such as participants in Medicare, Medicaid, employer-based health plans, and private health insurance plans. After enactment of the ACA, healthcare financing remains fragmented, with different sources of coverage for different groups of people. As one commentator has noted, "[U]nlike Medicare or Social Security, the ACA is not a single program. Rather, it is a collection of mandates, public insurance expansions, subsidies, and regulations that affect different groups of Americans in different ways and at different times."[21] Therefore, analyzing the ways in which the ACA affects these different groups of people is useful.

Medicare: As discussed in Chapter 8, the ACA made some improvements in coverage for beneficiaries. For example, the ACA provided for the reduction and eventual elimination of the "doughnut hole," which was the gap in coverage under Medicare prescription drug plans after the beneficiary exhausts the standard amount of coverage and before she qualifies for catastrophic coverage. In addition, the ACA includes many initiatives to reduce costs, improve efficiency, and increase the quality of care for Medicare beneficiaries. As one example, the ACA promotes the development of accountable care organizations (ACOs) under the Shared Savings Program, in which groups of healthcare providers deliver quality care to Medicare patients in a coordinated manner and share the cost savings resulting from those efforts. In addition, the ACA makes some adjustments to Medicare payment on the basis of quality by reducing the level of payment to hospitals that have a high rate of hospital-acquired conditions and an excessive rate of readmissions.

The ACA also provides for an Independent Payment Advisory Board (IPAB) to be established in 2014 to review excessive Medicare spending and submit legislative proposals for cutting spending. Some critics of the IPAB have argued that it would evaluate decisions about treatment options as a sort of "death panel." However, the ACA explicitly limits the power of the IPAB by providing that its proposals "shall not include any recommendation to ration health care, raise revenues or Medicare beneficiary premiums . . . increase Medicare beneficiary cost-sharing (including deductibles, coinsurance, and copayments), or otherwise restrict benefits or modify eligibility criteria."[22]

Medicaid: The ACA expands the Medicaid program by providing coverage for many poor adults under age 65 who have no dependent children and who had been unable to qualify for Medicare or Medicaid. However, as discussed in Chapter 8, the U.S. Supreme Court held in 2012 that the federal government cannot withdraw existing Medicaid funds from states that decline to participate in the ACA's expansion of Medicaid.[23] Thus, expansion of Medicaid is optional for the states. As of this writing, some state governments have decided to expand their Medicaid programs, while others have refused to participate in the expansion.

Employer-based coverage: Under the ACA, employers may continue to provide health insurance benefits for their employees. The ACA does not explicitly require employers to provide health insurance for their employees. However, employers that have at least 50 employees must pay penalties if any of their employees obtain subsidized insurance through an exchange, as discussed later. That requirement was delayed until 2015.[24]

The ACA also imposes requirements in regard to coverage and benefits in health insurance plans, including the health insurance plans that employers provide for their employees. As discussed in Chapter 13, one of the most controversial requirements is the mandate for most employers to provide insurance coverage for contraceptives, as one type of preventive service, with no copayment or deductible. This requirement does not apply to employees of churches, but it does apply to employees of some church-affiliated organizations, such as universities and hospitals. This requirement also applies to private, for-profit businesses that are owned by religious individuals. At the time of this writing, legal challenges to this mandate were pending in federal courts, and courts have disagreed among themselves about the legal issues.

Exchange
An entity established under the Affordable Care Act where individuals may buy health insurance regardless of their health status.

Individual coverage: The ACA establishes new **exchanges** where individuals may purchase health insurance regardless of their current health status. For some individuals, government subsidies are available on the basis of income. Under the ACA, each state may choose to operate its own exchange, partner with the federal government in operating the exchange, or let the federal government operate it alone. Many states have refused to establish an exchange, and, therefore, the federal government will operate the exchange in those states.

Some opponents of the ACA argue that, under the statutory language, federal subsidies may not be provided for coverage purchased through a federally operated exchange. However, the IRS, which is responsible for implementing the health insurance premium tax credits under the ACA, takes the position that subsidies are indeed available.[25] As of this writing, the issue is subject to litigation in federal courts.[26] Because this is an issue of statutory interpretation rather than constitutional law, most courts would be likely to give deference to the interpretation of the IRS as the agency responsible for implementing the statute.

The ACA also increases the regulation of health insurance companies and prohibits specific practices that have an adverse effect on consumers. For example, health insurance companies may not "rescind" (cancel) a health insurance policy because a person becomes sick. Health insurance companies may not refuse to cover people who have preexisting medical conditions or charge higher rates to people who are sick or have preexisting medical conditions.

Finally, the ACA provides that most individuals will be required to pay a penalty if they do not have health insurance. The individual mandate to have insurance—and the penalty for failure to do so—provided the basis for legal challenges to the ACA and a ruling by the Supreme Court in 2012 on the law's constitutionality.

Legal Challenges and the Supreme Court's Decision

Together with some private parties, state officials from 26 states challenged the federal government's authority to adopt the ACA, including the individual mandate to obtain health insurance and the penalty for failing to have insurance. On June 28, 2012, the U.S. Supreme Court held in *National Federation of Independent Business v. Sebelius* that the individual mandate to buy health insurance is not a valid regulation of interstate commerce, but the penalty for failure to do so is valid under Congress' power to tax.[27]

The individual mandate from Congress to buy health insurance is *not* analogous to requiring owners of automobiles to buy insurance because automobile insurance mandates are state laws. As discussed in Chapter 5, state governments have police power to protect the public.[28] Thus, state governments clearly have the power to require their residents to buy health insurance, as the state of Massachusetts has done. In contrast, a dispute arose over whether Congress has the power to require individuals to buy health insurance under its constitutional power to regulate interstate commerce.

Parties challenging the ACA argued that refusing to buy health insurance is merely "inactivity," and, therefore, cannot be regulated as conduct affecting interstate commerce. Supporters of the ACA argued that refusing to buy insurance is really an "activity" of imposing one's inevitable healthcare costs on other people, and, therefore, can be regulated as conduct affecting interstate commerce. Parties challenging the ACA responded that, if the federal government could require people to buy health insurance, Congress could also require people to buy broccoli or other healthy foods.[29]

As seen in the following excerpt from the opinion of the Supreme Court, the court agreed with those challenging the ACA that Congress may not regulate inactivity under its constitutional power to regulate interstate commerce. However, the court also held that Congress may use its constitutional taxing power to impose taxes on those individuals who remain inactive by refusing to buy health insurance.

National Federation of Independent Business v. Sebelius, 132 S. Ct. 2566 (2012)[30] (CITATIONS, FOOTNOTES, AND SOME TEXT OMITTED).

Today we resolve constitutional challenges to two provisions of the Patient Protection and Affordable Care Act of 2010: the individual mandate, which requires individuals to purchase a health insurance policy providing a minimum level of coverage; and the Medicaid expansion, which gives funds to the States on the condition that they provide specified health care to all citizens whose income falls below a certain threshold. We do not consider whether the Act embodies sound policies. That judgment is entrusted to the Nation's elected leaders. We ask only whether Congress has the power under the Constitution to enact the challenged provisions. . . .

The same does not apply to the States, because the Constitution is not the source of their power. The Constitution may restrict state governments—as it does, for example, by forbidding them to deny any person the equal protection of the laws. But where such prohibitions do not apply, state governments do not need constitutional authorization to act. The States thus can and do perform many of the vital functions of modern government—punishing street crime, running public schools, and zoning property for development, to name but a few—even though the Constitution's text does not authorize any government to do so. Our cases refer to this general power of governing, possessed by the States but not by the Federal Government, as the "police power." . . .

(continued)

(continued from previous page)

Congress may tax and spend. This grant gives the Federal Government considerable influence even in areas where it cannot directly regulate. The Federal Government may enact a tax on an activity that it cannot authorize, forbid, or otherwise control. And in exercising its spending power, Congress may offer funds to the States, and may condition those offers on compliance with specified conditions. These offers may well induce the States to adopt policies that the Federal Government itself could not impose. . . .

Our permissive reading of these powers is explained in part by a general reticence to invalidate the acts of the Nation's elected leaders. . . . Members of this Court are vested with the authority to interpret the law; we possess neither the expertise nor the prerogative to make policy judgments. Those decisions are entrusted to our Nation's elected leaders, who can be thrown out of office if the people disagree with them. It is not our job to protect the people from the consequences of their political choices. . . .

I

In 2010, Congress enacted the Patient Protection and Affordable Care Act, 124 Stat. 119. The Act aims to increase the number of Americans covered by health insurance and decrease the cost of health care. The Act's 10 titles stretch over 900 pages and contain hundreds of provisions. This case concerns constitutional challenges to two key provisions, commonly referred to as the individual mandate and the Medicaid expansion.

The individual mandate requires most Americans to maintain "minimum essential" health insurance coverage. . . .

Beginning in 2014, those who do not comply with the mandate must make a "[s]hared responsibility payment" to the Federal Government. That payment, which the Act describes as a "penalty," is calculated as a percentage of household income, subject to a floor based on a specified dollar amount and a ceiling based on the average annual premium the individual would have to pay for qualifying private health insurance. In 2016, for example, the penalty will be 2.5 percent of an individual's household income, but no less than $695 and no more than the average yearly premium for insurance that covers 60 percent of the cost of 10

(continued)

(continued from previous page)

specified services (e.g., prescription drugs and hospitalization). The Act provides that the penalty will be paid to the Internal Revenue Service with an individual's taxes, and "shall be assessed and collected in the same manner" as tax penalties, such as the penalty for claiming too large an income tax refund. The Act, however, bars the IRS from using several of its normal enforcement tools, such as criminal prosecutions and levies. And some individuals who are subject to the mandate are nonetheless exempt from the penalty—for example, those with income below a certain threshold and members of Indian tribes. . . .

II

Before turning to the merits, we need to be sure we have the authority to do so. The Anti-Injunction Act provides that "no suit for the purpose of restraining the assessment or collection of any tax shall be maintained in any court by any person, whether or not such person is the person against whom such tax was assessed." 26 U.S.C. § 7421(a). This statute protects the Government's ability to collect a consistent stream of revenue, by barring litigation to enjoin or otherwise obstruct the collection of taxes. Because of the Anti-Injunction Act, taxes can ordinarily be challenged only after they are paid, by suing for a refund.

The penalty for not complying with the Affordable Care Act's individual mandate first becomes enforceable in 2014. The present challenge to the mandate thus seeks to restrain the penalty's future collection. Amicus contends that the Internal Revenue Code treats the penalty as a tax, and that the Anti-Injunction Act therefore bars this suit. . . .

The Affordable Care Act does not require that the penalty for failing to comply with the individual mandate be treated as a tax for purposes of the Anti-Injunction Act. The Anti-Injunction Act therefore does not apply to this suit, and we may proceed to the merits.

III

The Government advances two theories for the proposition that Congress had constitutional authority to enact the individual mandate. First, the Government argues that Congress had the power to enact the mandate under the Commerce Clause. Under that theory, Congress may order individuals to buy health insurance because the failure to do so

(continued)

(continued from previous page)

affects interstate commerce, and could undercut the Affordable Care Act's other reforms. Second, the Government argues that if the commerce power does not support the mandate, we should nonetheless uphold it as an exercise of Congress's power to tax. According to the Government, even if Congress lacks the power to direct individuals to buy insurance, the only effect of the individual mandate is to raise taxes on those who do not do so, and thus the law may be upheld as a tax.

A

The Government's first argument is that the individual mandate is a valid exercise of Congress's power under the Commerce Clause. . . . According to the Government, the health care market is characterized by a significant cost-shifting problem. Everyone will eventually need health care at a time and to an extent they cannot predict, but if they do not have insurance, they often will not be able to pay for it. Because state and federal laws nonetheless require hospitals to provide a certain degree of care to individuals without regard to their ability to pay, hospitals end up receiving compensation for only a portion of the services they provide. To recoup the losses, hospitals pass on the cost to insurers through higher rates, and insurers, in turn, pass on the cost to policy holders in the form of higher premiums. Congress estimated that the cost of uncompensated care raises family health insurance premiums, on average, by over $1,000 per year.

In the Affordable Care Act, Congress addressed the problem of those who cannot obtain insurance coverage because of preexisting conditions or other health issues. It did so through the Act's "guaranteed-issue" and "community-rating" provisions. These provisions together prohibit insurance companies from denying coverage to those with such conditions or charging unhealthy individuals higher premiums than healthy individuals.

The guaranteed-issue and community-rating reforms do not, however, address the issue of healthy individuals who choose not to purchase insurance to cover potential health care needs. In fact, the reforms sharply exacerbate that problem, by providing an incentive for individuals to delay purchasing health insurance until they become sick, relying on the promise of guaranteed and affordable coverage. The reforms also threaten to impose massive new costs on insurers, who are

(continued)

(continued from previous page)

required to accept unhealthy individuals but prohibited from charging them rates necessary to pay for their coverage. This will lead insurers to significantly increase premiums on everyone.

The individual mandate was Congress's solution to these problems. By requiring that individuals purchase health insurance, the mandate prevents cost-shifting by those who would otherwise go without it. In addition, the mandate forces into the insurance risk pool more healthy individuals, whose premiums on average will be higher than their health care expenses. This allows insurers to subsidize the costs of covering the unhealthy individuals the reforms require them to accept....

1

The Government contends that the individual mandate is within Congress's power....

But Congress has never attempted to rely on that power to compel individuals not engaged in commerce to purchase an unwanted product. ...

The power to regulate commerce presupposes the existence of commercial activity to be regulated. If the power to "regulate" something included the power to create it, many of the provisions in the Constitution would be superfluous....

Our precedent also reflects this understanding. As expansive as our cases construing the scope of the commerce power have been, they all have one thing in common: They uniformly describe the power as reaching "activity." ...

The individual mandate, however, does not regulate existing commercial activity. It instead compels individuals to become active in commerce by purchasing a product, on the ground that their failure to do so affects interstate commerce. Construing the Commerce Clause to permit Congress to regulate individuals precisely because they are doing nothing would open a new and potentially vast domain to congressional authority. Every day individuals do not do an infinite number of things. In some cases they decide not to do something; in others they simply fail to do it. Allowing Congress to justify federal regulation by pointing to the effect of inaction on commerce would bring countless decisions an individual could potentially make within the scope of federal

(continued)

(continued from previous page)

regulation, and—under the Government's theory—empower Congress to make those decisions for him. . . .

Indeed, the Government's logic would justify a mandatory purchase to solve almost any problem. To consider a different example in the health care market, many Americans do not eat a balanced diet. That group makes up a larger percentage of the total population than those without health insurance. The failure of that group to have a healthy diet increases health care costs, to a greater extent than the failure of the uninsured to purchase insurance. Those increased costs are borne in part by other Americans who must pay more, just as the uninsured shift costs to the insured. Congress addressed the insurance problem by ordering everyone to buy insurance. Under the Government's theory, Congress could address the diet problem by ordering everyone to buy vegetables.

People, for reasons of their own, often fail to do things that would be good for them or good for society. Those failures—joined with the similar failures of others—can readily have a substantial effect on interstate commerce. Under the Government's logic, that authorizes Congress to use its commerce power to compel citizens to act as the Government would have them act.

That is not the country the Framers of our Constitution envisioned. . . . Congress already enjoys vast power to regulate much of what we do. Accepting the Government's theory would give Congress the same license to regulate what we do not do, fundamentally changing the relation between the citizen and the Federal Government.

To an economist, perhaps, there is no difference between activity and inactivity; both have measurable economic effects on commerce. But the distinction between doing something and doing nothing would not have been lost on the Framers. . . . The Framers gave Congress the power to regulate commerce, not to compel it, and for over 200 years both our decisions and Congress's actions have reflected this understanding. There is no reason to depart from that understanding now. . . .

The Government, however, claims that this does not matter. The Government regards it as sufficient to trigger Congress's authority that almost all those who are uninsured will, at some unknown point in the future, engage in a health care transaction. . . .

(continued)

(continued from previous page)

The proposition that Congress may dictate the conduct of an individual today because of prophesied future activity finds no support in our precedent. We have said that Congress can anticipate the effects on commerce of an economic activity. But we have never permitted Congress to anticipate that activity itself in order to regulate individuals not currently engaged in commerce. . . .

Everyone will likely participate in the markets for food, clothing, transportation, shelter, or energy; that does not authorize Congress to direct them to purchase particular products in those or other markets today. The Commerce Clause is not a general license to regulate an individual from cradle to grave, simply because he will predictably engage in particular transactions. Any police power to regulate individuals as such, as opposed to their activities, remains vested in the States.

The Government argues that the individual mandate can be sustained as a sort of exception to this rule, because health insurance is a unique product. According to the Government, upholding the individual mandate would not justify mandatory purchases of items such as cars or broccoli because, as the Government puts it, "[h]ealth insurance is not purchased for its own sake like a car or broccoli; it is a means of financing health-care consumption and covering universal risks." Reply Brief for United States 19. But cars and broccoli are no more purchased for their "own sake" than health insurance. They are purchased to cover the need for transportation and food. . . .

The proximity and degree of connection between the mandate and the subsequent commercial activity is too lacking to justify an exception of the sort urged by the Government. The individual mandate forces individuals into commerce precisely because they elected to refrain from commercial activity. Such a law cannot be sustained under a clause authorizing Congress to "regulate Commerce." . . .

B

That is not the end of the matter. Because the Commerce Clause does not support the individual mandate, it is necessary to turn to the Government's second argument: that the mandate may be upheld as within Congress's enumerated power to "lay and collect Taxes."

(continued)

(continued from previous page)

The Government's tax power argument asks us to view the statute differently than we did in considering its commerce power theory. In making its Commerce Clause argument, the Government defended the mandate as a regulation requiring individuals to purchase health insurance. The Government does not claim that the taxing power allows Congress to issue such a command. Instead, the Government asks us to read the mandate not as ordering individuals to buy insurance, but rather as imposing a tax on those who do not buy that product.

The text of a statute can sometimes have more than one possible meaning. To take a familiar example, a law that reads "no vehicles in the park" might, or might not, ban bicycles in the park. And it is well established that if a statute has two possible meanings, one of which violates the Constitution, courts should adopt the meaning that does not do so. . . .

The most straightforward reading of the mandate is that it commands individuals to purchase insurance. After all, it states that individuals "shall" maintain health insurance. Congress thought it could enact such a command under the Commerce Clause, and the Government primarily defended the law on that basis. But, for the reasons explained above, the Commerce Clause does not give Congress that power. Under our precedent, it is therefore necessary to ask whether the Government's alternative reading of the statute—that it only imposes a tax on those without insurance—is a reasonable one.

Under the mandate, if an individual does not maintain health insurance, the only consequence is that he must make an additional payment to the IRS when he pays his taxes. That, according to the Government, means the mandate can be regarded as establishing a condition—not owning health insurance—that triggers a tax—the required payment to the IRS. Under that theory, the mandate is not a legal command to buy insurance. Rather, it makes going without insurance just another thing the Government taxes, like buying gasoline or earning income. And if the mandate is in effect just a tax hike on certain taxpayers who do not have health insurance, it may be within Congress's constitutional power to tax.

The question is not whether that is the most natural interpretation of the mandate, but only whether it is a "fairly possible" one. . . .

(continued)

(continued from previous page)

The Government asks us to interpret the mandate as imposing a tax, if it would otherwise violate the Constitution. Granting the Act the full measure of deference owed to federal statutes, it can be so read, for the reasons set forth below.

C

The exaction the Affordable Care Act imposes on those without health insurance looks like a tax in many respects. . . .

It is of course true that the Act describes the payment as a "penalty," not a "tax." But while that label is fatal to the application of the Anti-Injunction Act, it does not determine whether the payment may be viewed as an exercise of Congress's taxing power. It is up to Congress whether to apply the Anti-Injunction Act to any particular statute, so it makes sense to be guided by Congress's choice of label on that question. That choice does not, however, control whether an exaction is within Congress's constitutional power to tax. . . .

None of this is to say that the payment is not intended to affect individual conduct. Although the payment will raise considerable revenue, it is plainly designed to expand health insurance coverage. But taxes that seek to influence conduct are nothing new. . . .

While the individual mandate clearly aims to induce the purchase of health insurance, it need not be read to declare that failing to do so is unlawful. Neither the Act nor any other law attaches negative legal consequences to not buying health insurance, beyond requiring a payment to the IRS. The Government agrees with that reading, confirming that if someone chooses to pay rather than obtain health insurance, they have fully complied with the law.

Indeed, it is estimated that four million people each year will choose to pay the IRS rather than buy insurance. We would expect Congress to be troubled by that prospect if such conduct were unlawful. That Congress apparently regards such extensive failure to comply with the mandate as tolerable suggests that Congress did not think it was creating four million outlaws. It suggests instead that the shared responsibility payment merely imposes a tax citizens may lawfully choose to pay in lieu of buying health insurance. . . .

(continued)

(continued from previous page)

The Affordable Care Act's requirement that certain individuals pay a financial penalty for not obtaining health insurance may reasonably be characterized as a tax. Because the Constitution permits such a tax, it is not our role to forbid it, or to pass upon its wisdom or fairness. . . .

The Affordable Care Act is constitutional in part and unconstitutional in part. The individual mandate cannot be upheld as an exercise of Congress's power under the Commerce Clause. That Clause authorizes Congress to regulate interstate commerce, not to order individuals to engage in it. In this case, however, it is reasonable to construe what Congress has done as increasing taxes on those who have a certain amount of income, but choose to go without health insurance. Such legislation is within Congress's power to tax. . . .

The Framers created a Federal Government of limited powers, and assigned to this Court the duty of enforcing those limits. The Court does so today. But the Court does not express any opinion on the wisdom of the Affordable Care Act. Under the Constitution, that judgment is reserved to the people.

The judgment of the Court of Appeals for the Eleventh Circuit is affirmed in part and reversed in part.

It is so ordered.

The debate over health reform and the constitutionality of the ACA was often viewed in partisan terms as a dispute between Democrats and Republicans or between liberals and conservatives. Yet the deciding vote at the Supreme Court to uphold most of the ACA was provided by Chief Justice John Roberts, who is widely regarded as a conservative. The reason for this apparent anomaly is that conservative jurisprudence includes a profound respect for decisions that were made by the legislative branch of government.

In making predictions about the outcome of that litigation, some people had emphasized the tendency of conservative justices to limit federal authority vis-à-vis the authority of the states. That is accurate, but it is not the only principle of conservative legal analysis. Another important conservative principle is to defer to decisions of the people's elected representatives in Congress.

From a political perspective, many people had viewed the litigation over constitutionality of the ACA as a judgment on the work of President Barack Obama and his administration. From a constitutional perspective, however, the ACA was not simply the work of President Obama and his appointees, even though he signed the law and provided the leadership for its enactment. Rather, the ACA was an act of the United States Congress. That was the basis on which the Supreme Court reviewed the law, and that was the basis for the deference which was given to the law by the majority of justices.

The Supreme Court reasoned that the individual mandate was not a valid exercise of Congress' power to regulate interstate commerce because the law attempted to regulate inactivity rather than activity. If Congress could require inactive individuals to enter commerce and buy insurance, what else could Congress require individuals to buy?

When one party to litigation argues for a particular interpretation of a law, the other party often tries to point out the harmful consequences that would occur if that argument were to be taken to its logical extreme. Then, the party arguing in favor of that interpretation bears the burden of demonstrating how its proposed rule could be limited in a reasonable and practical manner.

In the dispute over the individual mandate, parties challenging the law argued that, if the federal government could make people buy health insurance, that principle would also allow the federal government to make people buy broccoli. Supporters of the ACA were not able to articulate a logical and practical limit to their interpretation of the Constitution's Commerce Clause. Instead, supporters were forced to insist that health insurance is simply unique, but the Supreme Court was not persuaded by that argument. The inability to identify and articulate a limit was a major reason for holding that the individual mandate was not a valid regulation of interstate commerce.

Nevertheless, the court reasoned that the penalty for failure to buy health insurance was a valid exercise of Congress' constitutional power to impose taxes. In that part of its opinion, the court relied on longstanding conservative principles, such as providing significant deference to acts of Congress.

Moreover, when a statute enacted by Congress can be interpreted in two different ways, courts should interpret the statute in the way that makes it constitutional. In this case, the federal government argued that the penalty provision in the ACA could be interpreted as a tax, in which case it would be constitutional. Although the ACA could be interpreted in other ways, the court concluded that the financial penalty could reasonably be described as a tax. That was sufficient to uphold the constitutionality of the penalty under conservative legal principles.

Significantly, the Supreme Court did *not* hold that Congress lacked the power to require individuals to participate in a health insurance system. The court merely held that Congress could not rely on its power to regulate interstate commerce as the basis for requiring individuals to buy insurance. As one possible alternative, Congress could use its taxing power to establish a new tax-supported health insurance system for the entire country or expand the existing, tax-supported Medicare program to cover all residents of the United States. In 1937, the Supreme Court held that, because Congress has the power to tax and spend, it may require individuals to contribute to the federal Social Security system.[31] On the same basis, Congress would have the power to establish a government health insurance system for all residents of the country and could require all individuals to pay taxes in support of that system.

As another possible alternative, Congress could use its conditional spending power to provide federal funding to those states that are willing to impose an individual mandate or adopt other reforms that would expand health insurance coverage in a particular state. Congress has the power to impose conditions on the use of specific federal funds, but it may not impose conditions that relate to the use of other federal funds, as discussed in Chapter 8. In another part of its opinion, the Supreme Court explained that "[n]othing in our opinion precludes Congress from offering funds under the Affordable Care Act to expand the availability of health care, and requiring that States accepting such funds comply with the conditions on their use."[32] In fact, beginning in 2017, the ACA will provide an option for states to implement their own systems to expand insurance coverage and receive federal funds for state systems that meet ACA requirements. Activity 15.1 provides an opportunity to evaluate various types of state alternatives under the criteria for waivers set forth in the ACA.

ACTIVITY 15.1: WAIVERS FOR STATE INNOVATION

The Affordable Care Act (ACA) provides at Section 1332 that a state may opt out of the ACA's system for expanding health insurance coverage, provided the state adopts its own system to achieve universal coverage.[33] This is called a "waiver for state innovation." States have the option of applying to the federal government for a five-year waiver of particular ACA requirements. According to the ACA, this option is available as of 2017, but some members of Congress have discussed the possibility of advancing that date.

If a state receives a waiver, the federal government will provide funding to that state in an amount that is comparable to what the federal government would have provided for residents of that state in tax credits under the ACA. As the Department of the Treasury and the

(continued)

(continued from previous page)

Department of Health and Human Services (HHS) explained in their proposed regulations,

"Section 1332(a)(3) of the Affordable Care Act requires that the Secretaries provide for an alternative means by which the aggregate amount of tax credits or cost-sharing reductions that would have been paid had the State not received a waiver, be paid to the State for purposes of implementing the waiver. This amount will be determined annually by the Secretaries, on a per capita basis, taking into consideration the experience of other States for participation in an Exchange and tax credits and cost-sharing reductions provided in such other States."[34]

The following excerpt from an HHS press release about this option describes the four conditions in Section 1332 that states must meet to qualify for this waiver.[35]

March 10, 2011

Obama Administration Takes New Steps to Support Innovation, Empower States

New regulations implementing the Affordable Care Act propose a process for how states can apply for Innovation Waivers

Building on President Obama's commitment to ensure states have the power and flexibility to innovate and implement the health care solutions that work best for them, the Departments of Health and Human Services (HHS) and Treasury today proposed new rules outlining the steps states may pursue in order to receive a State Innovation Waiver under the Affordable Care Act.

The Affordable Care Act gives states the flexibility to receive a State Innovation Waiver so they may pursue their own innovative strategies to ensure their residents have access to high quality, affordable health insurance. Under the law, State Innovation Waivers are available in 2017. President Obama supports bipartisan legislation that would make waivers available to states beginning in 2014.

"Innovation Waivers empower states to take the lead on implementing the Affordable Care Act," said HHS Secretary Kathleen

(continued)

(continued from previous page)

Sebelius. "Today's announcement demonstrates the flexibility available to states as they continue to move forward on fixing our broken health insurance marketplace."

State Innovation Waivers are designed to allow states to implement policies that differ from those in the Affordable Care Act so long as they:

- *Provide coverage that is at least as comprehensive as the coverage offered through Health Insurance Exchanges—new competitive, private health insurance marketplaces.*
- *Make coverage at least as affordable as it would have been through the Exchanges.*
- *Provide coverage to at least as many residents as otherwise would have been covered under the Affordable Care Act.*
- *Do not increase the federal deficit.*

States could use a variety of strategies to innovate through a waiver, provided they meet the above requirements. For example, they could develop a new system for providing tax credits, which links small business tax credits to the tax credits for moderate-income families. Or they could change the benefit levels or add new benefit levels for health plans offered in the Exchanges, providing consumers and employers even more choices.

The proposed regulation announced today describes the content of the waiver application and how such proposals may be disclosed to the public, monitored, and evaluated. The administration welcomes suggestions for improving this process from states, patients, health care providers, and the general public. As the President said in his State of the Union address, he is open to ideas on how to improve the Affordable Care Act.

For purposes of this activity, please assume the following additional facts. Four state governments have submitted applications to the federal government to request waivers for state innovation under Section 1332. These four proposals are described below. For each of these proposals, please answer the following questions:

(continued)

(continued from previous page)

1. Is the state proposal likely to meet all of the requirements in Section 1332, as described in the excerpt from the HHS press release?
2. Apart from the requirements of the ACA, is it likely that the state government has the legal authority to adopt the state laws that would be required to implement its proposal?
3. Would the state proposal be an effective way to meet the goals of health policy?

State No. 1: This state proposes to enact a law that would require every state resident to have health insurance that meets standards comparable to those in the ACA. Individuals who are covered by Medicare or Medicaid will not be required to obtain other coverage. The state government would use its allotment of federal funds to provide subsidies for the purchase of health insurance by residents whose income is below a specified level.

State No. 2: This state proposes to enact a law that would require all employers in the state to provide health insurance coverage for all of their employees who are state residents. The coverage must meet standards comparable to those in the ACA. This requirement would not apply to employees who are covered by Medicare or Medicaid. The state government would use its allotment of federal funds to provide subsidies to small businesses to help them provide coverage for their employees.

State No. 3: This state proposes to enact a law that would establish a modified single-payer plan (SPP) for health insurance coverage in that state. This SPP would not apply to individuals who are covered by Medicare or Medicaid. (That is the reason this proposal is described as a *modified* SPP.) All other residents of the state would be required to have health insurance coverage through the SPP. Standards would be comparable to those in the ACA. State law would prohibit the sale of health insurance that would cover any of the services covered by the modified SPP. However, health insurance companies could sell policies that provide coverage for gaps in the SPP, such as copayments, deductibles, noncovered services, and amenities such as private hospital rooms. The modified SPP would be financed by state taxes on employers

(continued)

(continued from previous page)

and employees as well as by some general state tax revenues. Some residents of the state are unemployed. Therefore, the state would not receive employer or employee contributions for those individuals. Instead, the state would use its allotment of federal funds to provide additional financial support for its modified SPP.

State No. 4: This state proposes to rely on the free market to provide health insurance coverage for its residents. Under this proposal, no individual would be legally required to have health insurance, and no employer would be legally required to provide health insurance for its employees. The state proposes to enact a law that would provide state tax deductions to individuals who purchase health insurance and employers who provide health insurance for their employees. Individuals would have the right to choose the level and type of benefits that meet their individual or family needs. Thus, individuals would have the right to make their own trade-off between cost of coverage and amount of coverage. The state would use its allotment of federal funds to help offset the loss of state tax revenue from providing these state tax deductions.

Notes

1. See, e.g., 103rd Cong., S. 1770, Tit. I, Subtitle F, § 1501 (1993) (sponsored by Senator John Chafee and cosponsored by Senators Robert Dole, Orrin Hatch, *et al.*).
2. 15 U.S.C. §§ 1011–15 (2006).
3. See *Humana, Inc. v. Forsyth*, 525 U.S. 299, 302–306 (1999) ("When federal law is applied in aid or enhancement of state regulation, and does not frustrate any declared state policy or disturb the State's administrative regime, the McCarran-Ferguson Act does not bar the federal action").
4. 29 U.S.C. §§ 1001 *et seq.* (2006).
5. C. Lee (2007). "Universal Health Coverage Attracts New Support." *Washington Post*, January 22, A03.
6. *New York State Conference of Blue Cross & Blue Shield Plans v. Travelers Insurance Company*, 514 U.S. 645, 667 n.6 (1995) (analyzing the legislative history of the federal Medicare program).

7. Fair Share Act, Md. Code. Ann., Lab. & Empl. § 8.5-103(a)(1) (2006).

8. *Retail Industry Leaders Association v. Fielder*, 435 F. Supp. 2d 481, 485 and n.3 (D. Md.), *aff'd*, 475 F.3d 180, 2007 U.S. App. LEXIS 920 (4th Cir. 2007).

9. *Retail Industry Leaders Association v. Fielder*, 475 F.3d 180 (4th Cir. 2007).

10. *Golden Gate Restaurant Association v. City and County of San Francisco*, 546 F.3d 639 (9th Cir. 2008).

11. General Court of the Commonwealth of Massachusetts, Chapter 58 of the Acts of 2006. www.mass.gov/legis/laws/seslaw06/sl060058.htm.

12. See E. F. Haislmaier and N. Owcharenko, "The Massachusetts Approach: A New Way to Restructure State Health Insurance Markets and Public Programs," *Health Affairs* (2006), 25 (6): 1580–90.

13. Pub. L. No. 104-191, 110 Stat. 1936 (1996) (codified at 29 U.S.C. §§ 1181 *et seq.*).

14. 29 U.S.C. 1162 (2006).

15. See U.S. General Accounting Office, *Private Health Insurance: Progress and Challenges in Implementing 1996 Federal Standards*, GAO/HEHS-99-100 (May 1999): 12.

16. See The Department of Veterans Affairs and Housing and Urban Development and Independent Agencies Appropriations Act of 1997, Pub. L. No. 104-204, § 711, 110 Stat. 2874, 2935–36 (1996) (codified at 29 U.S.C. § 1185).

17. The Paul Wellstone and Pete Domenici Mental Health Parity and Addiction Equity Act of 2008, Pub. L. No. 110-343, Division C, §§ 511 and 512 of the Tax Extenders and Alternative Minimum Tax Relief Act of 2008 (2008).

18. U.S. Department of Labor, Employee Benefits Security Administration, "Fact Sheet: The Mental Health Parity and Addiction Equity Act of 2008 (MHPAEA)" (January 29, 2010). www.dol.gov/ebsa/newsroom/fsmhpaea.html.

19. Pub. L. No. 111-148 (2010).

20. Pub. L. No. 111-152 (2010).

21. J. Oberlander (2010). "Beyond Repeal—The Future of Health Care Reform." *New England Journal of Medicine* 363 (24): 2277–79.

22. Pub. L. No. 111-148, § 3403 (c)(2)(A)(ii), 10320(b) (changing the name of the board).

23. *National Federation of Independent Business v. Sebelius*, 132 S. Ct. 2566 (2012).

24. U.S. Department of the Treasury, "Continuing to Implement the ACA in a Careful, Thoughtful Manner" (July 2, 2013). www.treasury.gov/connect/blog/pages/continuing-to-implement-the-aca-in-a-careful-thoughtful-manner.aspx.

25. 77 Fed. Reg. 30377 (May 23, 2012) (final regulations), at 30378.

26. See, e.g., *Halbig v. Sebelius*, 2014 U.S. Dist. LEXIS 4853 (D.D.C. 2014).

27. 132 S. Ct. 2566 (2012).

28. *Jacobson v. Massachusetts*, 197 U.S. 11, 25 (1905).

29. See, e.g., W. K. Mariner, G. J. Annas, and L. H. Glantz, "Can Congress Make You Buy Broccoli? And Why That's a Hard Question," *New England Journal of Medicine* (2011), 364 (3): 201–203.

30. *National Federation of Independent Business v. Sebelius*, 132 S. Ct. 2566 (2012).

31. *Helvering v. Davis*, 301 U.S. 619 (1937) (upholding mandatory Social Security contributions under the taxing power).

32. 132 S. Ct. at 2607.

33. Pub. L. No. 111-148 (2010), § 1332.

34. 76 Fed. Reg. 13553, at 13555 (March 14, 2011).

35. U.S. Department of Health and Human Services, "Obama Administration Takes New Steps to Support Innovation, Empower States" (March 10, 2011). www.hhs.gov/news/press/2011pres/03/20110310a.html.

GLOSSARY

Accreditation. A voluntary process of industry self-regulation, such as evaluation of healthcare facilities by a private, nongovernmental organization.

Accountable care organization (ACO). A group of healthcare providers that delivers quality care to patients in a coordinated manner and shares the cost savings resulting from those efforts, such as a group established under Medicare's Shared Savings Program.

Adjudication. The procedure by which administrative agencies decide cases that involve a specific party, such as whether to revoke a license or impose an administrative penalty.

Affirmative obligations. Requirements to perform specific activities.

Agent. A person who acts on behalf of another person or organization without being an employee of that person or organization.

Alternative dispute resolution (ADR). Procedures for handling controversies other than through litigation in court.

Answer. The document that sets forth the defendant's response to the complaint.

Appellate court. A court that hears appeals from decisions of lower courts. It has the power to affirm, reverse, or modify the decisions of those lower courts, and may establish legal precedents that are binding on the lower courts in a particular jurisdiction.

Beneficence. The ethical principle of helping others.

Boycott. An unlawful agreement to refuse to deal with another party.

Breach of contract. Failure to meet the obligations of a contract.

Cert. denied. The designation in citation form to indicate that the U.S. Supreme Court declined to hear that case. Abbreviation of "the petition for writ of certiorari is denied."

Certificate-of-need (CON) laws. State laws that prohibit development of new healthcare facilities and services unless officials determine that the proposed facilities and services are needed and meet other criteria in statutes or regulations.

Certification. The process through which healthcare facilities are accepted for participation in government payment programs. For individual healthcare professionals, certification is a voluntary, nongovernmental process of professional self-regulation, such as the process for designating physicians as board certified in a particular specialty.

Citation form. The standardized method of identifying and labeling sources of legal authority, such as court decisions, statutes, and rules.

Civil law. In contrast to criminal law, these legal rules cover the private rights and obligations of specific parties, as in contracts, torts, or some violations of statutes.

Collateral source rule. The legal principle that plaintiffs may recover damages from defendants to compensate for losses even if they have already received compensation for those losses from other sources, such as insurance.

Common law. The body of legal principles and precedents that were established by courts in a particular jurisdiction, modified by those courts over time, and subject to change by those courts in the future.

Community health needs assessment. A process for a tax-exempt hospital with significant input from its community to determine and document the health needs of the community it serves.

Community rating. A method of pricing health insurance in which premiums do not vary on the basis of individual health status.

Complaint. The document that sets forth the plaintiff's allegations and requests particular types of legal relief.

Conditional spending power. The authority of Congress to impose conditions on the use of federal funds it provides to state governments.

Conditions of participation. Standards developed by the federal government for healthcare organizations in Medicare.

Contract. A voluntary agreement between two or more parties that meets the requirements for a binding and legally enforceable obligation.

Corporate Integrity Agreement. A contract between the OIG and a healthcare organization in the context of settlement, in which the OIG agrees to permit the organization to continue participating in federal programs and the organization agrees to take specific actions to promote compliance.

Corporate negligence. Liability for breach of a hospital's duty to a patient, such as the duty to exercise reasonable care in allowing a physician to treat patients at the hospital.

Corporation. A legal entity whose owners or members have limited liability for its debts.

Cost shifting. Charging higher rates to private payers to make up for low payment rates from government programs such as Medicare and Medicaid.

Covered entities. Health plans, healthcare clearinghouses, and healthcare providers that transmit information by electronic means.

Criminal law. Legal prohibitions and penalties for wrongs against society as a whole, even if the wrong harms an individual member of that society.

Deemer clause. A provision of ERISA that self-insured ERISA plans are *not* deemed to be insurance companies or to be in the business of insurance.

Diagnosis-related groups. The federal government's categories of medical conditions that Medicare uses to determine the amount of payment for each patient.

Directed verdict. A decision by a judge during a trial that the plaintiff has not introduced sufficient evidence to support her claim under applicable law and, therefore, entering a verdict in favor of the defendant without the need for a decision by the jury.

Discovery. The procedure for pretrial exchange of information in a civil lawsuit, in which each party may compel the disclosure of information from another party.

Diversity jurisdiction. The authority of a federal court to hear a civil case on the ground that the parties are diverse in citizenship (e.g., citizens of different states), even if the case does not arise under a federal statute or protect a constitutional right.

Exchange. An entity established under the Affordable Care Act where individuals may buy health insurance regardless of their health status.

Exhaustion of administrative remedies. The doctrine that a person opposed to a specific action of an agency must go through that agency's internal review process before challenging the agency in court.

Federalism. The relationship between federal and state governments, in which the powers of each level of government are subject to constitutional principles.

Fiduciary duties. Duties imposed by law in specific relationships to serve the interests of another person or organization rather than one's individual interests.

Gainsharing. An agreement by a hospital to give physicians part of the hospital's savings on patient care costs, thereby creating a risk that physicians might reduce the level of services for patients.

Guaranteed issue. A legal requirement that health insurance companies provide coverage to all applicants regardless of their health status.

Horizontal merger. A combination of entities at the same level of production or distribution, such as a merger of competing sellers of the same product or service.

Hospital cooperation act. A state statute that establishes a process for regulatory approval and supervision of particular activities by healthcare providers in an attempt to obtain state action immunity.

Hospitalists. Physicians employed by hospitals and specializing in the care of inpatients.

Informed consent. The legal doctrine that individuals have the right to make their own decisions about medical treatment after receiving the relevant information about risks, benefits, and alternatives.

Intentional tort. A civil wrong committed deliberately by one person against another for violation of a legal duty other than a contract between the parties.

Intermediate sanctions. Penalties for violation of the legal requirements for tax-exempt organizations that are less severe than revocation of an organization's tax-exempt status.

Judicial bypass procedure. A process to obtain court approval to perform an abortion on a woman who is under the age of 18 and not legally emancipated, as an alternative to consent of a parent or guardian.

Licensing board. A state agency that regulates practitioners of a specific profession.

Limited liability company (LLC). A form of business organization in which none of its members are liable for debts of the organization.

Limited liability partnership (LLP). A form of business organization in which partners are generally not liable for debts of the organization or for actions of other partners.

Limited partnership. A form of business organization in which some of the partners have limited liability for debts of the organization, but at least one partner has unlimited liability.

Managed care. A method of cost containment in which third-party payers use various techniques to reduce healthcare costs.

Mandated benefit laws. Laws that require all health plans to provide coverage for particular procedures and conditions.

Market allocation. An unlawful agreement among competitors to assign particular products and services or particular territories to each of the competing sellers.

Monopolization. The unlawful possession of monopoly power that was willfully acquired or maintained.

Motion. An oral or written request for a particular action from the court.

Negative obligations. Requirements to refrain from specific conduct or action.

Negligence. A civil wrong based on a failure to meet the duty imposed by law to exercise reasonable care under the circumstances.

Noerr-Pennington immunity. A defense from antitrust liability that is based on the First Amendment to the U.S. Constitution and protects parties in requesting action from an agency of government.

Nonmaleficence. The ethical principle of not harming others.

Objective test. The legal standard to evaluate the element of causation in a claim for lack of informed consent on the basis of whether a reasonable person, in the circumstances of the patient, would have consented to the medical procedure if the risks had been disclosed.

Ostensible agency. The legal doctrine that organizations may be held liable for the negligent acts of individuals who are not employees or agents if the organizations made it appear to the public that they were employees or agents, and the public reasonably assumed they were.

Per se rule. The rule in antitrust cases that some types of restraint have an adverse effect on competition without the need for any evidence.

Police power. The authority of state government to protect public health, safety, and welfare.

Practice acts. State statutes that regulate provision of specific professional services and create professional licensing boards.

Predatory pricing. Setting prices below cost to drive out a competitor with a plan to raise prices after the competitor is gone.

Preempt. The effect of a federal law that supersedes a contrary provision of state law.

Preemption clause. A provision of ERISA specifying that ERISA preempts state laws insofar as they relate to employee benefit plans regulated by ERISA.

Price fixing. An unlawful agreement between competitors on prices, such as an agreement on raising, lowering, or maintaining prices.

Private, nonprofit corporation. A type of corporation that is not operated for the purpose of profit but is a private organization rather than a government entity.

Professional limited liability company (PLLC) or professional limited liability partnership (PLLP). Specialized forms of LLC or LLP for professionals, such as physicians.

Prospective payment system. The federal government's method of paying hospitals for treatment of Medicare patients on the basis of prices determined before treatment regardless of the hospital's costs.

Quick look analysis. An intermediate standard for evaluating the effect on competition in an antitrust case, rather than categorizing the conduct as per se unlawful or subject to the rule of reason.

Remand. To send a case back to a lower court for further action.

Reports, reporters. Books or sets of books that contain decisions of particular courts.

Respondeat superior. The legal doctrine that organizations may be held liable for the negligent acts of their employees or agents who are acting within the scope of their employment or agency relationship.

Rule of reason. The rule in antitrust cases of determining the effect on competition on the basis of evidence in each case.

Rulemaking. The procedure by which administrative agencies propose and adopt regulations to implement a statute enacted by the legislature.

Safe harbor. Laws that provide a safety zone from liability if all of the requirements are satisfied.

Saving clause. A provision of ERISA that exempts some types of state laws from preemption.

Section 501(c)(3). The section of the federal Internal Revenue Code that sets forth the basic requirements for qualifying as a tax-exempt organization.

Selective contracting. A technique of cost containment in which third-party payers make contracts with healthcare providers that are willing to reduce their prices and agree to the payer's utilization review procedures.

Separation of powers. The division of authority among legislative, executive, and judicial branches of government, at both the federal and state levels.

Standard of care. The routine practice of similar professionals under similar circumstances in the same or similar communities.

State action immunity. The rule that federal antitrust laws do not apply to the acts of a state or under some circumstances the conduct of private parties acting under the authority and supervision of a state.

Statutes. Laws enacted by legislatures. Also called *acts*.

Subchapter S corporation. A hybrid form of business organization that combines the tax advantages of a partnership and the limited liability of a corporation, as described in Subchapter S of the federal Internal Revenue Code.

Subjective test. The legal standard to evaluate the element of causation in a claim for lack of informed consent on the basis of the patient's testimony in hindsight about whether he would have undergone the medical procedure if the risks had been fully disclosed.

Substituted judgment doctrine. The legal principle that a court should make a decision on behalf of an incompetent person by trying to determine what she would have decided.

Summary judgment. An order of a trial court that no genuine issue of material fact exists for determination at trial, and, therefore, the party that filed the motion is entitled to judgment in its favor as a matter of law.

Summons. The document that notifies the defendant about the suit and gives the deadline for the defendant to respond.

Tort. A civil wrong committed by one person against another for violation of a legal duty other than a contract between the parties.

Trial court. The court that hears a case first and determines the facts, before any appeal to a higher court.

Upcoding. Submitting a claim under an inappropriate diagnostic or procedural code to obtain a higher rate of reimbursement.

Utilization review. A technique of cost containment in which a third-party payer determines whether it will pay for treatment under the terms of the applicable plan, including retrospective review for services already rendered and prospective review for authorization of proposed services.

Vertical merger. A combination of entities at different levels of production or distribution, such as a manufacturer and a retailer.

INDEX

ABOUT THE AUTHOR

Dean M. Harris, JD, is a clinical associate professor in the Department of Health Policy and Management, Gillings School of Global Public Health, University of North Carolina (UNC) at Chapel Hill. For more than 20 years, he has taught courses on health law at UNC's Department of Health Policy and Management. Previously, he taught courses at UNC School of Law and an executive MBA program at The Fuqua School of Business at Duke University. He currently teaches courses on health law, ethics, and comparative health systems.

Professor Harris received his BA degree from Cornell University in 1973; he received his JD degree with high honors from UNC School of Law in 1981. He is a member of the American Health Lawyers Association, the European Association of Health Law, and the World Association for Medical Law.

He has written extensively about issues of healthcare law and policy, such as regulation of health systems, healthcare antitrust law, and Medicare. In addition, he was the lead author on a published article about China's regulation on the handling of medical accidents, and he is working with colleagues to update that research.

He frequently travels to Asia and Europe to give lectures and seminars. His interests include reform of medical malpractice laws, improving systems for handling medical disputes, using law and regulation as tools for health system reform, capacity building for regulation in public health, and health reform in the United States.

In addition, Professor Harris is a licensed attorney. He practiced law from 1981 to 1999, with a primary focus on representation of healthcare organizations and providers. In his work in the healthcare field, he provided legal advice and representation in areas such as antitrust, certificate of need and other regulatory matters, mergers and acquisitions, joint ventures and corporate reorganization, medical staff membership and clinical privileges, Medicare and Medicaid, professional licensure, and patient care issues.

ACF4806   5/29/91